Obstetric Emergencies
A Practical Manual

T0303866

Edited by

Sanjeewa Padumadasa, MBBS, MD, FSLCOG, FRCOG

Professor and Head, Department of Obstetrics and Gynaecology
Faculty of Medicine, University of Kelaniya, and
Former Member of Board of Study in Obstetrics and Gynaecology
Postgraduate Institute of Medicine, University of Colombo, Sri Lanka

Malik Goonewardene, MBBS, MS, FSLCOG, FRCOG

Consultant, Department of Obstetrics and Gynaecology
Sabaragamuwa University of Sri Lanka
Professor Emeritus, Former Senior Professor and
Head of Obstetrics and Gynaecology
Faculty of Medicine, University of Ruhuna
Past President of Sri Lanka College of Obstetricians and Gynaecologists, and
Former Chairperson, Board of Study in Obstetrics and Gynaecology
Postgraduate Institute of Medicine, University of Colombo, Sri Lanka

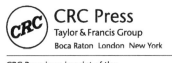

CRC Press
Taylor & Francis Group
Boca Raton London New York

CRC Press is an imprint of the
Taylor & Francis Group, an **informa** business

First edition published 2021
by CRC Press
2 Park Square, Milton Park, Abingdon, Oxon, OX14 4RN

and by CRC Press
6000 Broken Sound Parkway NW, Suite 300, Boca Raton, FL 33487-2742

© 2021 Taylor & Francis Group, LLC

CRC Press is an imprint of Taylor & Francis Group, LLC

Library of Congress Cataloging-in-Publication Data
Names: Padumadasa, Sanjeewa, editor. | Goonewardene, Malik, editor.
Title: Obstetric emergencies : a practical manual / edite by Sanjeewa Padumadasa, Malik Goonewardene.
Other titles: Obstetric emergencies (Padumadasa)
Description: First edition. | Boca Raton : CRC Press, 2021. | Includes bibliographical references and index.
Identifiers: LCCN 2021011680 (print) | LCCN 2021011681 (ebook) | ISBN 9780367543655 (hardback) | ISBN 9780367543648 (paperback) | ISBN 9781003088967 (ebook)
Subjects: MESH: Pregnancy Complications | Emergency Medicine--methods | Emergencies
Classification: LCC RG571 (print) | LCC RG571 (ebook) | NLM WQ 240 | DDC 618.3--dc23
LC record available at https://lccn.loc.gov/2021011680
LC ebook record available at https://lccn.loc.gov/2021011681

ISBN: 978-0-367-54365-5 (hbk)
ISBN: 978-0-367-54364-8 (pbk)
ISBN: 978-1-003-08896-7 (ebk)

Typeset in Times
by MPS Limited, Dehradun

Contents

Contributors

Professor Sabaratnam Arulkumaran
Professor Emeritus
St. George's University of London
Past President, Royal College of Obstetricians and Gynaecologists
Past President, International Federation of Gynaecology and Obstetrics
Past President of the British Medical Association
London, UK

Mr Amarnath Bhide
Consultant in Obstetrics and Fetal Medicine
Fetal Medicine Unit, St. George's Hospital
London, UK

Dr Asantha de Silva
Senior Lecturer in Anaesthesiology
Faculty of Medicine
University of Kelaniya
Colombo, Sri Lanka

Professor Janaka de Silva
Senior Professor and Chair of Medicine
Former Dean, Faculty of Medicine
University of Kelaniya
Past President, Ceylon College of Physicians
Former Director, Postgraduate Institute of Medicine, University of Colombo
Former Chairperson, National Research Council
Colombo, Sri Lanka

Professor Tiran Dias
Professor of Fetal Medicine
Department of Obstetrics and Gynaecology
University of Kelaniya
Kelaniya, Sri Lanka

Mr Ruwan Fernando
Consultant Obstetrician and Gynaecologist, Urogynaecology Subspecialist, and Honorary Senior Lecturer
Imperial College Healthcare NHS Trust
London, UK

Professor Malik Goonewardene
Consultant, Department of Obstetrics and Gynaecology
Sabaragamuwa University of Sri Lanka
Professor Emeritus

Former Senior Professor and Head of Obstetrics and Gynaecology
Faculty of Medicine
University of Ruhuna
Past President of Sri Lanka College of Obstetricians and Gynaecologists
Former Chairperson, Board of Study in Obstetrics and Gynaecology
Postgraduate Institute of Medicine
University of Colombo
Colombo, Sri Lanka

Professor Kapila Gunawardana
Professor of Obstetrics and Gynaecology
Faculty of Medicine
University of Peradeniya
Past President, Sri Lanka College of Obstetricians and Gynaecologists
Former Chairperson, Board of Study in Obstetrics and Gynaecology
Postgraduate Institute of Medicine, University of Colombo
Colombo, Sri Lanka

Dr Bhaagya Gunetilleke
Senior Lecturer in Anaesthesiology, Faculty of Medicine
University of Kelaniya
Colombo, Sri Lanka

Dr Amit Gupta
Consultant Neonatologist and Senior Lecturer
Oxford University Hospitals NHS Trust
Oxford, UK

Professor Sanjeewa Padumadasa
Professor and Head, Department of Obstetrics and Gynaecology
Faculty of Medicine
University of Kelaniya
Former Member of Board of Study in Obstetrics and Gynaecology
Postgraduate Institute of Medicine
University of Colombo
Colombo, Sri Lanka

Dr Anshuman Paria
Consultant Neonatologist
Lancashire Women and Newborn Centre

East Lancashire Hospitals NHS Trust
Blackburn, UK

Dr Sanjeewa Rajapakse
Consultant Cardiologist
North Colombo Teaching Hospital
Former Member, Board of Study in Cardiology
Postgraduate Institute of Medicine, University of Colombo
Former Secretary, Sri Lanka College of Cardiology
Colombo, Sri Lanka

Dr Udya Rodrigo
Consultant Intensivist
North Colombo Teaching Hospital
Colombo, Sri Lanka

Dr Aflah Sadikeen
Consultant Respiratory Physician
National Hospital
Colombo, Sri Lanka

Professor Hemantha Senanayake
Former Senior Professor and Chair of Obstetrics and Gynaecology
Faculty of Medicine
Past President, Sri Lanka College of Obstetricians and Gynaecologists
Former Chairperson, Board of Study in Obstetrics and Gynaecology
Postgraduate Institute of Medicine, University of Colombo
Colombo, Sri Lanka

Mr Austin Ugwumadu
Consultant Obstetrician and Gynaecologist,
St George's Hospital
Senior Lecturer, St George's University
London, UK

Professor Prasantha Wijesinghe
Senior Professor and Chair of Obstetrics and Gynaecology
Former Dean, Faculty of Medicine
University of Kelaniya
Past President, Sri Lanka College of Obstetricians and Gynaecologists
Former Deputy Director, Postgraduate Institute Medicine
University of Colombo
Colombo, Sri Lanka

Dr Nilmini Wijesuriya
Consultant Anaesthesiologist, North Colombo Teaching Hospital
National Co-ordinator, Working Committee on Resuscitation
College of Anaesthesiologists and Intensivists of Sri Lanka
Course Director, Immediate Life Support in Obstetrics
Accredited ERC and UK ALS Trainer
Colombo, Sri Lanka

_____

Illustrations by

Devmi Padumadasa
Shanika Madurapperuma
Dilanka Madhushan
Archana Padumadasa

1

Overview of Obstetric Emergencies

Sanjeewa Padumadasa and Malik Goonewardene

An emergency is a serious and often unforeseen situation that demands immediate action. Obstetric emergencies can occur anytime during pregnancy, during delivery or after delivery. Therefore, it is important for healthcare givers to be aware of these life-threatening conditions and be prepared to manage them, if they do occur. Moreover, an obstetric emergency differs from other emergencies. Because pregnancy is physiological, the woman would have most probably been well before the emergency ensued, and there are two lives involved – that of the woman and the fetus. Although pregnant women are generally young, fit and able to recoup well, the physiological demands of pregnancy can reduce their vitality. While fetal survival depends mainly on the optimal management of the woman, the obstetrician may have to sacrifice the fetus by delivering at gestations below or around the threshold of viability, in order to save the woman, because the woman's wellbeing takes precedence over that of the baby's.

Early Identification, Communication and Teamwork in Obstetric Emergencies

Early recognition of a potential problem, as well as early involvement of experienced practitioners, are vital factors when it comes to the management of obstetric emergencies. The 'Modified Early Obstetric Warning System' (MEOWS) is a tool used to recognise early signs of complications, so that timely and appropriate interventions can be adopted before the woman deteriorates further, possibly resulting in a major catastrophic event.

Excellent communication and teamwork are pivotal to the success of management in a demanding situation, such as an obstetric emergency. The primary aim of communication is to exchange critical information about the woman in order to formulate a reasonable management plan promptly. The use of standardised communication protocols such as 'Situation-Background-Assessment-Recommendation' (SBAR) has led to an improvement when dealing with obstetric emergencies. Effective teamwork requires a team leader who is capable of bringing the best out of the team to ensure that the woman receives the best possible care in a given emergency scenario. Lack of communication and teamwork have been implicated as major contributors to perinatal and maternal morbidity and mortality.

Early activation of a rapid response team, which comprises a diverse range of clinicians and stakeholders, has been associated with a decrease in the incidence of maternal cardiac arrest and admission to intensive care units, as well as an improvement in the survival rate of hospitalised patients. In addition to the routine critical care team, there should be a practitioner who is competent in performing delivery and a practitioner who is competent in the resuscitation of the neonate. If the transfer of a critically ill pregnant woman to a specialised centre is deemed necessary, then arranging facilities for delivery of the fetus if needed during transit, is an important aspect of management of an emergency.

Many obstetric emergencies are extensively known, and management strategies are widely accepted. However, the chance of conferring substandard care is still possible when managing a stressful and time-sensitive situation, such as an emergency, even in the presence of a multitude of healthcare personnel. Developing and adhering to a clear, evidence-based plan of response that is tailor-made for the particular setting ensures that no essential tasks are omitted, and this also creates a relatively more controlled environment. However, as clinical management needs to be individualised, management guidelines may need to be modified according to the individual needs of different women.

Simulation-Based Training

In the management of obstetric emergencies, Simulation-Based Training (SBT) has a vital role in a background of compromised exposure of trainees to emergencies and increasing concerns about patient safety. It is an invaluable accompaniment, although it is not a substitute for a proper apprenticeship and clinical experience. In-house training is comparably more effective than outbound training. In-house training, if combined with drills, also provides a means of identifying strengths and weaknesses in the infrastructure within a particular unit, so that the administration can address possible existing practical issues. Regular drills are immensely helpful in increasing awareness and skills in rare obstetric emergencies.

Managing an emergency under the guidance of an experienced obstetrician provides the ideal platform for learning as well as ensuring that both lives concerned, that of the woman and the fetus, are in safe hands. A trainee must aspire to learn around the subject whenever dealing with an emergency. This will undoubtedly equip him/her with the skills necessary in dealing with an emergency better the next time around. The best textbook on obstetric emergencies is the situation itself, provided that the wellbeing of both the woman and the fetus are ensured.

Consent, Debriefing and Documentation

Obtaining informed written consent is preferable, but this may not be feasible when managing obstetric emergencies, and in some instances, verbal consent may be the most practical. However, in certain situations such as in perimortem caesarean delivery, obtaining any consent may not be possible, and the obstetrician is expected to act in the best interests of the woman. Debriefing the woman, the relatives and the staff involved forms a vital aspect of management of any emergency. The aim of good documentation is not only as a means of providing good defence against litigation, but also to provide a stimulus to promote safe practice, and its importance cannot be underestimated.

> *'Good documentation – good defence, some documentation – some defence, no documentation – no defence, because if you did not document, you did not do it'.*

Risk Management and Audit

Risk management in healthcare is a systematic effort to uncover, mitigate and prevent risks in healthcare institutions. Sentinel events, which are unanticipated events in a healthcare setting resulting in death or serious physical or psychological injury to a patient or patients and which are unrelated to the natural course of the patient's illness, need thorough investigation in an atmosphere of non-blame to prevent the event from recurring. Severe Acute Maternal Morbidity (also referred to as near misses), where a woman could have died but instead survived, also requires thorough investigation. There should be a robust and efficient system that encourages these incidents to be reported so that preventive measures and best practices can be instituted. Regular audits ensure that appropriate measures are in place for preventing and managing emergencies.

Conclusion

Medical practitioners are bound by the Hippocratic Oath, which states *'primum non nocere'* – first, do no harm. Harm not only results from errors of commission, but also from errors of omission, such as failure to take preventive action. Although problems are anticipated and preventive measures are adopted, emergencies still occur unexpectedly. The need to be conversant with the skills and be equipped with the infrastructure in dealing with such emergencies cannot be undervalued. Although the rates of assisted vaginal breech delivery, instrumental vaginal delivery, internal podalic version and breech extraction, internal iliac artery ligation and emergency obstetric hysterectomy have dwindled in the recent past, it is imperative that an obstetrician is competent with these techniques which may be needed in both under-resourced and well-resourced settings. Obstetrics is an art as well as a science, and both aspects are equally important. An evidence-based and pragmatic approach to the management of obstetric emergencies is therefore presented in this book.

> *'Skill is something one never knows when one may need it. It is better for one to have the skill and never get to use it than not have it and one day need it'.*

2

Umbilical Cord Prolapse

Sanjeewa Padumadasa and Prasantha Wijesinghe

Umbilical cord prolapse is defined as the descent of the umbilical cord through the cervix, alongside (occult) or past (overt) the presenting part, in the presence of ruptured membranes. The incidence of umbilical cord prolapse has dramatically declined over the last century and ranges from approximately 1–6/1,000 live births today. It is believed that the increased use of caesarean delivery for unstable lie at term, reduction in rates of grand multiparity, increased use of prostaglandins for ripening of the cervix and a policy of delivering footling breeches by caesarean delivery have led to the decrease in the prevalence of umbilical cord prolapse today.

Umbilical cord prolapse could either be overt (complete) when the umbilical cord lies below the presenting part (Figure 2.1A), or occult (incomplete), when it lies adjacent to the presenting part but not below it (Figure 2.1B) and in the presence of ruptured membranes. Cord presentation refers to the situation in which the umbilical cord lies below the presenting part but above the cervix (Figure 2.1C). In cord presentation, the membranes are usually intact but, occasionally, the membranes could be ruptured yet the cord may not have prolapsed out as the cervix is not dilated. Cord prolapse is a more acute problem than cord presentation, and the danger of cord presentation is the risk of cord prolapse along with its serious consequences.

Pathophysiology

The loop of the umbilical cord is compressed between the maternal pelvis and the presenting part, resulting in fetal hypoxia. This occurs even in occult cord prolapse. The degree of compression is greater in a cephalic presentation than in a non-cephalic presentation of the fetus. Furthermore, the umbilical cord vessels that are exposed to the colder temperature outside the vagina undergo vasospasm, which further reduces blood supply to the fetus. Total cord compression for more than 10 minutes can cause fetal cerebral damage, and more than 20 minutes of this can cause fetal death. The fetal condition can rapidly deteriorate if the fetus is already compromised, as in prematurity and fetal growth restriction.

Risk Factors for Umbilical Cord Prolapse

Umbilical cord prolapse can occur when the maternal pelvis is not completely filled by the fetal presenting part, e.g. in fetal malpresentation, such as breech or abnormal lie, i.e. transverse, oblique, unstable, or when the presenting part is not engaged. It may arise in the presence of multiparity, a small fetus, preterm labour, preterm prelabour rupture of membranes, fetal malformations, polyhydramnios, a low lying placenta and in the second twin.

In addition, obstetric interventions such as external cephalic version (as discussed in Chapter 27), internal podalic version and breech extraction (as discussed in Chapter 28), artificial rupture of membranes in the presence of a high presenting part, vaginal manipulation of the fetus with ruptured

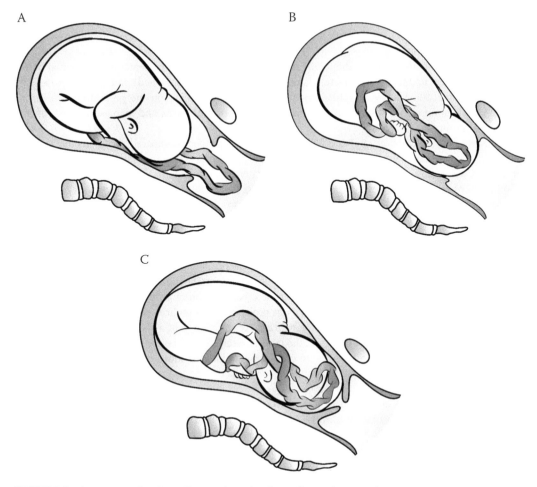

FIGURE 2.1 A – overt cord prolapse, B – occult cord prolapse, C – cord presentation.

membranes and insertion of an intrauterine pressure catheter and Foley catheter induction of labour are associated with the risk of umbilical cord prolapse.

What is common among these risk factors is that these prevent the presenting part from being closely applied to the lower part of the uterus or pelvic brim, thereby leaving room between the presenting part of the fetus and the uterus in order for the umbilical cord to descend through.

Prevention of Umbilical Cord Prolapse

Awareness about the risk of umbilical cord prolapse in the presence of risk factors should prevent this complication from occurring. Women with abnormal fetal lie, e.g. transverse, oblique or unstable, should be advised immediate admission to a hospital in case of the onset of labour or rupture of membranes, because prelabour rupture of membranes, especially in the presence of a high presenting part, carries a high risk of umbilical cord prolapse. A sterile speculum examination is indicated in the presence of ruptured membranes, especially with any evidence of fetal heart rate abnormalities, to exclude umbilical cord prolapse. Amniotomy should be avoided in the presence of a high presenting part, and if it is absolutely necessary, a stabilising induction should be performed. Stabilising induction entails commencing an oxytocin infusion to initiate uterine contractions, performing amniotomy once uterine contractions are established and releasing liquor slowly while an assistant stabilises the presenting part over the pelvis, stabilising the presenting part at the pelvis for some time until the presenting part descends further and maintaining uterine contractions with the oxytocin infusion.

In all women, palpation through the membranes and excluding a cord presentation is essential before amniotomy. If the umbilical cord is felt, amniotomy should be abandoned, and caesarean delivery should be carried out. Undue upward pressure should not be applied on the presenting part during vaginal examination, as this could displace the presenting part upwards and increase the risk of umbilical cord prolapse.

As the risk of umbilical cord prolapse is higher in a footling breech compared to that in other types of a breech, a caesarean delivery is usually carried out in a case of a footling breech presentation. Ultrasound with colour Doppler can be used to detect cord presentation in women with risk factors for umbilical cord prolapse. However, its predictive value is debatable, as the cord may revert to a normal position prior to the onset of labour in a significant proportion of such women.

Diagnosis of Umbilical Cord Prolapse

Vaginal examination (digital or speculum) is the most important method used in diagnosing cord prolapse, and this should be performed whenever there is suspicion of cord prolapse or in situations in which the risk of cord prolapse is high. With overt prolapse, the umbilical cord can be seen protruding from the introitus, or loops of the cord can be palpated, or in the case of a speculum examination, seen, within the vaginal canal. In occult prolapse, the cord is rarely felt on pelvic examination, and the only indication may be fetal heart rate changes. In cord presentation, the loops of the cord may be palpable through the membranes. A speculum examination is mandatory when membranes rupture in a woman with risk factors for umbilical cord prolapse.

If the woman has been connected to a cardiotocograph, then abnormalities in the fetal heart rate pattern may be observed in case of cord prolapse. The fetal heart rate patterns can vary from subtle changes, such as decelerations with uterine contractions in the initial stages of cord compression, to more obvious signs of fetal distress, such as fetal bradycardia, with prolonged compression of the cord.

Diagnosis of Cord Presentation

Occasionally, the loop of the umbilical cord can be felt below the presenting part through the intact membranes. Ultrasound, especially when combined with colour Doppler, can be used to detect cord presentation in women with risk factors for the aforementioned condition. However, the umbilical cord may revert to a normal position prior to the onset of labour in a significant proportion of such women.

Management of Umbilical Cord Prolapse

Assess for Fetal Viability

Umbilical cord prolapse is an obstetric emergency, and prompt action is required to save the life of the fetus. Examining for cord pulsations is a practical and quick method of ascertaining fetal viability, but this may give rise to false positives and false negatives, and therefore, is not a reliable indicator of fetal viability. The pulsations in the clinician's own fingers may be confused with those of the fetus, while fetal heart activity may still be present even in the absence of umbilical artery pulsations or non-detection of a fetal heartbeat by a hand-held Doppler Fetal Heart Detector. Accordingly, fetal viability should be ideally confirmed by visualising the heartbeat by abdominal ultrasound examination. Cardiotocography is time-consuming and unnecessary. If the fetus is confirmed dead or has a lethal abnormality, then vaginal delivery should be anticipated or labour should be induced.

Expedite Delivery

In case of a viable fetus, delivery should be expedited. The decision of delivery time has been shown to affect the neonatal outcome. Usually, caesarean delivery is performed, unless the cervix is fully dilated and the presenting part has descended, to enable a vaginal delivery. The urgency of the situation may demand rapid induction of general anaesthesia. However, spinal anaesthesia may be administered if the fetal condition is satisfactory.

The principles of management until the fetus is delivered are:

- Relieve compression of the umbilical cord.
- Relieve vasospasm of the umbilical cord vessels.

The methods to relieve compression of the umbilical cord are:

- Digital elevation of the presenting part.
- Filling the bladder.
- Positioning the woman in such a way that gravity helps relieve the compression of the umbilical cord.

Digital Elevation of the Presenting Part

The presenting part of the fetus should be elevated using tips of the index and middle fingers inserted into the vagina, in an attempt to relieve compression of the umbilical cord caught between the presenting part of the fetus and the maternal pelvis (Figure 2.2). Care must be taken to not exert pressure on the umbilical cord while pushing the presenting part upwards. One must also be mindful of not elevating the presenting part excessively, as this may cause more of the umbilical cord to prolapse. The hand should remain inside the vagina, and the presenting part should be elevated until the incision is made on the lower segment of the uterus.

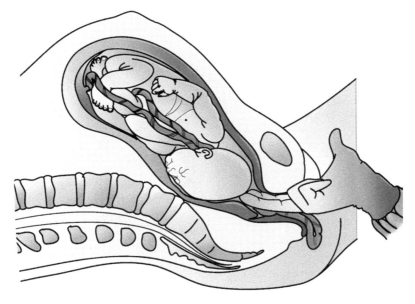

FIGURE 2.2   Digital elevation of the presenting part.

Filling the Bladder

An alternative to the digital elevation of the presenting part is filling the urinary bladder, which should help in the elevation of the presenting part, thereby preventing compression of the umbilical cord (Figure 2.3). This can be achieved by inserting a urinary catheter to fill the bladder with approximately 500 ml of normal saline and then clamping the catheter. Bladder filling is particularly helpful if there is a delay in performing caesarean delivery. A full bladder also has the advantage of inhibiting uterine contractions. The bladder should be emptied by removing the clamp on the catheter right before entering the abdominal cavity at caesarean delivery in order to avoid damage to the bladder.

Positioning the Woman

Cord compression can be reduced by placing the woman in either knee-chest, i.e. patient is facing the bed at chest-level with knees tucked under chest and buttocks elevated (Figure 2.4), or the exaggerated Sim's, i.e. left lateral with a pillow under the hip, position (Figure 2.5). Gravity helps to relieve compression of the umbilical cord between the fetal presenting part and the maternal pelvis when a woman is placed in either of these positions. The knee-chest position, as compared to the exaggerated Sim's position, provides greater elevation of the presenting part, but this could be tiring when there is a delay in delivery, in which case the exaggerated Sim's position would be more feasible and comfortable for the woman. The exaggerated Sim's position is also the most practical position to use when a woman with an umbilical cord prolapse is transferred to the operating room for caesarean delivery, from one hospital to another or from her home to a hospital. A head-low (Trendelenburg) left lateral position could also be used. This is a relaxed position for the woman and is especially useful when there is a delay in performing a caesarean delivery.

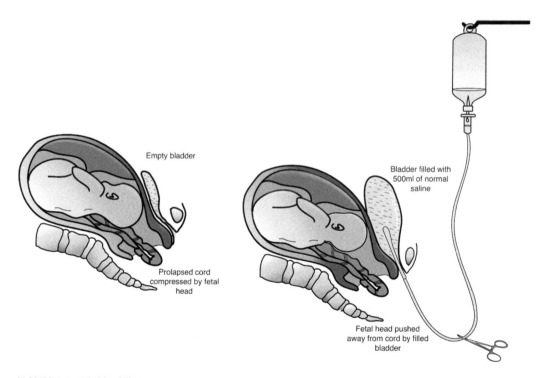

FIGURE 2.3   Bladder filling.

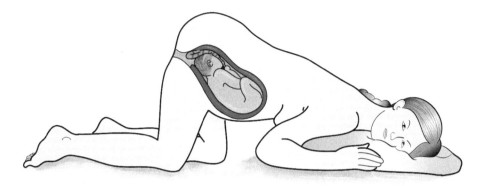

FIGURE 2.4   Knee-chest position.

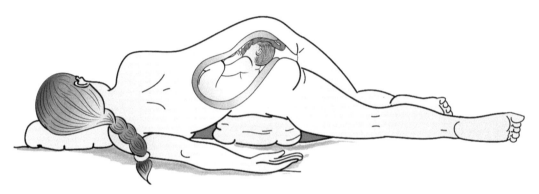

FIGURE 2.5   Exaggerated sim's position.

Other Measures

Tocolytics

If the woman is on an intravenous oxytocin infusion, then it should be stopped immediately. Tocolytics can be considered when there are abnormalities in the fetal heart rate, even after attempts to relieve cord compression by mechanical methods have been employed and especially if there is a delay in performing caesarean delivery. However, there is an increased risk of uterine atony after delivery following the administration of tocolytics.

Intrauterine Resuscitation Measures

Intrauterine fetal resuscitation measures, such as the administration of oxygen and intravenous fluids, may be adopted, but these should not hinder the immediate transport of the woman to the operating room.

Relieving of Spasms of the Umbilical Cord Vessels

If the umbilical cord has prolapsed through the introitus, then it should be gently placed within the vagina as soon as possible and with minimal handling (Figure 2.6A). This should be followed by the insertion of a moist gauze into the vagina below the cord to help hold it in place (Figure 2.6B). Excessive handling can aggravate vasospasm and further impair the fetal blood

A

B

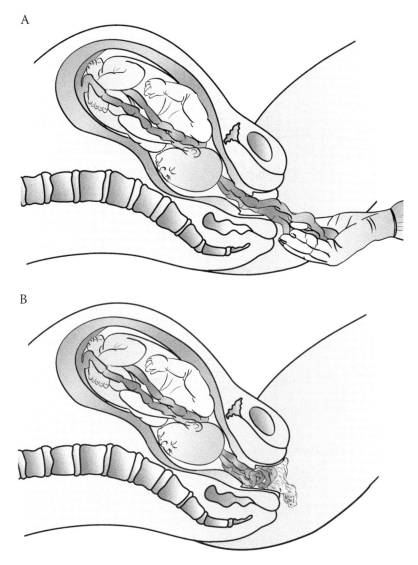

FIGURE 2.6   A – placement of umbilical cord inside the vagina, B – insertion of a moist gauze into the vagina.

supply. Keeping the cord moist is important when the interval from diagnosis to delivery is prolonged, as the umbilical cord could dry out when exposed to the outside environment and lead to spasms of umbilical cord vessels. Replacing the prolapsed umbilical cord above the presenting part, i.e. funic reduction, is not recommended.

Choice of Manoeuvres in Umbilical Cord Prolapse

The above-mentioned manoeuvres should be selected according to the clinical situation. If the woman is in the second stage of labour, then an immediate instrumental vaginal delivery or assisted vaginal breech delivery or breech extraction may possibly be the most appropriate management option, provided that the usual criteria are met (Figure 2.7) (discussed in Chapters 9 and 25). As much as possible, care must be taken to prevent the impingement of the cord when performing instrumental vaginal delivery.

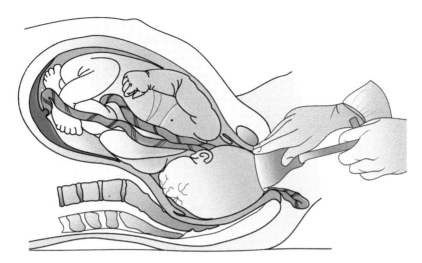

FIGURE 2.7   Instrumental vaginal delivery for cord prolapse in a woman during the second stage of labour.

If there is a delay in performing caesarean delivery, then a combination of filling the bladder and placing the woman in the exaggerated Sim's position is the most practical manoeuvre to relieve cord compression. The placement of the umbilical cord inside the vagina and the insertion of a moist gauze can be carried out, especially in the absence of uterine contractions. If immediate caesarean delivery is feasible, then digital elevation of the presenting part and placing the woman in the knee-chest position would suffice.

Care of the Newborn

The neonatal team should be prepared for the resuscitation of the newborn. Although delayed cord clamping may be advocated when the baby is not compromised, immediate resuscitation should be prioritised over delayed cord clamping if the baby needs intubation and ventilation.

Prognosis of Umbilical Cord Prolapse

The outcome following umbilical cord prolapse is generally satisfactory. However, prematurity and congenital abnormalities could contribute to perinatal mortality. The serious morbidities associated with cord prolapse, mainly hypoxic brain injury and cerebral palsy, are due to birth asphyxia. The outcome is more favourable if cord prolapse occurs while the woman is in hospital as compared to when it occurs in the community.

Umbilical Cord Prolapse under Special Circumstances

If umbilical cord prolapse occurs at pre-viable gestations, then expectant management anticipating vaginal delivery is the most reasonable management option, as the neonatal outcome is poor, and the maternal morbidity as a result of caesarean delivery at these gestations is high. Vaginal delivery should also be awaited in case of umbilical cord prolapse in the presence of a dead fetus or one with a lethal abnormality, as discussed earlier. However, an abnormal lie in such situations may necessitate delivery by caesarean delivery, a decision that should be taken according to the clinical situation.

The management of umbilical cord prolapse is summarised in Figure 2.8.

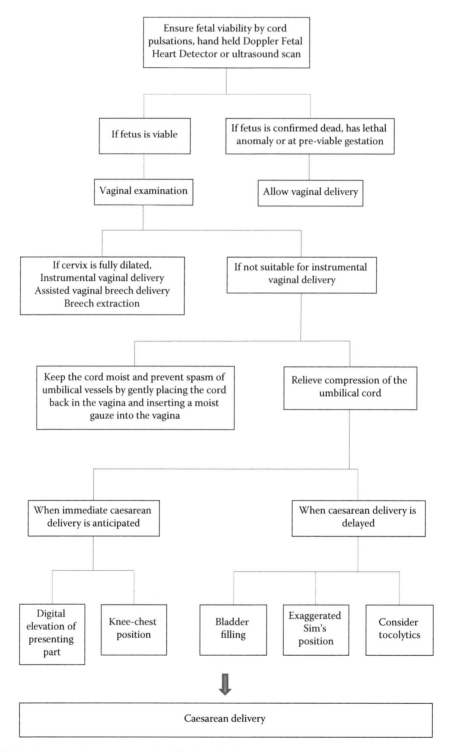

FIGURE 2.8 Summary of management of umbilical cord prolapse.

Key Points

- Awareness about risk factors is essential in reducing the incidence of umbilical cord prolapse.
- A category 1 caesarean delivery should be performed in most cases of umbilical cord prolapse.
- Measures to relieve cord compression, such as digital elevation of the presenting part, bladder filling, maternal positioning (knee-chest or exaggerated Sim's) and gentle replacement of the umbilical cord in the vagina, either individually or in combination, are employed until the fetus is delivered.

BIBLIOGRAPHY

1. Altaras M, Potashnik G, Ben-Adereth N, Leventhal H. The use of vacuum extraction in cases of cord prolapse during labor. *Am J Obstet Gynecol* 1974;118:824–30.
2. Bord I, Gemer O, Anteby EY, Shenhav S. The value of bladder filling in addition to manual elevation of presenting fetal part in cases of cord prolapse. *Arch Gynecol Obstet* 2011;283:989–91.
3. Holbrook BD, Phelan ST. Umbilical cord prolapse. *Obstet Gynecol Clin North Am* 2013; 40(1):1–14.
4. Jones G, Grenier S, Gruslin A. Sonographic diagnosis of funic presentation: implications for delivery. *BJOG* 2000;107:1055–57.
5. Katz Z, Lancet M, Borenstein R. Management of labor with umbilical cord prolapse. *Am J Obstet Gynecol* 1982;142:239–41.
6. Lin MG. Umbilical cord prolapse. *Obstet Gynecol Surv* 2006;61:269–77.
7. McDonald SJ, Middleton P. Effect of timing of umbilical cord clamping of term infants on maternal and neonatal outcomes. *Cochrane Database Syst Rev* 2008;2:CD004074.
8. Murphy DJ, MacKenzie IZ. The mortality and morbidity associated with umbilical cord prolapse. *BJOG* 1995;102:826–30.
9. Vago T. Prolapse of the umbilical cord: a method of management. *Am J Obstet Gynecol* 1970; 107:967–69.

3

Eclampsia and Pre-Eclampsia with Severe Features

Sanjeewa Padumadasa and Malik Goonewardene

Hypertensive disorders of pregnancy remain a major cause of maternal and perinatal morbidity and mortality despite advances in diagnosis and treatment. Pre-eclampsia accounts for over 500,000 fetal and neonatal deaths and over 70,000 maternal deaths globally every year.

Classification of Hypertensive Disorders of Pregnancy

A systolic blood pressure (BP) of ≥140 mmHg and/or a diastolic BP of ≥90 mmHg is considered indicative of hypertension in pregnancy. The BP should be confirmed by repeated measurements over a few hours or repeated after 15 minutes if a systolic BP of ≥160 mmHg and/or a diastolic BP of ≥110 mmHg is detected. Table 3.1 gives the classification of hypertensive disorders of pregnancy as recommended by the International Society for the Study of Hypertension in Pregnancy (ISSHP). There are important differences from the previous classification.

- Proteinuria is no longer mandatory for the diagnosis of pre-eclampsia. Pre-eclampsia is currently defined as the presence of de novo hypertension after 20 weeks of gestation accompanied by proteinuria and/or evidence of maternal acute kidney injury, liver dysfunction, neurological features, haemolysis or thrombocytopaenia and/or fetal growth restriction. In rare cases, there may be instances in which blood pressure is normal in the presence of other features of pre-eclampsia. A future definition of pre-eclampsia without a reference made to blood pressure is a possibility. The term 'pre-eclampsia' itself may not be the ideal term to describe this condition, as the occurrence of eclampsia is uncommon with early identification and management.
- Pre-eclampsia is not graded from mild to severe, as it can deteriorate rapidly, and if labelled as 'mild', then it can lead to complacency in the management.
- The HELLP syndrome (Haemolysis, Elevated Liver Enzymes and Low Platelets) is a serious manifestation of pre-eclampsia and is not considered a separate disorder.

White-coat hypertension is hypertension that is evident only at clinic visits, and although considered a benign condition, it carries an increased risk of pre-eclampsia. Masked hypertension is a form of chronic hypertension that is characterised by a BP that is considered normal in the clinic, but with evidence of target organ damage that suggests that the BP may be elevated at other times. The diagnosis of transient gestational hypertension, gestational hypertension or pre-eclampsia implies that the BP must have been normal before pregnancy or during the first trimester of pregnancy. A normal BP after 12 weeks of gestation does not exclude preexisting hypertension, because the blood pressure may decrease to normal levels even if it has been high before this time due to the physiological changes that occur during pregnancy. Gestational hypertension occurs de novo after 20 weeks in the absence of the features of pre-eclampsia. Although the outcome in gestational hypertension is generally good, about a quarter of women with gestational hypertension, especially those who develop the disease early, could progress

TABLE 3.1

Classification of hypertensive disorders of pregnancy

Hypertension known before pregnancy or hypertension that presents in the first 20 weeks
- Chronic hypertension
  ○ Essential
  ○ Secondary
- White-coat hypertension
- Masked hypertension

Hypertension arising de novo at or after 20 weeks
- Transient gestational hypertension
- Gestational hypertension
- Pre-eclampsia – de novo or superimposed on chronic hypertension

into pre-eclampsia, in which case the outcome is poor. It is important to monitor even cases in which the BP is transiently elevated for the first time during pregnancy after 20 weeks, i.e. transient gestational hypertension, as there is an approximately 40% risk of developing true gestational hypertension or pre-eclampsia. About a quarter of women with chronic hypertension develop pre-eclampsia. Eclampsia is defined as the new onset of generalised tonic-clonic seizures in a woman with pre-eclampsia.

Pathophysiology of Pre-Eclampsia

Pre-eclampsia has been referred to as a 'disease of theories', and the exact aetiology and pathogenesis have been enigmas for both clinicians and researchers for centuries. Among the theories postulated are: trophoblastic invasion of only the decidual segments of the spiral arterioles leaving the intramyometrial segments intact; an exaggerated maternal inflammatory response to the allogenic trophoblast (which contains a 'foreign' paternal component) due to a maternal immune maladaptation; a consumptive coagulopathy involving the microvasculature of the placenta, kidneys and liver; uteroplacental ischaemia associated with an abnormal response of uteroplacental vessels to vasoactive substances; endothelial dysfunction associated with impaired release of nitric oxide; and genetic factors. It is possible that some or all of these factors are interlinked and at least partially associated with pre-eclampsia. However, it is unclear as to what extent these have an aetiological role.

Recent evidence suggests that a tilt of the balance towards anti-angiogenic factors produced by the placenta in the first trimester could play a central role in the systemic vascular dysfunction characteristic of pre-eclampsia. It is hypothesised that excessive production of soluble FMS-like tyrosine kinase 1 (sFlt1), which inhibits signalling of vascular endothelial growth factor (VEGF) and placental growth factor (PlGF), and also excessive production of soluble endoglin, which inhibits signalling of trans-forming growth factor-β (TGF-β), may lead to the endothelial dysfunction, impaired production of nitric oxide and vasoconstriction observed in pre-eclampsia. More importantly, measurement of these factors could be useful in predicting the severity of the disease, especially in ruling out those who are unlikely to develop complications. Therefore, their application in clinical practice has the potential in differentiating women with pre-eclampsia who would develop complications from those who would not, a dilemma that has tormented clinicians throughout the years. Late-onset pre-eclampsia, which apparently is a different clinical entity from early-onset pre-eclampsia, may stem from an interaction between the placenta and a maternal genetic predisposition to cardiovascular and metabolic disease.

Prediction of Pre-Eclampsia

Currently, screening for pre-eclampsia involves a history-based risk assessment approach, and the risk factors for pre-eclampsia are widely recognised (Table 3.2). The BP at booking and the sonographic detection of uterine artery notching has also been associated with early-onset (prior to 34 weeks gestation)

TABLE 3.2

Risk factors for pre-eclampsia

Major risk factors

    Previous hypertensive disorder of pregnancy

    Chronic hypertension

    Diabetes mellitus

    Chronic kidney disease

    Autoimmune disease

    Multiple pregnancy

    Receipt of assisted reproductive therapy

Moderate risk factors

    Nulliparity

    Maternal age ≥ 40 years

    Body mass index at booking ≥ 35 kg/m^2

    Inter-pregnancy interval >10 years

    Family history of pre-eclampsia

---

pre-eclampsia, but not with late onset pre-eclampsia. Biochemical parameters, such as decreased levels of PlGF, alpha-fetoprotein and pregnancy-associated plasma protein A and increased levels sFlt1, inhibin A and activin A, have been associated with early-onset pre-eclampsia. However, using only these parameters, especially the PlGF or sFLT-1/PlGF ratio to rule in or rule out women who are suspected to have preterm pre-eclampsia, is currently not recommended by the ISSHP, except as a part of a clinical trial.

Recently, the use of a first-trimester multimodal algorithm has been described by the fetal Medicine Foundation (FMF) of the UK. This includes maternal factors, mean arterial pressure, first-trimester uterine artery pulsatility index Doppler and measurement of pregnancy-associated plasma protein A. The use of this method and aspirin prophylaxis has been found to be feasible and effective in a public health setting. In comparison with the use of the risk-based assessment recommended by the National Institute of Clinical Excellence – UK, the use of the FMF algorithm has been shown to result in a 50% reduction in the proportion of women labelled as being at risk for the development of preterm pre-eclampsia, doubling of pre-eclampsia detection, almost total physician compliance of aspirin use and a significant reduction in the prevalence of preterm pre-eclampsia.

Prevention of Pre-Eclampsia

Aspirin inhibits thromboxane A2 (TXA2) production by platelets, thereby increasing prostacyclin/TXA2 ratio and reducing platelet aggregation and, therefore, protects against vasoconstriction and pathological blood coagulation in the placenta. It is recommended that aspirin should be commenced at a dose of 150 mg/day in women with at least one major high-risk factor or two moderate high-risk factors for pre-eclampsia ideally before 16 weeks and definitely before 20 weeks of gestation, and continued until delivery to reduce the risk of pre-eclampsia. The number needed to treat is approximately 70. It is also recommended to administer calcium at a dose of 1.2–2.5 g/day if a pregnant woman's daily consumption of calcium is low or if it cannot be assessed. Calcium supplements are unnecessary if dietary calcium intake is adequate. Administration of low molecular weight heparin or the vitamins C, E or D, is not recommended. General measures such as exercise should be encouraged to maintain health and appropriate body weight as well as to reduce the likelihood of developing hypertension. If a woman's BP is consistently >140/90 mmHg, then she should be treated with oral methyldopa, labetalol, oxprenolol or nifedipine to decrease the likelihood of developing severe maternal hypertension and other complications. However, the BP should not be allowed to fall below 130/80 mmHg.

Clinical Features

Pre-eclampsia is a multi-organ disease, and there is a wide spectrum of clinical features which could vary depending on the organs involved, as well as the severity of their involvement. One woman may be asymptomatic despite severe hypertension or proteinuria. On the other hand, another woman may develop serious complications of pre-eclampsia despite having a normal BP. A woman may develop warning prodromal symptoms such as a headache and an aura prior to developing seizures. As the majority of women with pre-eclampsia are asymptomatic and the course of pre-eclampsia is highly unpredictable, it is important to advise every pregnant woman to seek help if they develop symptoms of pre-eclampsia.

Apart from hypertension, these women may have: neurological symptoms such as frontal headache, double vision, blurred vision, scotoma; nausea and vomiting; epigastric or right hypochondrial pain; fainting spells; a general feeling of being unwell. The development of these symptoms towards the latter part of pregnancy should alert the clinician with the possibility of pre-eclampsia, irrespective of blood pressure information or the presence/absence of proteinuria. The signs they may bear are: irritability and restlessness; epigastric or right hypochondrial tenderness; clonus; papilloedema; features of pulmonary oedema; oliguria; non-dependent oedema. If any of these symptoms or signs are present, then the diagnosis should be 'pre-eclampsia with severe features'.

The occurrence of seizures shifts the diagnosis from pre-eclampsia to eclampsia. Approximately 40% of eclamptic seizures occur in the antepartum period, 20% during the intrapartum period and 40% in the postpartum period. Therefore, even after delivery, which is part of the treatment, it is important to monitor the woman for the development of seizures and other complications of pre-eclampsia.

Investigations

Evidence of Target Organ Damage

Neither the BP nor the degree of proteinuria is directly proportional to organ dysfunction in pre-eclampsia. Serious organ dysfunction may occur at seemingly harmless levels of hypertension. Investigations that detect target organ damage include:

- Tests for proteinuria. This is performed with dipstick urinalysis, which is automated in well-resourced settings. If the results are positive, then a urine protein/creatinine ratio should be performed. Accordingly, if it turns out to be 30 mg/mmol or greater, then it is considered abnormal. Although the adverse outcomes in pre-eclampsia may not be directly proportionate to the degree of proteinuria, massive proteinuria of >5 g/24 hours has been associated with more severe neonatal outcomes and with early delivery, while a spot urine protein/creatinine ratio of >900 mg/mmol has been associated with worse maternal outcomes. If a urine protein/creatinine ratio cannot be obtained, then the traditional 24-hour urinary protein of 300 mg or more is used as the diagnostic criterion.
- Full blood count, which indicates the haemoglobin level and the haematocrit (to identify haemoconcentration) and the platelet count (to look for thrombocytopaenia)
- Alanine transaminase and aspartate transaminase (as markers of liver function)
- Blood urea, serum electrolytes and serum creatinine (as markers of renal function)
- Serum uric acid (not a diagnostic criterion but associated with worse maternal and fetal outcomes and may indicate the need for a detailed assessment of fetal growth)

Evidence of Fetal Growth and Wellbeing

In women who are managed conservatively, fetal assessment should be done with fetal biometry, which includes biparietal diameter (BPD), head circumference (HC), abdominal circumference (AC) and femur length (FL), that are used to calculate an estimated fetal weight (EFW) and also the amniotic fluid volume and umbilical artery Doppler. fetal growth is monitored at 2–3 weekly intervals with HC, AC and EFW, and the severity of fetal growth restriction (FGR) would dictate the frequency and type of Doppler assessments. Referral to a fetal medicine specialist is advised if any abnormality is detected, especially at gestations <34 weeks.

Special Investigations

Cerebral imaging is indicated if there are focal neurological signs, recurrent seizures and if there is a deterioration of the woman's condition. This is to exclude other differential diagnoses which include cerebrovascular accidents, brain tumours, aneurysms and cerebral vein thrombosis. Epilepsy, lupus, metabolic disorders, cerebral vasculitis, post-dural puncture, may also have to be excluded in a woman having recurrent seizures. Imaging of the liver is indicated in women presenting with features suggestive of liver disease as an accompaniment in the diagnosis of acute fatty liver of pregnancy (AFLP) and also to exclude focal lesions of the liver (discussed in Chapter 4).

Management of Eclampsia or Pre-Eclampsia with Severe Features

Figure 3.1 summarises the principles of management of a woman with eclampsia or pre-eclampsia with severe features. These women should be managed in a critical care setting, with the involvement of an experienced obstetrician, intensivist, anaesthesiologist and neonatologist, and if necessary, hepatic and renal physicians and a transfusion specialist. The primary aim of management would be to stabilise and deliver. The timing and the mode of delivery would depend on the gestational age, system/systems affected most and comprise of one or more of the following actions.

- Treat hypertension
- Prevent or control seizures
- Look for and treat renal, liver and haematological involvement
- Identify fetal compromise
- Achieve meticulous fluid balance
- Administer steroids for fetal lung maturity

Antihypertensive Therapy

The complications of hypertension in pregnancy that are related to blood pressure are cerebral hae-morrhage, cardiac failure and pulmonary oedema, retinal haemorrhage, haemorrhage under the capsule of the liver and placental abruption. Therefore, it is essential to control the BP using a rapidly acting antihypertensive if the blood pressure is ≥160/110 mmHg. Excessive reduction of blood pressure could cause a reduction of uteroplacental blood flow, thereby compromising the fetus. This is especially true if the fetus is growth-restricted. Therefore, the systolic BP should not be reduced to <140 mmHg and the diastolic BP to <90 mmHg. The severity of dysfunction in the other organs and systems is not directly proportional to the severity of hypertension.

Labetalol, a combined alpha and beta-adrenergic blocker, is used at a dose of 20 mg intravenous (IV) injection followed by 40 mg after 15 minutes, if the blood pressure remains ≥160/110 mmHg. Labetalol could be continued as an infusion, depending on the need to control the BP, using 200 mg in 200 ml Normal Saline (40 mg/hour, and doubled half-hourly up to 160 mg/hour). As labetalol can result in significant bradycardia, the pulse rate should be carefully monitored during labetalol therapy, and not

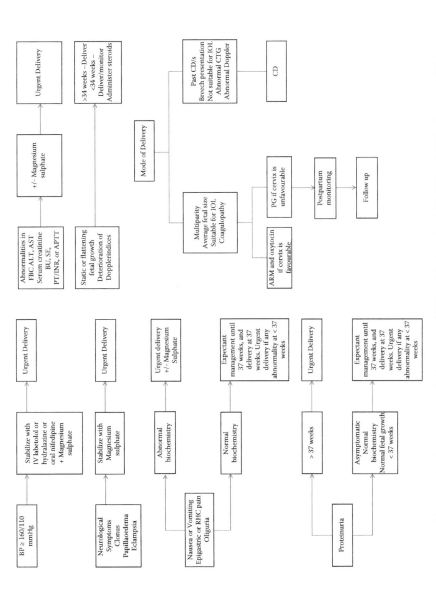

FIGURE 3.1 Summary of management of hypertension in pregnancy (IV – intravenous, RHC – right hypochondrial, FBC – full blood count, ALT-alanine transaminase, AST – aspartate transaminase, BU-blood urea, SE – serum electrolytes, PT/INR – prothrombin time/international normalised ratio, APTT – activated partial thromboplastin time, CTG – cardiotocograph, IOL – induction of labour, ARM – artificial rupture of membranes, PG – prostaglandin vaginally, CD – caesarean delivery).

allowed to decrease to <60/bpm. Labetalol should be avoided in women with bronchial asthma, cardiac failure and bradyarrhythmias.

Hydralazine, is another antihypertensive that could be used as a 5–10 mg IV bolus injection over two minutes and can be repeated, as 5 mg IV boluses every 15 minutes, up to a maximum total dose of 20 mg, depending on the blood pressure. Hydralazine can cause the blood pressure to drop drastically, and may even cause acute fetal compromise. To prevent this, a bolus of Normal saline 250 ml (5 ml/kg) should be administered over 30 minutes, before giving hydralazine, unless the woman already has pulmonary oedema. Hydralazine can also give rise to troublesome tachycardia and should be omitted (or reduced in dosage) if the pulse rate is >120/bpm. Hydralazine could be continued as an infusion depending on the need to control the BP, using 20 mg in 200 ml of Normal saline (2 mg/hour, increasing by 0.5 mg/hour and up to a maximum of 20 mg/hour). It should not be given as bolus injections.

The aim of therapy is to maintain the systolic BP between 140-150 mmHg and the diastolic BP between 90–100 mmHg. If the systolic BP decreases to <130 mmHg and/or the diastolic BP decreases to <90 mmHg, then the doses of the antihypertensives should be halved. If either IV hydralazine or labetalol is not available, 10 mg of oral nifedipine (as a normal tablet, not the slow release form) could be given and repeated after 30–45 minutes, depending on the response, up to a maximum of four doses, until the woman reaches a tertiary care centre. Headaches, which are a frequent side effect of nifedipine, could be mistaken for a symptom of neurological involvement.

Anticonvulsant Therapy

Magnesium sulphate is the anticonvulsant of choice and is indicated for eclampsia as well as if there are neurological features suggestive of impending eclampsia, such as frontal headache, double vision, blurred vision, scotoma or clonus. It is also indicated if the woman's systolic BP is ≥160 mmHg and/or the diastolic BP is ≥110 mmHg, in case of derangements in the liver and renal profile and in HELLP syndrome, even if there are no features of impending eclampsia. It has the additional benefit of providing fetal neuroprotection which is particularly important at gestations less than 32 weeks. It is usually administered with an initial dose of 4 g IV over 20 minutes, followed by a maintenance dose of 1 g/hour.

For recurrent convulsions, a repeat dose of magnesium sulphate 2 g in 20 ml should be given over 20 minutes, or the infusion rate should be increased to 1.5 g or 2.0 g/hour (7.5–10 ml/hour Infusion). If the woman does not respond to these measures, then she will need thiopentone sodium 250–300 mg IV, muscle relaxants, intubation and assisted ventilation in the intensive care unit. It is important to exclude intracranial haemorrhage in these cases. In the community or in a primary care setting, magnesium sulphate can also be administered intramuscularly as a loading dose of 10 g (5 g on each buttock) followed by 5 g every 4 hours, until the woman reaches a tertiary care centre. Magnesium sulphate should be continued for 24 hours following delivery or following the last seizure, whichever occurs later. The therapeutic range of serum magnesium is 2–3 mmol/L and although not routinely monitored, the serum magnesium level may need to be checked if there is uncertainty about overdose.

Magnesium toxicity can cause respiratory and cardiovascular depression which could prove to be fatal. Therefore, it is essential to monitor the woman's pulse rate, BP, respiratory rate, oxygen saturation, deep tendon reflexes, and urine output (as magnesium is excreted solely via the kidneys). In women with renal impairment (creatinine >1.2 mg/dl), magnesium sulphate at half of the usual dose may be used if the clinical situation demands so, provided that the urine output is more than 25 ml/hour. Magnesium sulphate should be discontinued if the respiratory rate falls below 12/minute, the oxygen saturation is <95%, the deep tendon reflexes are absent or the urine output is less than 25 ml/hour over 4 hours. The biceps tendon reflex should be checked instead of the usual patellar reflex if an epidural is sited. Magnesium sulphate overdose should be treated with 1 g of calcium gluconate (10 ml of 10% solution) given over the span of 10 minutes.

Liver, Renal and Haematological Involvement

It is important to investigate evidence of target organ damage by performing the investigations mentioned earlier. Derangement of liver enzymes in the presence of pre-eclampsia and in the absence of any other explanation for the abnormality indicates liver involvement and requires delivery before worsening of the condition. This is especially true if these are >70 IU/l. If the liver is involved, it is vital to perform a coagulation profile before delivery. Similarly, renal involvement, as evident by derangements in renal profile, especially a serum creatinine of >1.1 mg/dl, requires delivery. It is important that pregnancy-specific reference ranges are used for the interpretation of the results. Thrombocytopaenia, which is a platelet count less than 100,000/ml may occur. Spontaneous haemorrhage is unlikely if the platelet count is above 20,000/ml. However, delivery, either vaginally or abdominally, requires a platelet count of at least 50,000/ml, and peripartum or perioperative platelet transfusions should be given to achieve this. If the HELLP syndrome is suspected by liver enzymes and thrombocytopaenia, lactate dehydrogenase and blood picture can be performed to look for haemolysis, although this does not influence the management thereof.

Although the woman may not have features of impending eclampsia, it is advisable to administer magnesium sulphate if abnormalities exist in the biochemical parameters, especially liver and/or haematological, considering the safety of magnesium sulphate and the possibility of eclampsia in these cases. The use of magnesium sulphate in the case of abnormalities in the renal profile and the absence of features of impending eclampsia should be balanced against the risk of accumulation of magnesium sulphate and magnesium toxicity, and the decision must be taken on a case-by-case basis.

Identifying Fetal Compromise

Continuous cardiotocography (CTG) should be performed during the period of the woman's stabilisation. A pathological CTG may require an urgent caesarean delivery. However, optimisation of the maternal condition is vital before delivery. Delivery is indicated for fetal reasons when fetal growth is static or flattening across the centiles, or when there is a deterioration of umbilical, middle cerebral arterial and ductus venosus Doppler indices, depending on the period of gestation. The decision to deliver in these cases should be taken in consultation with the neonatologist, considering the prognosis at the particular gestation and the available neonatal facilities, after counselling the woman and her partner.

Fluid Balance

Meticulous attention should be paid to fluid balance. The woman is at risk of developing pulmonary oedema due to the reduced colloid osmotic pressure as a result of hypoalbuminaemia, increased capillary permeability and increased hydrostatic pressure. On the other hand, she may not tolerate fluid loss, as the plasma volume is depleted due to capillary leak and reduced colloid osmotic pressure. In addition, she is also at risk of acute kidney injury. Total fluids should be limited to 80 ml/hour, at least until postpartum diuresis occurs. The amount of fluid contained in the anticonvulsants and antihypertensives should be taken into consideration when calculating the input. An indwelling catheter should be inserted in order to monitor urine output, which should be at least 25 ml/hour. Central venous pressure (CVP), or rarely, pulmonary artery pressure monitoring may be needed in critical cases.

Delivery

The only known definitive management for eclampsia or pre-eclampsia with severe features at present is delivery, although the woman is not out of danger even after delivery is accomplished. Corticosteroids should be administered in order to improve the lung maturity of the fetus, although delivery cannot be deferred until the full effect of steroids is achieved. Urgent delivery is indicated in eclampsia, the HELLP syndrome, placental abruption and pulmonary oedema. The mode of delivery will depend on: parity, co-morbidities, gestational age, fetal size, presence or absence of FGR, fetal wellbeing, presentation, position, head level abdominally and vaginal station, how soon the delivery should be achieved, the favourability of the cervix for induction of labour (IOL), etc.

If the woman is in a centre without adult 'High Dependency and Intensive Care' facilities or if the fetus is grossly pre-term and the centre has no neonatal intensive care facilities, then the woman should be transferred to a tertiary care centre with these facilities. An attempt should be made to control the systolic BP to <150 mmHg and the diastolic BP to <100 with oral nifedipine, and a loading dose of magnesium sulphate (5g to each buttock) should be given, prior to transfer. The receiving centre should be informed about the transfer, and details of the medication given should accompany the woman.

A platelet count and a coagulation profile should be available on the day of delivery, and considering the rapidity of worsening of the condition, these should be monitored during delivery. Amniotomy and oxytocin or prostaglandins should be used for induction of labour (IOL), if it is considered appropriate depending on the clinical situation. As oxytocin is associated with fluid retention, it should be administered as a more concentrated infusion than normal. Continuous electronic fetal monitoring should be instituted during labour. Instrumental vaginal delivery is not routinely needed, but may be necessary to assist labour in case the maternal bearing-down phase is prolonged, as excessive maternal effort may give rise to increased blood pressure. Ergometrine can precipitate a hypertensive crisis, and therefore, oxytocin should be used instead of ergometrine or syntometrine during the active management of the third stage of labour. However, ergometrine can be used if postpartum haemorrhage occurs and the blood pressure drops (discussed in Chapter 14). Coagulopathy, if present, should be corrected before delivery, ideally with the use of rotational thromboelastometry and in consultation with a transfusion specialist. An uncomplicated vaginal delivery is preferable in case of coagulopathy, because it has the potential to cause less maternal trauma than a caesarean delivery.

Caesarean delivery is performed if IOL is not considered to be appropriate, e.g. absent or reversed umbilical artery end-diastolic flow, breech presentation, primigravida with a cervix unfavourable for IOL, delivery after IOL unlikely to occur within 12 hours, etc. Regional anaesthesia is advisable over general anaesthesia, and can be administered if the platelet count is >80 × 10^9/l and there is no evidence of any other coagulation abnormality. Epidural anaesthesia also offers the advantage of effective pain relief during the immediate postpartum period. Judicious fluid therapy for preloading before the administration of epidural analgesia is required to prevent acute hypotension (due to hypovolaemia) as well as pulmonary oedema (due to fluid overload and increased capillary permeability). General anaesthesia carries a risk of difficult intubation due to laryngeal oedema but may be required in the presence of coagulopathy. A sudden rise of blood pressure may occur at the time of intubation and also during recovery from general anaesthesia.

Management of a woman with pre-eclampsia with severe features at the threshold of fetal viability poses a clinical as well as an ethical dilemma to the clinician. Vaginal delivery which causes the least amount of trauma, but avoids a hysterotomy scar which has the potential to cause serious complications in subsequent pregnancies, should be the goal in these cases. However, the fetus who may already be compromised may not tolerate the stress of labour. The involvement of the neonatologist, the woman and her partner in the discussions on management is paramount.

Management during the Postpartum Period

If antihypertensives were administered prior to delivery, these will usually need to be continued during as well as after the delivery. If the patient is normotensive soon after delivery, a thorough evaluation should be carried out to exclude an undetected postpartum haemorrhage. Nifedipine, labetolol, Angiotensin-converting enzyme inhibitors, Angiotensin receptor blockers and even diuretics are safe during breastfeeding and can be used during the postpartum period. Methyldopa is avoided as it increases the risk of postpartum depression. Often, the BP will normalise within 3–4 days, but if it does not, then the woman could be discharged home on antihypertensives, provided her systolic BP is <150 mmHg and the diastolic BP is <100 mmHg, and she is reviewed after 10–14 days.

Platelet count may drop until day three of postpartum, and in the absence of bleeding, does not require any treatment. Similarly, the liver enzymes may elevate on the first day or two after delivery. As pre-eclampsia is a risk factor for thromboembolic disease, thrombo-embolic deterrent stockings should be used. However, the use of low molecular weight heparin should be balanced against the risk of bleeding that may be present due to coagulopathy. Non-steroidal anti-inflammatory agents as a form of postpartum analgesia should be avoided if there is acute kidney injury or coagulopathy.

Follow-Up

Follow-up depends on the severity of the disease antenatally and the recovery during the postpartum period. The aims of follow-up are to assess the recovery of target organs and to ascertain whether the antenatal development of hypertension and associated complications were part of a long-term disease process. If the woman is continuing antihypertensive therapy, then the aim of therapy is to maintain the systolic BP between 120–130 mmHg and the diastolic BP between 80–90 mmHg. It could take up to three months for the antihypertensives to be safely tailed off. At the end of three months, if the woman is not normotensive without therapy, then she should be referred to a physician for appropriate investigations and management. Up to approximately 13% could have underlying essential hypertension or chronic renal disease undetected antenatally, and depending on the clinical picture, screening for autoimmune diseases and thrombophilias may be indicated as well.

Any abnormality in the haematological and biochemical parameters warrants appropriate referral. As she is at a higher risk of developing cardiovascular complications and metabolic syndrome long-term, she should be advised on the importance of a healthy lifestyle including a balanced diet and exercise. The importance of spacing out the pregnancies should be stressed, and contraceptive advice should be given. Pre-conceptional counselling, including optimisation of blood pressure and any associated medical conditions before embarking on future pregnancies and antenatal aspirin therapy form a vital aspect of management.

Documentation, Debriefing, Risk management and Training

Proper documentation and debriefing of the woman, her partner and staff involved, as well as risk management are important. All maternity units must have a competent staff member, equipment and medication to deal with eclampsia or pre-eclampsia with severe features. Regular simulation-based training with multi-professional involvement is important.

Key Points

- Pre-eclampsia is characterised by hypertension (systolic blood pressure of ≥140 mmHg and/or diastolic blood pressure of ≥90 mmHg) occurring after 20 weeks of gestation and the presence of proteinuria, and/or evidence of maternal acute kidney injury, liver dysfunction, neurological features, haemolysis or thrombocytopaenia and/or fetal growth restriction.
- Proteinuria is not essential for the diagnosis of pre-eclampsia.
- Pre-eclampsia has the potential to progress into a severe form at any time, and a high degree of suspicion is required to detect women who present with atypical features.
- Neither the blood pressure nor the degree of proteinuria is predictive of the severity of the disease.
- Stabilisation and urgent delivery constitute the only definitive management for eclampsia and pre-eclampsia with severe features. However, complications could occur during the postpartum period as well.
- The main principles of management of eclampsia and pre-eclampsia with severe features are: antihypertensive therapy (primarily with intravenous hydralazine or labetalol); anticonvulsant therapy (primarily with magnesium sulphate); monitoring for liver, renal and haematological abnormalities; meticulous attention to fluid balance; ensuring fetal wellbeing; stabilisation and urgent delivery; close monitoring in the postpartum period; and follow-up.

- In the community and primary care settings, oral nifedipine and intramuscular magnesium sulphate could be given prior to transfer to a specialised centre.
- Dexamethasone is indicated, in order to improve fetal lung maturity, if the gestational age is less than 36 weeks.
- The mode of delivery will depend on several maternal and fetal factors, and this need not invariably be a caesarean delivery.

BIBLIOGRAPHY

1. Tomimatsu T, Mimura K, Endo M, Kumasawa K, Kimura T. Pathophysiology of preeclampsia: an angiogenic imbalance and long-lasting systemic vascular dysfunction. *Hypertens Res* 2017;40(4): 305–10.
2. Verlohren S. Pre-eclampsia is primarily a placental disorder. BJOG2017;124(11):1762.
3. Hurrell A, Beardmore-Gray A, Duhig K, Webster L, Chappell LC, Shennan AH. Placental growth factor in suspected preterm pre-eclampsia: a review of the evidence and practicalities of implementation. BJOG 2020;127(13):1590–97. https://doi.org/10.1111/1471-0528.16425
4. Guy GP, Leslie K, Diaz Gomez D, Forenc K, Buck E, Khalil A, Thilaganathan B. Implementation of routine first trimester combined screening for pre-eclampsia: a clinical effectiveness study. BJOG 2021;128(2):149–56. https://doi.org/10.1111/1471-0528.16361
5. Bartsch E, Medcalf KE, Park AI, Ray JG. Clinical risk factors for pre-eclampsia determined in early pregnancy: systematic review and meta-analysis of large cohort studies. *BMJ* 2016;353:i1753.
6. Brown MA, Magee LA, Kenny LC, Karumanchi SA, McCarthy FP, Saito S, Hall DR, Warren CE, Adoyi G, Ishaku S on behalf of the International Society for the Study of Hypertension in Pregnancy (ISSHP). The hypertensive disorders of pregnancy: ISSHP classification, diagnosis & management recommendations for international practice. *Pregnancy Hypertens* 2018;13:291–310.
7. Hawkins TL, Brown MA, Mangos GJ, Davis GK. Transient gestational hypertension: not always a benign event. *Pregnancy Hypertens* 2012;2(1):22–27.
8. Roberge S, Nicolaides K, Demers S, Hyett J, Chaillet N, Bujold E. The role of aspirin dose on the prevention of pre-eclampsia and fetal growth restriction: systematic review and meta-analysis. *Am J Obstet Gynecol* 2017;216(2):110–20.
9. Sakae C, Sato Y, Kanbayashi S, Taga A, Emoto I, Maruyama S, Mise H, Kim T. Introduction of management protocol for early-onset severe pre-eclampsia. *J Obstet Gynaecol Res* 2017;43:644–52.
10. Wang Y, Hao M, Sampson S, Xia J. Elective delivery versus expectant management for pre-eclampsia: a meta-analysis of RCTs. *Arch Gynecol Obstet* 2017;295:607–22.
11. ACOG. Hypertension in pregnancy: executive summary. *Obstet Gynecol* 2013;122(5):1122–31.

4

Acute Fatty Liver of Pregnancy

Janaka de Silva and Sanjeewa Padumadasa

Introduction

Acute fatty liver of pregnancy (AFLP) is a condition that is unique to pregnancy which may result in fulminant hepatic failure and, if untreated, carries a high risk of maternal and perinatal morbidity and mortality. First described by Sheehan in 1940 as 'acute yellow atrophy of the liver', it has an incidence of approximately 1 in 10,000–15,000 pregnancies. It typically occurs during the third trimester of pregnancy but may also occur as early as 26 weeks of gestation and as late as the immediate postpartum period. In the past, the maternal and perinatal mortality rates were reported to be over 75%. In recent times, the recognition of milder presentations, early intervention and delivery, and aggressive management of complications have reduced the maternal mortality rate to 10%–15% and perinatal mortality rate to approximately 20%.

Pathogenesis

Acute fatty liver of pregnancy is more frequent in primigravida, older women, women with low Body Mass Index, multiple pregnancy and apparently, also in the presence of a male fetus. The pathogenesis of AFLP, although still not completely elucidated, has been attributed to defective mitochondrial β-oxidation of fatty acids – a mitochondrial cytopathy. Mutations in genes coding fetal fatty acid oxidation have been found to be associated with AFLP. Levels of free fatty acids increase during pregnancy, especially during the third trimester, to ensure that the fetus has an adequate source of energy. When fetuses are either homozygous or heterozygous (to a lesser extent) for long-chain 3-hydroxyacyl-coenzyme A dehydrogenase (LCHAD) deficiency, they have deranged fatty acid metabolism that leads to impaired uptake and oxidation of fatty acids. In these instances, the unmetabolized medium and long-chain fatty acids re-enter the maternal circulation and overwhelm the fatty acid β-oxidation enzymes of the woman if she is heterozygous for LCHAD deficiency and brings about microvesicular fatty infiltration of her hepatocytes (steatosis).

Complications

Steatosis of the liver impairs liver function and can activate fulminant liver failure and multiorgan dysfunction, which may result in the death of the woman and the fetus. Liver injury can be complicated by haematoma, infarction or rupture. Renal dysfunction can occur due to direct fatty infiltration, hypoperfusion and hepatorenal syndrome. Fatty acid metabolites are toxic to pancreatic tissue and may cause pancreatitis, which can be complicated by pseudocysts with secondary infection, haemorrhage and necrosis. Placental dysfunction results from the deposition of fatty acids as well as fibrin in the placenta. The reduced levels of fibrinogen, coagulation factors and antithrombin III (due to reduced production by the liver) together with endothelial cell dysfunction leads to coagulopathy. Transient diabetes insipidus may develop as a result of elevated levels of vasopressinase, the enzyme that metabolises vasopressin and is normally cleared by the liver. Encephalopathy may occur, and can lead to convulsions and coma.

Diagnosis

Clinical Features

The following symptoms are usually seen.

- Nausea
- Vomiting
- Loss of appetite
- Feeling unwell
- Fatigue
- Abdominal pain
- Heartburn

The non-specificity of these symptoms and their resemblance to usual symptoms in pregnancy make an early diagnosis of AFLP difficult. Acute fatty liver of pregnancy should be considered in any woman who presents with these symptoms, especially during the third trimester.
The following clinical features may be found in advanced cases.

- Polydipsia
- Polyuria
- Fever
- Right hypochondrial or epigastric tenderness
- Jaundice
- Encephalopathy

Differential Diagnosis

The differential diagnosis of AFLP is given in Table 4.1.

TABLE 4.1

The differential diagnosis of acute fatty liver of pregnancy

Pregnancy-related acute causes
Pre-eclampsia with haemolysis, elevated liver enzymes and low platelets (HELLP syndrome)
Intrahepatic cholestasis of pregnancy
Non-pregnancy-related acute causes
Haemolytic uraemic syndrome
Antiphospholipid syndrome
Infective hepatitis
Drug-induced hepatitis
Bacterial sepsis
Gallstones
Non-pregnancy-related chronic causes
Alcoholic liver disease
Autoimmune hepatitis
Wilson's disease
Acute decompensation of cirrhosis due to any cause

Investigations

Haematological Investigations

It is important that reference values that are specific to the trimester of pregnancy are used when interpreting laboratory results. The majority of liver function tests remain within the non-pregnant range during pregnancy, except for alkaline phosphatase and alpha-fetoprotein which increase due to their production by the placenta and albumin which decreases due to haemodilution. Although hypoglycemia and derangements of the liver and renal function tests may be found in AFLP, these may not be always visible. Aspartate and Alanine Transaminase (AST/ALT) levels are often elevated, but these may not reflect the severity of the condition. The neutrophil leukocytosis, which is commonly observed during pregnancy, is usually more distinct in AFLP. As coagulopathy is usually present in AFLP, a coagulation screen should be performed. Serum ammonia is useful if encephalopathy is suspected.

It is crucial to exclude infective hepatitis in communities where it is prevalent, because in such cases, delivery is not indicated as it can lead to hepatic failure and massive postpartum haemorrhage. Infective hepatitis is suspected by high AST and ALT values and should be confirmed by hepatitis serology. If a diagnosis of infective hepatitis is made, then specialised medical input is essential.

Imaging Studies

Abdominal ultrasound may show a bright liver with increased echogenicity, usually with sparing of zone 1. However, abdominal ultrasound has limited diagnostic value in AFLP because of its low sensitivity and specificity, but this can be helpful in excluding other liver pathology such as tumours or rare complications of AFLP such as haemorrhage, rupture and necrosis. Computerised tomography and magnetic resonance imaging are not commonly used in the diagnosis of AFLP.

Histological Investigations

Although liver biopsy confirms the diagnosis, it is rarely performed due to the increased risk of bleeding in the presence of coagulopathy. A liver biopsy may be done in cases of doubt, where a diagnosis of AFLP is required to make a decision to deliver early and in cases that do not recover following delivery in order to differentiate AFLP from other causes of hepatic failure. If liver biopsy is considered necessary, then the percutaneous route with ultrasound guidance is preferred, but the transjugular route may have to be used in the presence of significant coagulopathy. Ch'ng et al proposed a set of clinical, biochemical, radiological and histopathological parameters known as the Swansea criteria for the diagnosis of AFLP (Table 4.2). The presence of six or more of the 14 features laid in the criteria, and in the absence of any other explanation, suggests a diagnosis of AFLP. In most instances, these criteria enable a diagnosis of AFLP, and a liver biopsy is not needed.

Acute fatty liver of pregnancy, the HELLP syndrome and intrahepatic cholestasis of pregnancy are conditions unique to pregnancy that typically occur during the third trimester of pregnancy. The distinguishing features among these conditions are summarised in Table 4.3.

Highlighted Main Distinguishing Features

Profound hypoglycaemia, marked hyperuricaemia and coagulopathy (in the absence of severe thrombocytopaenia) strongly support a diagnosis of AFLP over the HELLP syndrome. However, irrespective of the diagnosis, in both AFLP and the HELLP syndrome, early recognition, patient stabilising, delivery expediting and supportive therapy are crucial to a successful outcome for both the woman and the fetus.

Management

Initial Management

Acute fatty liver of pregnancy is best treated in an intensive care setting with multidisciplinary input from an obstetrician, a hepatologist, an intensivist, an obstetric anaesthesiologist, a transfusion medicine

TABLE 4.2

Swansea criteria to diagnose acute fatty liver of pregnancy

Clinical parameters
    Vomiting
    Abdominal pain
    Polydipsia/polyuria
    Encephalopathy
Biochemical parameters
    Elevated transaminases (>42 IU/l)
    Elevated bilirubin (>140 μmol/l)
    Elevated uric acid (>340 μmol/l)
    Elevated ammonia (>47 IU/l)
    Coagulopathy (PT >14 seconds or APTT >34 seconds)
    Hypoglycaemia (<4 mmol/l)
    Leukocytosis (>11×10^6/l)
    Creatinine (>150 μmol/l)
Radiological parameters
    Ascites or bright liver
Histological parameters
    Microvesicular steatosis on liver biopsy

specialist and a neonatologist. The woman should be stabilised before delivery. This involves treating hypertension (if present), and the correction of hypoglycaemia, electrolyte and coagulation abnormalities. The monitoring of maternal vital signs as well as the evaluation of the patient's mental status are crucial in initial management.

Assessment of Fetal Wellbeing

Acute fatty liver of pregnancy can be detrimental to the fetus and is compounded by preterm birth. However, the severity of maternal illness does not correlate well with fetal complications. The fetus should be continuously monitored with cardiotocography until plans are made for delivery. The correction of maternal acidosis and delivery improves the outcome for the fetus.

Administration of Corticosteroids and Magnesium Sulphate

The administration of corticosteroids for improving lung maturity should be considered in pregnancies that are less than 37 weeks and magnesium sulphate for neuroprotection of fetus in pregnancies that are less than 32 weeks. In addition, the administration of magnesium sulphate as a prophylactic agent against eclampsia is important in cases where an overlap occurs between AFLP and HELLP syndrome (discussed in Chapter 3). The dose of magnesium sulphate has to be reduced in case there is renal compromise, which may be a complication of AFLP.

Delivery

Acute fatty liver of pregnancy has an unpredictable course, and there is no place for expectant management. Delivery following stabilisation of the woman should be the norm. Additionally, vaginal delivery is preferred. Induction of labour with amniotomy followed by oxytocin, or with prostaglandin is a reasonable option if vaginal delivery is likely to be accomplished within 24 hours, and when the disease is not rapidly progressing within that time frame. However, the speed of deterioration of the maternal or fetal condition may necessitate a caesarean delivery. General anaesthesia may worsen hepatic encephalopathy, while regional anaesthesia carries a risk of spinal or epidural haematoma in the presence of coagulopathy. General anaesthesia is favoured over regional anaesthesia in the event of coagulopathy. Gentle intubation

TABLE 4.3

Differential diagnosis – pregnancy-related acute causes

	AFLP	HELLP syndrome	ICP
Symptoms			
Nausea	++	+	–
Vomiting	++	+	–
Epigastric pain	+	++	–
Right hypochondrial pain	+	++	–
Headache	+	++	
Loss of appetite	+	+/-	–
Malaise	+	+/-	–
Polydipsia/polyuria	+	–	–
Severe pruritus	–	–	++
Dark urine	–	–	++
Steatorrhoea	–	–	++
Signs			
Unwell	++	++	–
Jaundice	++	–	–
Hypertension	+ (in 50%)	++	–
Investigations			
Urine			
Proteinuria	+ (in 50%)	++	–
Haematological			
Transaminases	300–500 U/l	Raised	Normal to mild rise
Serum bilirubin	Markedly raised >8 mg/dl	Raised (unconjugated)/normal	May be elevated, but < 6 mg/dl
Bile acids	Normal	Normal	10–100 fold increase (>10 µmol/l)
Platelet count	Reduced	Markedly reduced	Normal
White cell count	Markedly raised	Raised	Normal
Prothrombin time	Raised	Normal	Normal
APTT	Raised	Normal	Normal
Fibrinogen	Reduced	Normal	Normal
Antithrombin III	Markedly reduced	Reduced	Normal
Uric acid	Markedly raised	Raised	Normal
Creatinine	Markedly raised	Raised/normal	Normal
LDH	Raised	Raised	Normal
Blood glucose	Hypoglycaemia	Normal	Normal
Ammonia	Raised	Normal	Normal
Imaging			
Ultrasound of liver	Fatty infiltration	Infarction/haematoma/rupture	Normal
Histology			
Liver biopsy	Microvesicular steatosis mainly in the central zone	Periportal patchy necrosis/ haemorrhage/rupture	Normal/mild cholestasis
Complications			
Coagulopathy	80%–100%	20%	–
PPH	++	+	+
Encephalopathy	+	–	–
Liver failure	++	+/–	–
Renal failure	++	+	–
Statistics			

(*Continued*)

TABLE 4.3 (Continued)
Differential diagnosis – pregnancy-related acute causes

	AFLP	HELLP syndrome	ICP
Maternal mortality	7–18%	1%	0%
Perinatal mortality	9–23%	10–60%	0.4–1.4%
Recurrence	Rare	4–19%	70%

Abbreviations: AFLP – Acute fatty liver of pregnancy; HELLP – Haemolysis Elevated Liver Enzymes Low Platelets; ICP – Intrahepatic cholestasis of pregnancy; APTT – Activated partial thromboplastin time; LDH – Lactate dehydrogenase; PPH – Postpartum haemorrhage
Note: + Usually present; − Usually absent; +/− Present or absent; ++ Markedly present

is advisable because of possible laryngeal oedema and the risk of bleeding in the airway due to coagulopathy. Caesarean delivery carries a higher risk of bleeding compared to vaginal delivery, and preparations should be in place to handle perioperative bleeding. Coagulopathy should be managed with transfusion of packed red cells, fresh frozen plasma and cryoprecipitate which is guided by rotational thromboelastometry, if available, and early administration of 1 g of intravenous tranexamic acid.

Postpartum Management

The woman should receive intensive care in the postpartum period. As coagulopathy is usually present, the woman must be closely monitored for bleeding irrespective of the mode of delivery. Coagulopathy is often the presenting feature in women who develop AFLP during the immediate postpartum period. Postoperative pain management is challenging because of the altered metabolism of opioids, the contraindication of paracetamol in liver failure and the contraindication of nonsteroidal anti-inflammatory agents in the presence of renal failure and coagulopathy. Fentanyl is relatively safe, but it is short-acting. Therefore, intravenous infusions of low-dose morphine are often used for postoperative analgesia in cases of AFLP.

Following delivery, most women recover within a few weeks with supportive treatment, as the stimulus for fatty acid overload is removed. Usually, there is a worsening of clinical and haematological parameters in the immediate postpartum period. Biochemical changes may persist for up to one week postpartum, while the histological changes in the liver may carry on for months. The postpartum clinical course is dependent on the interval between the development of symptoms and delivery.

Management of Complications

Cerebral oedema and intracranial hypertension contribute significantly to maternal morbidity and mortality in AFLP. Therefore, in case of hepatic encephalopathy, the elevation of head-end by 30° and treatment with mannitol or hypertonic saline are useful in reducing cerebral oedema and intracranial pressure and thereby improve cerebral perfusion. Avoidance of hypoxia and hypercarbia, both of which increase cerebral blood flow, which in turn leads to intracranial hypertension, is important. This could be achieved by giving oxygen via nasal prongs, and, if necessary, intubation and ventilation. In hepatic failure, protein intake should not be restricted. Laxatives, e.g. lactulose, should be administered in order to speed the evacuation of nitrogenous waste. Work extrapolated from acetaminophen-related toxicity shows that N-acetyl cysteine improves the outcome. N-acetyl cysteine, an antioxidant and glutathione precursor, promotes selective inactivation of free radicals. However, L-ornithine-L-aspartate (LOLA) which reduces ammonia levels by increasing hepatic ammonia disposal and its peripheral metabolism, does not improve survival in acute hepatic failure, and its use in AFLP cannot be recommended.

Plasma exchange has been shown to be successful in certain non-randomised trials. Liver transplantation may be required in the rare instances of worsening hepatic encephalopathy despite standard interventions, liver necrosis or rupture and severe metabolic acidosis. Patients must be kept under observation for pancreatitis which typically occurs after the onset of hepatic or renal dysfunction. Serial assessments of serum lipase and amylase coupled with imaging of the abdomen help identify women at risk of pancreatitis. Pseudocysts in the pancreas with secondary infection and haemorrhagic pancreatitis, with the potential to bleed into the retroperitoneal space, can be difficult to manage and carry a considerable risk of maternal morbidity and mortality.

Recurrence

As defective fatty acid oxidation (LCHAD deficiency) is an autosomal recessive condition, there is a 25% theoretical risk of recurrence of AFLP in a subsequent pregnancy. However, the actual figure is lower. This somewhat disputes the theory of defective fatty acid oxidation playing a pivotal role in the development of AFLP. Nevertheless, women should be counselled about the risk of recurrence of AFLP. Women with a history of AFLP should be closely monitored in a subsequent pregnancy. Baseline tests, ALT, AST and coagulation profile should be performed at the initial clinic visit. In addition to routine antenatal care, they should be informed about symptoms of AFLP, examined for jaundice and right hypochondrial or epigastric tenderness, and liver function tests should be performed regularly. It is prudent to begin close surveillance of these women four weeks before the gestational age at which AFLP occurred during the previous pregnancy.

Monitoring of Neonate

Neonates born to women who had AFLP should be screened for LCHAD deficiency and other genetic defects in fatty acid oxidation by a clinical geneticist, as they are at risk of failure to thrive and also liver failure, cardiomyopathy, myopathy, neuropathy and hypoglycaemia. This allows early identification before they manifest the disease and gives way to dietary intervention which includes an institution of a low fat, high carbohydrate diet and the substitution of long-chain fatty acids with medium-chain fatty acids.

Key Points

- Symptoms of nausea, vomiting and abdominal pain, although common in pregnancy, should be viewed seriously, and women presenting with these symptoms should be investigated for possible liver disease.
- Liver function tests, at least AST and ALT, should be performed in women presenting with such symptoms.
- Marked hypoglycaemia, hyperuricaemia and coagulopathy strongly support a diagnosis of AFLP.
- Early diagnosis, stabilisation and delivery and supportive care are pivotal in the management of AFLP.
- In cases of AFLP, vaginal delivery is favored over caesarean delivery, but the urgency of the clinical situation may necessitate a caesarean delivery.

BIBLIOGRAPHY

1. Ch'ng CL, Morgan M, Hainsworth I et al. Prospective study of liver dysfunction in pregnancy in Southwest Wales. *Gut* 2002;51:876–80.
2. Joshi D, James A, Quaglia A, Westbrook RH, Heneghan MA. Liver disease in pregnancy. *Lancet* 2010;375:594–605.
3. Liu J, Ghaziani TT, Wolf JL. Acute fatty liver disease of pregnancy: updates in pathogenesis, diagnosis, and management. *Am J Gastroenterol* 2017;112(6):838–46.
4. Tran TT, Ahn J, Reau NS. ACG clinical guideline: liver disease and pregnancy. *Am J Gastroenterol* 2016;111(2);176–94.
5. Westbrook RH, Dusheiko G, Williamson C. Pregnancy and liver disease. *Journal of Hepatology* 2016;64:933–45.

5

Cardiac Emergencies in Obstetrics

Sanjeewa Padumadasa and Sanjeewa Rajapakse

Cardiac disorders are the most common cause of maternal deaths in high-income countries. Hypertensive disorders constitute the most frequent cardiovascular disorder in pregnancy, and these are discussed in Chapter 3. While congenital heart disease is the prevailing cardiac disease in high-income countries, rheumatic heart disease is its counterpart in low-middle income countries. The incidence of cardiac disease in pregnancy is rising due to advancing maternal age and the increased number of women with congenital heart disease reaching childbearing age due to advances in medical and surgical management. Pulmonary hypertensive crisis, myocardial infarction and acute pulmonary oedema due to cardiomyopathy are the most frequent cardiac emergencies that occur in pregnancy, with aortic dissection and arrhythmias also contributing.

Physiological Changes in the Cardiovascular System during Pregnancy

The cardiac output increases from as early as ten weeks to reach a maximum of 40%–50% above the non-pregnant level at 32 weeks of gestation. There is a reduction of peripheral resistance by 20%–30% due to systemic vasodilatation. This usually results in a reduction of blood pressure, starting early during pregnancy, reaching a maximum in mid-pregnancy and returning to approximately pre-pregnancy level during the third trimester. Pregnancy is a hypercoagulable state which increases the risk of thromboembolism. Aortocaval compression by the gravid uterus which becomes significant after 20 weeks can lead to supine hypotension syndrome. These physiological changes that occur in pregnancy may either worsen preexisting cardiac disease or unmask previously undiagnosed conditions.

Management

Women with cardiac disease should be managed by a multidisciplinary team which includes an obstetrician, a cardiologist, an anaesthesiologist, an intensivist and a neonatologist with the additional involvement of a cardiothoracic surgeon, a fetal medicine specialist, a paediatric cardiologist and a haematologist, when necessary.

Prevention

The majority of women with preexisting cardiac disease can be identified by conducting a careful history and performing a thorough clinical examination. In addition, electrocardiogram (ECG), echocardiogram, exercise testing, and rarely, cardiac computerised tomography (CT) or magnetic resonance imaging (MRI) scan, are useful to risk stratify women with cardiac disease. Compared to the New York Heart Association (NYHA) classification of cardiac disease based on the functional capacity of a woman with cardiac disease, the modified WHO risk stratification model, which considers the cardiac condition itself, is more useful in pregnancy. The aims of the assessment are to identify women who will benefit from an operative intervention, to optimise management, to identify potential complications and to formulate a management plan during the antenatal period, delivery and the postpartum period. Women who are identified during the pre-pregnancy assessment to be at a significantly high risk of cardiac complications should be advised to not conceive, and if they do conceive, early therapeutic termination of pregnancy should be offered.

Acute Exacerbation of Preexisting Cardiac Disease

Mitral stenosis of rheumatic origin, which is probably the most commonly acquired cardiac condition observed in low-middle income countries, is associated with arrhythmias such as atrial fibrillation (AF) and acute pulmonary oedema. Anaemia, arrhythmias, hypertension and thyroid disease increase the risk of pulmonary oedema in these women, and the highest risk is during straining due to increased cardiac output and immediately following delivery due to the acute rise in plasma volume. In general, regurgitant lesions of the mitral and aortic valve are better tolerated than stenotic lesions. On the other hand, corrected congenital heart lesions pose a minimal risk during pregnancy.

Acute Heart Failure

Heart failure is the most prevalent complication and the most important cause of mortality due to cardiac disease in pregnant women. Women with shunt lesions, reduced cardiac function, pulmonary hypertension and left heart obstruction are at the highest risk, especially at the end of the second trimester or immediate postpartum period. The causes of heart failure in pregnancy are given in Table 5.1.

Clinical Features

Symptoms

A woman with heart failure may present with the following symptoms.

- Shortness of breath on exertion or at rest
- Paroxysmal nocturnal dyspnoea or orthopnoea
- Blackouts
- Palpitations
- Chest pain
- Cough, especially if it is nocturnal

TABLE 5.1

Causes of heart failure in pregnancy

Valvular heart disease
Peripartum cardiomyopathy
Pulmonary hypertension
Cardiac arrhythmias
Viral myocarditis
Myocardial infarction
Constrictive pericarditis
Thyrotoxicosis
Medications

While shortness of breath could be present even in normal pregnant women, pink frothy sputum is a dire symptom and may indicate underlying disease.

Signs

Sinus tachycardia, peripheral oedema, displaced apex beat and mildly elevated jugular venous pressure, in addition to most of the symptoms mentioned above, could also be present in normal pregnant women, making the diagnosis of heart failure difficult. Cyanosis, clubbing, tachycardia at rest, any arrhythmia, a collapsing pulse, hypertension or hypotension, tachypnoea or other clinical signs of respiratory distress, a pulsatile and significantly elevated JVP, a pansystolic or any diastolic murmur with or without associated thrill or any clinical signs of pulmonary oedema should prompt further testing in order to diagnose underlying cardiac disease.

Management

Management should be decided by a multidisciplinary team comprising of at least an obstetrician, a cardiologist, an anaesthesiologist and a neonatologist after assessing the maturity of the fetus, severity of heart failure and the woman's intentions.

Investigations

Useful investigations in women with heart disease are electrocardiogram, chest x-ray and echocardiogram. In a normal pregnancy, the electrocardiogram may show left axis deviation, transient ST elevation, a Q wave and an inverted T wave, while the echocardiogram may show a mild dilatation of heart chambers, a change in left ventricular wall thickness and an increase in valve gradient.

Pharmacological Treatment

Diuretics are the first-line of treatment for pulmonary oedema, and in pregnancy, it is no different. Diuretics are useful when there is left ventricular dysfunction. However, there is a risk of uteroplacental hypoperfusion due to depletion of maternal intravascular volume. Parenteral vasodilators, such as nitroglycerin, are used when heart failure is secondary to diastolic dysfunction as in hypertensive heart disease or pre-eclampsia.

Angiotensin-converting enzyme (ACE) inhibitors and angiotensin receptor blockers (ARB) are contraindicated in pregnancy due to fetal toxicity causing neonatal renal failure. However, these can safely be administered during breastfeeding. In women with AF, treatment with beta-blockers and digoxin, and anticoagulation to minimise the risk of thromboembolism, should be considered. In women with heart failure due to pulmonary hypertension, phosphodiesterase type 5 inhibitors such as sildenafil or tadalafil and prostaglandin therapy improve maternal survival. Endothelin receptor antagonists are contraindicated due to teratogenic effects.

Delivery

General aseptic measures are important in reducing the risk of infection. Prophylactic antibiotics are usually administered at the onset of labour, prelabour rupture of membranes and amniotomy, to prevent infective endocarditis, although strong evidence for its benefits is lacking. Uterine contractions cause a surge in the left ventricular workload by boosting the plasma volume, and a pain-induced rise in catecholamines increases the heart rate. The woman may also need to perform Valsalva during the second stage of labour. In addition, the intravascular blood volume further increases immediately following delivery, although this is offset to some extent by blood loss. On the other hand, caesarean delivery is associated with risks of anaesthesia, haemorrhage and postoperative complications. Therefore, the mode of delivery in these women has to be decided by an experienced obstetrician in consultation with a cardiologist while taking into account individual patient characteristics. Epidural analgesia is the ideal form of pain relief in these women. Induction or augmentation of labour may be carried out, as usual, taking care to not cause any fluid overload. Although routine instrumental vaginal delivery is not necessary, the second stage may be assisted by the use of forceps or a vacuum in case of poor maternal effort or a prolonged second stage. Oxytocin, and not ergometrine which leads to vasoconstriction and hypertension, should be administered during the active management of the third stage of labour.

Postpartum Period

Fluid overload should be avoided due to the risk of pulmonary oedema. Ergometrine should be used only in cases of severe postpartum haemorrhage. Thromboprophylactic measures such as early ambulation, thromboembolic deterrent stockings and low molecular weight heparin are important in minimising the risk of venous thromboembolic disease. In women with severe heart failure, breastfeeding is discouraged to reduce the high metabolic demand and to enable early optimisation of medical therapy.

Follow-Up

Pregnancy may have provided the opportunity to diagnose preexisting heart conditions in some women and optimise the management in others. The risk of future pregnancies has to be considered, and contraceptive advice should be offered. It is vital that long-term follow-up sessions are arranged with a cardiologist.

Peripartum Cardiomyopathy

Peripartum cardiomyopathy (PPCM), also referred to as pregnancy-associated cardiomyopathy or pregnancy-associated heart failure, is a condition unique to pregnancy. It is a rare type of heart failure that occurs during the last month of pregnancy and up to five months postpartum. It is a dilated form of heart muscle disease which causes the chambers of the heart to enlarge and the heart muscle to weaken. Despite recent advances in understanding the pathogenesis of PPCM and improvement in targeted treatment, PPCM still remains an underdiagnosed condition and carries a heightened risk of maternal and perinatal morbidity and mortality, especially in resource-poor settings.

Pathogenesis

Recent studies on animal models have shown that prolactin may play a role in the pathogenesis of PPCM. Due to oxidative stress, the hormone prolactin is cleaved into the anti-angiogenic, pro-inflammatory and pro-apoptotic fragment vasoinhibin, which directly impairs endothelial function and triggers the release of micro-RNA, which is detrimental to cardiomyocytes. This results in systolic heart failure. It is postulated that upregulated soluble FMS-like tyrosine kinase-1 (sFlt-1), which is implicated in the pathogenesis of pre-eclampsia as well, may play a role in the pathogenesis of PPCM.

Some women with PPCM display mutations in genes associated with dilated cardiomyopathy. These women are usually asymptomatic outside pregnancy. However, the profound haemodynamic changes that happen during the latter part of pregnancy, delivery and the early postpartum period may unmask these genetic cardiomyopathies.

Risk Factors

The risk factors for PPCM include the following.

- Obesity/poor nourishment
- History of pre-eclampsia

- History of cardiac disease, e.g. myocarditis
- Multiparity
- Multiple pregnancy
- Smoking and alcohol intake
- African-American descent

Clinical Features

The clinical features of PPCM are the same as heart failure due to any other cause. The clinical course ranges from mild symptoms to severe forms with acute heart failure and cardiogenic shock. The clinical features of PPCM may mimic normal features of pregnancy. Therefore, a high degree of care and scepticism is required in order to make a diagnosis of PPCM early, so that treatment can be initiated as early as possible.

The severity of PPCM can be classified according to the NYHA system as follows.

- Class I – Disease with no symptoms
- Class II – Mild symptoms/symptoms only with ordinary physical activity
- Class III – Symptoms with minimal exertion/less than ordinary activity
- Class IV – Symptoms at rest

Investigations

The following investigations are done in PPCM.

- Investigations that help distinguish PPCM from pre-eclampsia
  - Urine full report
  - Full blood count
  - Serum glutamic oxaloacetic transaminase (SGOT)/Serum glutamic pyruvic transaminase (SGPT)
  - Blood urea, serum electrolytes, serum creatinine

- ECG – This is a condition that usually reports repolarization abnormalities.
- 24-hour Holter monitoring, if arrhythmia is suspected
- Echocardiogram
- Brain Natriuretic Peptide (BNP) – This is a screening biomarker for heart failure. Although its specificity is low, a negative test can rule out the disease.

In some cases, additional tests may need to be performed in order to arrive at a diagnosis.

- Cardiac magnetic resonance imaging (MRI) scan – This procedure is used to look for thrombi and exclude infection or inflammation of the heart when findings from the echocardiogram are not clear.
- Coronary angiogram – This technique is done to look for coronary artery disease.
- Endomyocardial biopsy – This is not usually required.

Diagnosis

In order to make a diagnosis of PPCM, the following three criteria should be met.

- Heart failure that develops during the last month of pregnancy and up to five months postpartum
- Ejection fraction of less than 45%
- Absence of another cause for heart failure

Management

The principles of management are the treatment of heart failure as well as supportive treatment. Women with acute heart failure should be transferred to an intensive care unit and managed in a multidisciplinary setting involving a cardiologist, an obstetrician and an intensivist. Pharmacological treatment includes ACE inhibitors, ARB, beta-blockers, diuretics, digitalis and anticoagulants. Treatment with bromocriptine, a dopamine 2 agonist that blocks the release of prolactin, has shown promising results. In addition to being a disease-specific treatment, it also has the advantage of inhibiting lactation, which in turn, reduces the metabolic demands of the woman. A low salt diet with restriction of fluids is advised. In women who present during the antenatal period, therapy should be aimed at optimising maternal haemodynamics and fetal monitoring. Steroids are administered to improve fetal lung maturity. While vaginal delivery is possible, a caesarean delivery may be required for a woman in poor health.

Prognosis and Follow-Up

Many women recover spontaneously with no residual damage. A few progress to severe heart failure which requires mechanical ventilation and heart transplantation. Echocardiography should be performed after six weeks and thereafter, every six months in order to inspect for recovery.

Heart failure can worsen in a subsequent pregnancy. Most drugs used in heart failure are contra-indicated in pregnancy and breastfeeding. Hence, advice on contraception is important. Oestrogen containing contraceptives can be detrimental in heart failure, and therefore, should be avoided.

Pregnancy-Associated Acute Myocardial Infarction

There is a 3–4 fold increase in the risk of acute myocardial infarction (AMI) in pregnancy and the post-partum period compared to that in non-pregnant women of similar age. The risk factors for the development of AMI in pregnancy are increased maternal age, obesity, chronic hypertension, pre-eclampsia, hyperch-olesterolaemia, diabetes mellitus and smoking. The majority of acute coronary syndrome is due to spon-taneous coronary artery dissection in late pregnancy or early postpartum period. Coronary thrombosis is known to occur in pregnancy without atherosclerosis, probably as a result of the hypercoagulable state.

Diagnosis

Diagnostic criteria in AMI are similar to those outside pregnancy and include history, ECG changes and increased troponin levels. An echocardiogram is helpful when an ECG is not diagnostic. A high degree of suspicion for AMI is required for any pregnant woman bearing chest pain.

Management

Primary percutaneous coronary intervention (PCI) is preferred in patients with ST-elevation myocardial infarction (STEMI). Early PCI is indicated in unstable patients with Non-ST elevation myocardial in-farction (NSTEMI), while a noninvasive approach is preferred in stable patients with NSTEMI. Thrombolytic therapy is considered relatively contraindicated in pregnancy. However, available evidence from the use of thrombolytic therapy in women with stroke, pulmonary embolism or deep vein throm-bosis suggests that there is only minimal placental transfer of streptokinase or tissue-type plasminogen activator, and that there are the slightest effects on the fetus. However, there have been occasional complications such as miscarriage, placental abruption, preterm delivery, intrauterine fetal demise and major obstetric haemorrhage. As some women with AMI have normal coronary anatomy, ill-considered use of thrombolytic therapy is discouraged. Thrombolysis is useful in thrombosis, but it can worsen the situation in spontaneous coronary dissection which is the cause of 40% of STEMI in pregnancy.

Low-dose aspirin is safe during pregnancy, but there is limited evidence available regarding the safety of clopidogrel. Beta-blockers can be used, and nifedipine is the drug of choice when coronary spasm is suspected. Newer antiplatelets and statins are contraindicated in pregnancy.

Aortic Dissection in Pregnancy

Aortic dissection in pregnancy is rare and is associated with Marfan syndrome, vascular type Ehlers-Danlos syndrome, aortic root diameter of 40 mm or more, bicuspid aortic valve disease, coarctation of aorta, hypertension, older age and trauma. However, pregnancy itself may be an independent risk factor, and therefore, aortic dissection may occur in women with no known risk factors. This is potentially devastating to both the woman and the fetus.

Pathogenesis

Aortic dissection in pregnancy occurs most commonly in the third trimester and also in the early post-partum period due to the hyperdynamic circulation and hormonal effects on the vasculature. Oestrogen suppresses the synthesis of collagen and elastin, leading to a weakening of vascular walls. Systolic hypertension is a key factor in the causation of aortic dissection. This emphasises the importance of monitoring for and treatment of hypertension in pregnancy. The ascending aorta is the commonest site affected accounting for 65% of cases, followed by the descending aorta, aortic arch and abdominal aorta.

Diagnosis

Aortic dissection presents with severe ripping or tearing type of chest pain radiating to the back, vomiting and syncope. Bronchospasm may also happen due to vagal stimulation resulting from tearing of the intima. Bedside ultrasound which shows evidence of pericardial effusion and intramural haematomas is the most practical and efficient tool for the detection of aortic dissection. An electrocardiogram may be normal or it may show the dissection flap, a grossly dilated vascular lumen, a false lumen and a haemopericardium suggestive of aortic dissection as well as evidence of left ventricular hypertrophy or AMI. A chest x-ray has a sensitivity of only around 85%. A computerised tomography angiogram is preferred in diagnosis, but carries a risk of radiation to the unborn child. However, the risk of radiation must be weighed against the risk of missing a potentially lethal vascular catastrophe. Trans-oesophageal echocardiography and MRI are other useful noninvasive tests for the diagnosis of aortic dissection, but these may not be feasible in an acute setting.

Management

Whatever the diagnosis is, resuscitation should be of foremost priority in a collapsed obstetric patient. Pericardiocentesis is the initial treatment in relieving external pressure on the heart and establish cardiac output, if there is associated pericardial effusion with features of impending tamponade. An open thoracotomy is an option if pericardiocentesis fails. However, open thoracotomy carries a poor prognosis in a collapsed patient. Once diagnosed with aortic dissection, the woman should be treated with intravenous nitroprusside and a beta-blocker. Urgent caesarean delivery followed by aortic repair is essential in some women with DeBakey type 1 dissection involving the aortic root in order to avoid haemodynamic stress, progressive aortic expansion and rupture and also in cases of fetal distress. In other types of aortic dissections, emergency aortic repair is performed with the fetus in situ when it is not mature enough, but this carries significant risk to the fetus. If the woman is stable, then initial medical management followed by caesarean delivery and elective aortic repair on a later date is feasible.

Key Points

- The consequences of cardiac emergencies in the pregnant woman can be catastrophic for both the woman and the fetus.
- Initial diagnosis of cardiac emergencies may be difficult due to an overlap of clinical features as those present in a normal pregnancy.
- Prompt recognition, effective resuscitation and coordinated multidisciplinary management can make the difference between life and death for both the woman and the fetus.

BIBLIOGRAPHY

1. Regitz-Zagrosek V, Roos-Hesselink JW, Bauersachs J, Blomström-Lundqvist C, Cífková R, De Bonis M, et al. ESC Scientific Document Group. 2018 ESC Guidelines for the management of cardiovascular diseases during pregnancy: The Task Force for the Management of Cardiovascular Diseases during Pregnancy of the European Society of Cardiology (ESC), *Eur Heart J* 2018;39(34):3165–241.
2. Mulubrhan FM, Mariann RP, Barbara LM, Jason LS, Kylea LL, Joan EB. Heart failure in pregnant women: A concern across the pregnancy continuum. *Circ Heart Fail* 2018;11:e004005.
3. Heart Failure Association of the European Society of Cardiology Study Group on peripartum cardiomyopathy. Pathophysiology, diagnosis and management of peripartum cardiomyopathy: A position statement. *Eur J Heart Fail* 2019;21:827–43.
4. Elkayam U, Jalnapurkar S, Barakkat MN, et al. Pregnancy-associated acute myocardial infarction: A review of contemporary experience in 150 cases between 2006 and 2011. *Circulation* 2014;129:1695–702.
5. Yuan SM. Aortic dissection during pregnancy: A difficult clinical scenario. *Clin Cardiol* 2013;36(10):576–84.

6

Maternal Sepsis

Sanjeewa Padumadasa and Udya Rodrigo

Sepsis is the third most common direct cause of maternal mortality and contributes to a significant proportion of other maternal deaths in both low-middle income and high-income countries. It accounts for approximately 10% of maternal deaths worldwide. The physiological changes that take place make pregnant women more susceptible to deterioration following infection as compared to non-pregnant women. Sepsis may not only lead to death and cause considerable maternal morbidity, but it may also result in miscarriage, intrauterine fetal demise, neonatal death or serious morbidities such as encephalopathy and cerebral palsy. The development of symptoms can be insidious, and the woman can misleadingly appear well before the development of septic shock, multiorgan dysfunction and death. Early detection, identification of the source of sepsis and targeted therapy are key to the successful management of maternal sepsis.

Definitions

The definition of sepsis has evolved over time, and currently, there is no gold standard test for its diagnosis. Maternal sepsis is defined as organ dysfunction caused by a dysregulated host response to infection during pregnancy, childbirth, post-abortion or postpartum period. Septic shock is characterised by hypotension refractory to fluid resuscitation and requiring vasopressor support to maintain a mean arterial pressure (MAP) of >65 mmHg, and a lactic acid of >2 mmol/L.

Puerperal pyrexia is relatively prevalent and is defined as a temperature of more than 38°C on more than one occasion in the puerperium. The majority of cases present within ten days of delivery. Puerperal sepsis is an important cause of puerperal pyrexia, and one should have a high degree of suspicion of sepsis in any woman with puerperal pyrexia. Endometritis, which is an important cause of puerperal sepsis, is discussed in detail in Chapter 15.

Prevention

Avoiding unnecessary interventions during pregnancy and childbirth, minimising vaginal examinations during labour, attention to aseptic measures and strengthening infection prevention and control measures in health facilities, reduce the risk of maternal sepsis. Cleaning the vagina with iodine-based or chlorhexidine-based antiseptic solution prior to caesarean delivery, especially in women who are in labour, is recommended to reduce the risk of postoperative infection. Control or treatment of conditions that increase the risk of infection, such as malnutrition, anaemia, diabetes mellitus, is vital. Increased awareness about sepsis among first contact healthcare providers such as general practitioners, midwives and accident and emergency personnel would lead to early detection and initiation of appropriate management.

Prophylactic antibiotic administration in women with preterm prelabour rupture of membranes (PPROM), in those following instrumental vaginal delivery, third and fourth-degree perineal tears or manual removal of placenta and preoperatively for caesarean delivery is recommended.

Although antibiotics are commonly used to prevent or treat infection, their misuse leads to the emergence of resistant bacterial strains and may have implications on curtailing infection in the global context. Therefore, whenever possible, the use of antibiotics should be based on local guidelines. Polymerase chain reaction (PCR) and mass spectrometry which can identify the pathogen/s quickly are promising as an alternative to the standard cultures which take at least 24 hours and can alleviate the need for empirical antibiotic therapy.

Causes

The causes of maternal sepsis are listed in Table 6.1. Antepartum sepsis is likely to be of non-pelvic origin, while intrapartum or postpartum sepsis is likely to be of pelvic origin.
The differential diagnosis of maternal sepsis is shown in Table 6.2.

TABLE 6.1

Causes of maternal sepsis

Antepartum
- Septic abortion
- Cystitis
- Acute pyelonephritis
- Intra-amniotic infection
- Pneumonia
- Infective hepatitis
- Ruptured appendix
- Acute cholecystitis

Postpartum
- Endometritis
- Pelvic abscess
- Peritonitis
- Infection of episiotomy site/perineal tears
- Wound abscess
- Mastitis
- Meningitis
- Thrombophlebitis

TABLE 6.2

Differential diagnosis of maternal sepsis

- Pulmonary embolism
- Amniotic fluid embolism
- Acute fatty liver of pregnancy
- Acute pancreatitis
- Drug and transfusion reactions
- Acute adrenal insufficiency
- Acute pituitary insufficiency
- Autoimmune conditions
- Concealed haemorrhage
- Disseminated malignancy

Microbiology

Although bacterial infections predominate, maternal sepsis may also occur due to viruses and other infections. Organisms commonly associated are beta-haemolytic streptococci (Group A), *Escherichia coli*, *Streptococcus pneumoniae* and influenza A and B. Less common causes include Group B Streptococcus, *Klebsiella pneumoniae*, *Staphylococcus aureus*, *Listeria monocytogenes*, *Clostridium* species, *Varicella zoster* and *Herpes simplex*. Although the impact of the COVID-19 outbreak on the global burden of sepsis is yet to emerge, pregnancy does not appear to be associated with increased disease severity. Opportunistic organisms can cause infection in immunocompromised women, such as those with human immunodeficiency virus (HIV) infection, diabetes mellitus or those on steroids.

Group A Streptococcus is responsible for the majority of deaths due to maternal sepsis, although *Escherichia coli* is the most common cause of bacterial infection in pregnancy. Sepsis due to Group A Streptococcus can present during pregnancy and postpartum period with nonspecific symptoms, such as fever, sore throat, diarrhoea and vomiting. Therefore, a high degree of suspicion is necessary to diagnose this extremely virulent infection. It is critical to note that the aetiological agent for sepsis varies depending on the geographical location, and it is of paramount importance to consider infections that are prevalent in a given area, e.g. dengue, when dealing with sepsis.

Pathophysiology

Sepsis occurs when the body's response to infection causes injury to its own tissues and organs. As a result of the stimulus presented by toxins of the infecting agent, the body's defence cells release large amounts of pro-inflammatory cytokines, which activate the endothelial tissue. This results in the production of various inflammatory mediators and causes a wide range of systemic changes across the body. Furthermore, this leads to an imbalance between oxygen supply and consumption, which is followed by generalised tissue hypoperfusion, cell hypoxia, anaerobic metabolism, hyperlactataemia and acidaemia that culminate in multiple organ dysfunction.

The excessive inflammatory response that occurs with sepsis includes extravasation of albumin and fluid; the result is intravascular hypovolaemia. This is compounded by the decreased systemic vascular resistance which occurs as a result of cytokines. These factors, along with microvascular occlusion due to thrombi resulting from disseminated intravascular coagulation, contribute to tissue hypoxia. Cardiac oedema and lowered myocardial compliance lead to decreased diastolic filling and less stroke volume. Together with reduced oncotic pressure, these predispose to the development of pulmonary oedema, especially with aggressive fluid resuscitation.

Fever during the first trimester has been discovered to be associated with a heightened incidence of neural tube defects, oral clefts and congenital heart disease. Antipyretic therapy with paracetamol is beneficial. However, aspirin should not be used until infections that cause haemorrhage, e.g. dengue, are eliminated, especially in countries in which these infections are prevalent.

Diagnosis

The clinical features in sepsis are listed below.

- Observably ill
- Warm extremities
- Increased respiratory rate (more than 20/minute), which is often overlooked but is an important sign of sepsis
- Tachycardia and pounding pulse
- Hypotension
- Low urine output/anuria

- Signs of shock
- Altered mental state: drowsiness, confusion, restlessness
- Fetal distress, i.e. Fetal tachycardia, acidosis, if antepartum

Fever, which is a common feature of infection, may be absent in sepsis. Sometimes, there could be hypothermia. The clinical features may be insidious and nonspecific, and sepsis may be undetected until its advanced stages, at which time the disease process might even already be irreversible. In addition, as these signs may be obscured due to the physiological changes during pregnancy, a high degree of suspicion is imperative for early diagnosis and treatment.

The obstetrically modified quick Sequential Organ Failure Assessment (omqSOFA), proposed by the Society of Obstetric Medicine of Australia and New Zealand is a scoring system based on easily identifiable bedside clinical features that can be used to screen for sepsis, as well as to assess the severity of the condition. As it does not depend on results of laboratory investigations, it is a rapid test used to identify women who need urgent attention (Table 6.3). A score of two or more is significant.

Management

Sepsis should be considered an obstetric emergency, and early diagnosis and aggressive treatment have demonstrated considerable effectiveness in improving maternal and perinatal morbidity and mortality rates. Women with sepsis should be managed in an intensive care setting by a multidisciplinary team, which includes an experienced obstetrician, an intensivist, a microbiologist and, in antepartum cases, a neonatologist. Cardiorespiratory compromise (systolic BP < 90 mmHg or mean arterial pressure <65 mmHg), evidence of organ dysfunction, proof of tissue hypoperfusion (lactate > 2 mmol/L) and any other serious clinical concerns necessitate admission to an intensive care unit.

The aims of management are as follows.

- Initial resuscitation with maintenance of tissue perfusion with the administration of intravenous fluids and, when necessary, vasoactive substances
- Adequate oxygenation
- Identification of the source of infection and, if considered appropriate, its removal
- Commencement of broad-spectrum intravenous (IV) antibiotics
- Effective support for multiorgan dysfunction
- Thromboprophylaxis
- Assessment and maintenance of fetal health

Initial Stabilisation

Effective resuscitation with attention to **A**irway, **B**reathing and **C**irculation, assessment of **D**isability and **E**xposure, is important. A left lateral tilt is advised in order to prevent supine hypotension syndrome. Intravenous fluids should be administered at 30 ml/kg, but with care to avoid fluid overload. Despite the

TABLE 6.3

Obstetrically modified quick sequential organ failure assessment (omqSOFA)

Parameter	omqSOFA Score	
	0	**1**
Systolic Blood pressure	90 mmHg or greater	Less than 90 mmHg
Respiratory Rate	Less than 25/minute	25/minute or greater
Altered Mentation	Alert	Not alert

emergence of more conservative fluid therapy regimes in the management of sepsis in non-pregnant patients, a more aggressive approach for fluid therapy is advocated in most current guidelines on the management of sepsis in pregnant women, in whom it is even more important to prevent fluid overload and the consequent development of pulmonary oedema and myocardial dysfunction.

Although vasopressors and inotropic agents are not contraindicated during pregnancy, it should be borne in mind that noradrenaline and vasopressin may cause a reduction of uteroplacental blood flow, thus compromising the fetus. However, noradrenaline is considered the first-line therapy to treat hypotension in sepsis. Vasopressors are indicated if fluid therapy fails to improve hypotension, or if the presence of pulmonary oedema precludes further fluid therapy. Taking into consideration the physiological changes which occur in pregnancy, a lower blood pressure may be acceptable in the pregnant woman compared to a non-obstetric patient, provided that there are no indicators of hypoperfusion such as oliguria, cold extremities, altered mental state or elevated serum lactate levels.

Investigations

Investigations to assess organ damage include the following.

- Normal white blood cell count with >10% immature forms
- Increased C reactive protein (CRP) levels - Although a non-specific investigation, this can be used to monitor the efficacy of treatment.
- Hyperglycaemia (blood glucose > 110 mg/dL)
- Increase in serum creatinine
- International normalised ratio > 1.5 or Activated partial thromboplastin time > 60 seconds
- Platelet count < 100×10^9/L
- Raised alanine transaminase and aspartate transaminase
- Plasma total bilirubin > 4 mg/dL or 70 mmoL/L
- Lactate > 2 mmoL/L
- Arterial blood gases

Although an increased white cell count (greater than 11×10^9/L) is considered useful to diagnose sepsis outside pregnancy, this data could be a physiological finding during pregnancy, and a count of less than 4×10^9/L is more useful.

The obstetrically modified Sequential Organ Failure Assessment (omSOFA) is a scoring system based on laboratory investigations, that assesses end-organ damage and identifies women at risk of death and those who would require intensive treatment (Table 6.4). A score of two or more in its equivalent in the non-pregnant population is associated with a mortality rate of 10%, but it is yet to be validated for the obstetric population. Pregnancy-specific ranges should be used when interpreting the results of laboratory investigations.

TABLE 6.4

Obstetrically modified sequential organ failure assessment (omSOFA) score

System	Parameter	omSOFA Score		
		0	1	2
Respiration	PaO$_2$/FiO$_2$	400 or greater	300–399	Less than 300
Coagulation	Platelets ×10^6/L	150 or greater	100–149	Less than 100
Liver	Bilirubin µmol/L	20 or less	20–32	Greater than 32
Cardiovascular	Mean Arterial Pressure mmHg	70 or greater	Less than 70	Vasopressors required
Central Nervous System		Alert	Arousable by voice	Arousable by pain
Renal	Creatinine µmol/L	90 or less	90–120	Greater than 120

The physiological changes which occur in pregnancy pose difficulties in the diagnosis and management of sepsis (Table 6.5).

Microbiological Studies

Samples for microbiological studies should ideally be obtained before commencing antibiotic treatment, as the presence of antibiotics may inhibit the growth of pathogens in cultures and reduce the chances of identifying the hostile organism. Even in situations where antibiotics have been commenced without culture studies and the woman develops sepsis, relevant cultures should be performed, as these may bring about the presence of virulent organism/s. However, a negative result does not exclude an infective organism. Two sets of blood cultures should be obtained from different sites. Other samples should be obtained depending on clinical features.

- Mid-stream urine
- Wound swab from episiotomy site or skin incision
- Placental swabs
- Amniotic fluid
- Sputum
- Naso-pharyngeal swab/aspirate

TABLE 6.5

Physiological changes in pregnancy and their impact on the diagnosis and management of sepsis

System	Changes	Impact
Cardiovascular	Increased heart rate	Masking of initial signs of sepsis
	Increased cardiac output	Aggravation of tissue hypoperfusion
	Reduced peripheral resistance	
	Reduced blood pressure	
Respiratory	Reduced residual volume	Rapid onset of hypoxia
	Alkalosis	
Blood	Anaemia	Impaired oxygenation
	Increased white cell count	Delayed diagnosis of sepsis
Coagulation	Increased factors VII, VIII, IX, X, XII, von Willebrand and fibrinogen	Increased risk of thrombotic events Increased risk of disseminated intravascular coagulation
	Reduced fibrinolysis	
	Reduced protein S	
Renal	Dilatation of pelvicalyceal system	Predisposition to pyelonephritis
	Decreased peristalsis	
	Increased vesicoureteric reflex	
	Mechanical compression by the uterus	
	Reduced urea and creatinine	Delayed identification of renal injury
Liver	Reduced serum albumin and colloid osmotic pressure	Increased susceptibility to pulmonary oedema
Vaginal	Reduced vaginal pH	Increased risk of intraamniotic infection
	Increased glycogen in the vaginal epithelium	
Gastrointestinal	Reduced muscle tone of the tract	Increased risk of bacterial translocation
	Delayed gastric emptying Changes in the composition of bile	Increased risk of cholestasis, hyperbilirubinaemia and jaundice
		Increased risk of aspiration

- Cerebrospinal fluid
- Vaginal swab
- Stool culture
- Any other tests that may be done according to the history and clinical examination (e.g. laboratory testing for infective hepatitis, varicella-zoster, herpes simplex, HIV, COVID-19)

Imaging

Maternal health should gain prominence over that of the fetus or the neonate, and imaging, if required for diagnosis, should not be withheld during pregnancy or breastfeeding.

Antibiotic Therapy

Polymicrobial infections in pregnancy are common and need coverage with broad-spectrum intravenous (IV) antimicrobials. Combination therapy is more effective than monotherapy until the causative organism is found. Locally prevalent infections and antibiotic resistance patterns should be considered when starting empiric antibiotic therapy, and the input of a microbiologist is paramount. Ideally, antibiotic therapy should be initiated within one hour of presentation, as a delay considerably increases the risk of death. Antibiotic therapy can be modified once the results of microbiological tests are available. In up to 60% of patients, the causative agent/s may be undetermined. The pharmacokinetics of several antibiotics are altered in pregnancy, including a greater distribution volume and modifications in their absorption and excretion, which eventually lead to a reduction of serum drug levels. In addition, some antibiotics are contraindicated during pregnancy and breastfeeding. These factors may influence the type and use of antibiotic therapy during pregnancy or breastfeeding.

Thromboprophylaxis

Pregnancy and sepsis are independent risk factors for venous thromboembolism. Therefore, low molecular weight heparin (LMWH), as well as mechanical methods of preventing thromboembolism, such as graduated elastic compression stockings, should be used. As LMWH is excreted via kidneys, dose adjustments should be made in case of renal dysfunction. Low molecular weight heparin should not be used in the presence of coagulopathy.

Maternal Monitoring

Monitoring of vital signs, cardiopulmonary status and capillary refill complimented by central venous pressure, central venous oxygen saturation, and echocardiography should be performed to assess the response to treatment and to detect any deterioration in the maternal condition. This should be combined with biochemical investigations to assess the recovery or any decline of organ function.

Fetal Monitoring

The balance between fetal oxygen supply and consumption might be severely altered in the presence of maternal sepsis. Therefore, assessing fetal condition forms a vital part of management at viable gestations. In these cases, electronic fetal monitoring (EFM) should be instituted and in the intrapartum period, continuous EFM. Usually in maternal sepsis, there is fetal tachycardia which would improve with fluid therapy and antipyretic treatment. However, the presence of reduced or absent variability and decelerations may be suggestive of fetal acidosis and possibly necessitate urgent delivery, provided that the woman is stable to undergo delivery. In pre-viable gestations, ultrasound assessment for fetal heart activity may be all that is required to monitor the fetus. Preterm delivery may occur following maternal sepsis, although the source may not be the uterus. Steroids are not contraindicated in sepsis, and should be administered before 36 weeks of gestation, to improve fetal lung maturity.

Delivery

The decision for delivery in severe sepsis and septic shock is a challenging one. The fetal condition will usually improve with the stabilisation and improvement of the condition of the woman. If the source of sepsis is the uterus, then this necessitates delivery of the fetus or the evacuation of the uterus, irrespective of the period of gestation. In rare circumstances, hysterectomy is required, and this requires considerable skill due to intra-abdominal adhesions and extremely friable necrotic tissue. The decision to deliver or not, if the source of infection is not the uterus, is based on several factors which include the feasibility of adequate treatment of sepsis while undelivered, the likelihood of improvement of the maternal condition with delivery, the impact of delivery on the maternal condition and the risk of neonatal infection. Vaginal delivery, which is less stressful to the woman as compared to a caesarean delivery, is preferred. Epidural or spinal anaesthesia should be avoided, and general anaesthesia is usually required for caesarean delivery.

The Place of Perimortem Caesarean Delivery

In cardiorespiratory arrest at gestations >20 weeks, perimortem caesarean delivery should be considered, to aid resuscitation of the woman as well as to save the fetus (discussed in Chapter 7). The management of maternal sepsis, including that during the critical first hour, is summarised in Figure 6.1.

Intraamniotic Infection

Intraamniotic infection, commonly referred to as chorioamnionitis, is the infection of the chorion, amnion, amniotic fluid and the placenta, or a combination. Maternal complications include endometritis, peritonitis, sepsis, postpartum uterine atony with haemorrhage, and rarely, death. Perinatal adverse outcomes include stillbirth, prematurity and neonatal infections, and long-term adverse outcomes include chronic lung disease, cerebral palsy and neurodevelopmental abnormalities of the baby.

Risk Factors

Prolonged rupture of membranes, prolonged labour, multiple vaginal examinations, internal monitoring during labour, invasive intrauterine procedures (including amniotomy and artificial separation of membranes), genital tract infections, Group B Streptococcus colonisation, meconium-stained amniotic fluid, smoking, alcohol or drug abuse and immunocompromised states are known risk factors for the development of intraamniotic infection.

Prevention

Although the use of the combination of amoxicillin and clavulanic acid is not recommended, the use of ampicillin and erythromycin has been shown to reduce the incidence of intraamniotic infection and

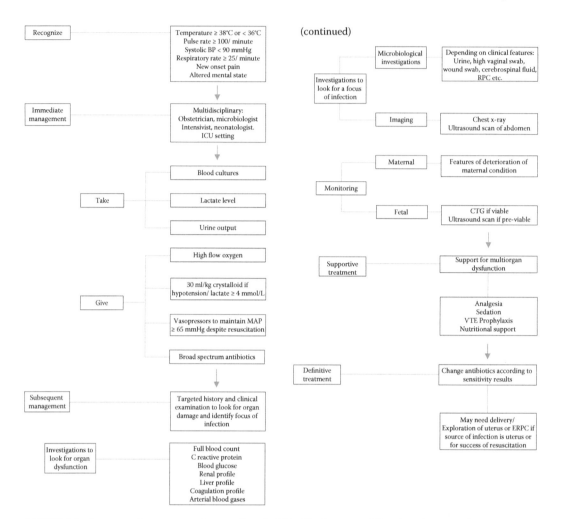

FIGURE 6.1 Summary of management of maternal sepsis. BP – blood pressure, ICU – intensive care unit, MAP – mean arterial pressure, RPC – retained products of conception, CTG – cardiotocograph, VTE – venous thromboembolism, ERPC – evacuation of retained products of conception.

neonatal sepsis and to prolong time-to-delivery in women with PPROM who are being managed expectantly, but not in those with preterm labour and intact membranes. Induction of labour is recommended for PPROM after 34 weeks of gestation. Obstetric interventions, including vaginal examinations, should be performed only if indicated and under strict aseptic conditions. Screening for Group B Streptococcus colonisation and prophylactic intrapartum antibiotic therapy with penicillin or clindamycin in women with risk factors are essential.

Pathogenesis

Intraamniotic infection is often polymicrobial in origin, and develops due to ascending infection from the vagina following the rupture of membranes. Infrequently, it can occur via haematogenous spread (especially with *Listeria monocytogens*), anterograde spread from the peritoneum through the fallopian tubes and following obstetric procedures such as amniocentesis. The common isolates are *Ureaplasma* species and *Mycoplasma hominis,* which can be found in the lower genital tract of 70% of women. Other isolates include the vaginal flora, anaerobes such as *Gardnerella vaginalis* and bacteroides, as well as aerobes including Group B streptococcus (GBS) and enteric flora, gram-negative rods including *Escherichia coli* and enterococci.

The presence of infectious agents in the chorioamnion initiates a maternal and fetal inflammatory response characterised by the release of pro-inflammatory and inhibitory cytokines and chemokines in the woman and the fetus. The inflammatory response may produce clinical intraamniotic infection and/ or lead to release of prostaglandins resulting in ripening of the cervix, membrane injury, and labour at term or preterm. In addition, the fetal inflammatory response may induce cerebral white matter injury which may result in cerebral palsy and other neurodevelopmental disabilities of the baby.

Diagnosis

Intraamniotic infection is a clinical diagnosis, and the common features include maternal temperature of more than 38°C, foul-smelling liquor, uterine tenderness and maternal and fetal tachycardia. Although abdominal pain and maternal and fetal tachycardia are considered normal during labour, the presence of fever and/or foul-smelling liquor in intraamniotic infection helps in differentiating it from epidural-induced fever. Non-infectious conditions such as placental abruption, thrombophlebitis of pelvic veins and colitis should be considered in a woman with abdominal pain but without fever. Appendicitis should be suspected if a woman in advanced gestation presents with right-sided abdominal pain, and abdominal ultrasound helps in its diagnosis as well as in the diagnosis of pyelonephritis.

Maternal leukocytosis and increased C reactive protein levels, although non-specific, often support a diagnosis of intraamniotic infection, in the presence of clinical features. High vaginal and endocervical swabs together with blood culture should be obtained for microbiological studies. Urine culture should be performed in women with urinary symptoms.

Management

Prompt administration of broad-spectrum IV antibiotics, e.g. ceftriaxone, metronidazole and genta-micin, is essential to prevent both maternal and fetal complications. Neonatal sepsis is reduced by up to 80% with intrapartum antibiotic treatment. The currently used standard antibiotic regimens do not cover *Ureaplasma urealyticum,* which is one of the most rampant microorganisms implicated in the pathogenesis of intraamniotic infection. At the same time, specific coverage against *ureaplasma* (with macrolide antibiotics) has not been found to improve the outcome in intraamniotic infection. Antipyretics, e.g. paracetamol, should be administered.

Urgent delivery on both fetal and maternal grounds is often needed. Emergency caesarean delivery is not indicated unless there are other obstetric indications. It is advisable to induce labour if the woman is not in labour, and expedite delivery with oxytocin in case of dysfunctional labour. Communication with the neonatal team is important to optimise neonatal management. Antibiotics should be continued in the postpartum period in order to prevent endometritis and the development of antibiotic resistance.

Although little data exists in regard to the management of women with isolated fever during labour in the absence of other features of intraamniotic infection, antibiotics should be considered in this instance, given its potential benefits for the woman as well as the newborn.

Key Points

- Early recognition of maternal sepsis is vital. A delay in diagnosing and initiating therapy considerably increases the risk of death.
- Furthermore, fever or hypothermia may not be present in sepsis.
- A quick bedside clinical assessment using a respiratory rate of >25/minute, blood pressure of <90 mmHg and a mental state that is anything less than alert, is useful to screen for maternal sepsis and also to identify women who need intensive treatment.
- Initial stabilisation using oxygen and judicious intravenous therapy, early empiric antibiotic therapy as soon as samples are obtained for microbiological studies, multidisciplinary management and effective support for multiorgan dysfunction are key items necessary to the successful management of sepsis.
- Thromboprophylactic measures which include graduated elastic compression stockings and LMWH should be instituted to prevent venous thromboembolism.
- Close monitoring of the woman is crucial, because deterioration to an irreversible state may occur rapidly.
- Fetal monitoring with cardiotocography should be performed at viable gestations in case plans are made for urgent delivery in the event of fetal compromise.
- Antenatal steroids should be administered for improving fetal lung maturity at gestations < 36 weeks.
- Lastly, perimortem caesarean delivery should be considered to aid maternal resuscitation as well as to save the fetus, in case of cardiorespiratory arrest at >20 weeks of gestation.

BIBLIOGRAPHY

1. Bowyer L, Robinson H, Barrett H, Crozier T, Giles M, Idel I, Lowe S, Lust K, Marnoch C, Morton M, Said J, Wong M and Makris A. SOMANZ Guidelines for sepsis in pregnancy, 2017. Society of Obstetric Medicine Australia and New Zealand.
2. WHO recommendations for prevention and treatment of maternal peripartum infections. 2015; Geneva: World Health Organization. PMID: 26598777.
3. Haas DM, Morgan S, Contreras K, Kimball S. Vaginal preparation with antiseptic solution before cesarean section for preventing postoperative infections. *Cochrane Database Syst Rev* 2020 Apr 26;4(4):CD007892. doi: 10.1002/14651858.CD007892.pub7. PMID: 32335895; PMCID: PMC7195184.
4. Dellinger RP, Levy MM, Rhodes A, Annane D, Gerlach H, Opal SM, et al. Surviving Sepsis Campaign Guidelines Committee including The Pediatric Subgroup Surviving Sepsis Campaign: international guidelines for management of severe sepsis and septic shock, 2012. *Intensive Care Med* 2013;39(2): 165–228.
5. Frankling CC, Finfer S, Lissauer D, Perner A, Patel JM, Gao F. The dark ages of maternal sepsis: time to be enlightened. *Br J Anaes* 2018;120(4):626–28.
6. Kenyon SL, Taylor DJ, Tarnow-Mordi W, ORACLE Collaborative Group. Broad-spectrum antibiotics for preterm, prelabour rupture of fetal membranes: the ORACLE I randomised trial. ORACLE Collaborative Group. *Lancet* 2001;357(9261):979–88.
7. Royal College of Obstetricians and Gynaecologists. Bacterial sepsis following pregnancy. Green-top guideline. 2012: 64b.
8. Rhodes A, Evans LE, Alhazzani W, Levy MM, Antonelli M, Ferrer R, et al. Surviving sepsis campaign: international guidelines for management of sepsis and septic shock: 2016. *Intensive Care Med* 2017;43:304–377. doi: 10.1007/s00134-017-4683-6.

9. Rudd KE, Johnson SC, Agesa KM, Shackelford KA, Tsoi D, Kievlan DR, Colombara DV, Ikuta KS, Kissoon N, Finfer S, Fleischmann-Struzek C, Machado FR, Reinhart KK, Rowan K, Seymour CW, Watson RS, West TE, Marinho F, Hay SI, Lozano R, Lopez AD, Angus DC, Murray CJL, Naghavi M. Global, regional, and national sepsis incidence and mortality, 1990-2017: analysis for the Global Burden of Disease Study. *Lancet* 2020 Jan 18;395(10219):200–11. doi: 10.1016/S0140-6736(19)32 989-7. PMID: 31954465; PMCID: PMC6970225.

10. Committee on Obstetric Practice. Committee Opinion No. 712: Intrapartum Management of Intraamniotic Infection. *Obstet Gynecol* 2017 Aug; 130(2):e95–101. doi: 10.1097/ AOG.0000000000002236. PMID: 28742677.

7

Maternal Cardiorespiratory Arrest

Sanjeewa Padumadasa and Nilmini Wijesuriya

Maternal cardiorespiratory arrest (CRA) is defined as an acute event involving the cardiorespiratory systems and/or the brain, resulting in absent or reduced consciousness level and potentially cardiac arrest and death at any stage during pregnancy and up to six weeks following delivery. Although it is said that there is one maternal death globally every minute, maternal CRA is extremely rare. Managing a maternal cardiac arrest is a challenging task, as there are two lives involved, that of the woman and the fetus, and both probably would have been healthy before the incident. Although the woman's life takes priority over that of the fetus, the best chance for fetal survival would be with maternal survival during resuscitation, and the outcome for both depends on timely and effective resuscitation.

Causes of Maternal Cardiorespiratory Arrest

The common causes of maternal CRA can be classified according to the popular mnemonic Hs and Ts (which have been modified to cover causes that are unique to pregnancy) and are given in Table 7.1.

Identification of Women at Risk of Cardiorespiratory Arrest

The Modified Early Obstetric Warning Scoring (MEOWS) chart, which utilises simple physiological features such as pulse rate, blood pressure and respiratory rate, has been developed to identify women at risk of an adverse event, including CRA. These charts are recommended to be used in all hospitalised pregnant and postpartum women. The rationale behind the usage of this chart is that derangement of simple physiological vital signs precedes significant deterioration, and therefore, women at risk can be identified early. Once a risk is determined, a system should be available to trigger a response depending on the grade of risk (Track-Trigger-Response). The response may be more frequent and vigilant monitoring for further damage, simple interventions such as administering oxygen, fluid bolus, among others or an immediate assessment by a consultant. It is also important to be vigilant for warning features of deterioration apart from those found in the MEOWS chart in order to find women at risk of CRA. It must be noted that some cases of maternal CRA occur without prior warning. Therefore, it is essential that every healthcare provider is competent with initial resuscitation techniques.

Cardiopulmonary Resuscitation in a Pregnant Woman

Proper management of Airway, Breathing, Circulation, Disability and Exposure (ABCDE), is important as in any other patient in order to maximise the chances of survival when managing CRA in pregnancy. An AVPU (alert, verbal stimulus, pain stimulus and unresponsive) assessment,

TABLE 7.1

The common causes of cardiorespiratory arrest in pregnancy

Cause	Cause in pregnancy
H	
Haemorrhage (possibly concealed)	Antepartum haemorrhage
	Postpartum haemorrhage
	Ruptured ectopic pregnancy
	Liver rupture
	Splenic artery rupture
Hypovolaemia (Non-Haemorrhagic)	Relative hypovolaemia of dense spinal block, total spinal after epidural block
	Septic shock
	Neurogenic shock, including uterine inversion
	Anaphylactic shock
Hypoxia	Cardiac events
	Peripartum cardiomyopathy
	Myocardial infarction
	Aortic dissection
	Acute left ventricular failure
	Cardiac arrhythmias
	Infective endocarditis
	Large-vessel aneurysm
	Airway obstruction due to aspiration
	Status asthmaticus
Hypo/hyperkalaemia	Similar to that of non-obstetric patients
Hyponatraemia	Use of oxytocin
Hypoglycaemia	Use of insulin
Hypothermia	Similar to that of non-obstetric patients
Hypertensive (and related disorders)	Pre-eclampsia
	Eclampsia
	Intracranial haemorrhage
	Acute fatty liver of pregnancy
T	
Thromboembolism	Amniotic fluid embolism
	Pulmonary embolism
	Air embolism
	Cerebrovascular event
Toxicity	Local anaesthetic
	Magnesium
	Illicit drug overdose, etc.
Tension Pneumothorax	Traumatic/following suicide attempt
Tamponade (Cardiac)	Traumatic/following suicide attempt

should be performed, because an altered state of consciousness can be a sign of critical illness. The basic principles of resuscitation in a pregnant woman are more or less similar to those in a non-pregnant woman. However, the physiological and anatomical changes that occur during pregnancy should be taken into consideration (Table 7.2), and resuscitation must be modified accordingly.

TABLE 7.2

Physiological and anatomical changes during pregnancy and their impact on maternal resuscitation

Parameter	Changes during pregnancy	Impact on resuscitation
Cardiovascular system		
Plasma volume	Increased by 50%	Dilutional anaemia and reduced oxygen-carrying capacity
Heart rate	Increased by 15–20 beats/min	Increased CPR demands
Cardiac output	Increased by 40%	Increased CPR demands
Venous return	Reduced by the pressure of the gravid uterus on the inferior vena cava	Only 10% of cardiac output achieved
Blood pressure	Reduced by 10–15 mmHg	Reduced reserve
Uterine blood flow	Increased and constitutes 10% of cardiac output at term	Potential for massive uterine haemorrhage
Respiratory system		
Respiratory rate	Not changed	
Oxygen consumption	Increased by 20%	Increased tendency to develop hypoxia
Residual capacity	Reduced by 25% as a result of the enlarged uterus pushing the diaphragm upwards	Increased tendency to develop hypoxia
Arterial PCO_2	Reduced	Mild respiratory alkalosis
Laryngeal oedema	Increased	Difficult and failed intubation
Chest wall compliance	Reduced due to enlarged uterus and breasts	Difficult mechanical ventilation
Gastrointestinal system		
Gastric motility	Reduced	Increased risk of aspiration
Lower oesophageal sphincter	Relaxed	Increased risk of aspiration
Intra-abdominal pressure	Increased due to the enlarged uterus	Increased risk of aspiration
Reproductive system		
Uterus	Enlarged and causes aortocaval compression leading to reduced venous return	15° left lateral tilt or manual displacement of uterus required during CPR
Breasts	Enlarged	Difficult intubation
Skin		
Skin oedema	Increased chest wall resistance	Need for stronger chest compressions

Abbreviation: CPR – Cardiopulmonary resuscitation

The important aspects of resuscitation in a pregnant woman are further described in detail below.

Activate Teams

When a maternal CRA occurs, it is important to activate the maternal cardiac arrest teams. This includes the resident obstetrician, the resident obstetric anaesthesiologist, the resident neonatologist and the nurses in addition to the general cardiac arrest team of the hospital. A team leader from within the aforementioned team should take the responsibility of managing all of this personnel. Moreover, there should be regular simulated skills training in CPR as a team. Equipment necessary for the resuscitation of both the woman and the neonate should always be ready. Ideally, an antiseptic solution, a few sterile towels and gauze, a scalpel and a few cord clamps should also be available for an emergency perimortem caesarean delivery (PMCD).

Relieve Aortocaval Compression by the Gravid Uterus

It has been shown that chest compressions can achieve only 10% of cardiac output if the woman in advanced gestation is supine due to reduced venous return resulting from aortocaval compression by the gravid uterus, as opposed to 30% of the cardiac output in a non-pregnant patient. Two methods are used to overcome this, i.e. manual uterine displacement or tilting the woman. Before 20 weeks of gestation, the degree of aortocaval compression by the gravid uterus is minimal, and therefore, these methods are unnecessary.

Manual Left Uterine Displacement

This could be achieved either by a pushing motion using one hand or by a pulling motion using both hands (Figure 7.1), and it adjusts the woman in a supine position, which improves airway access and the effectiveness of chest compressions and facilitates defibrillation. However, it is important to note that this must be discontinued during defibrillation.

Tilt

A tilt of 15° to the left relieves aortocaval compression by the gravid uterus. Effectiveness of chest compressions declines with greater angles of inclination. According to the situation, the tilt can be achieved by: the tilting of the operating table, a Cardiff wedge or an upturned chair back used as a wedge below the woman. Alternatively, the tilt can be achieved by someone kneeling on the right side of the woman and then placing their knees underneath the woman's thorax. Rolled-up towels or pillows underneath the woman do not provide the desired firm surface suitable for counter-pressure when performing chest compressions, and therefore, should not be employed. In cases of major trauma, if a wedge is used, it should be placed below the spinal board.

Airway and Breathing

As the risk of aspiration is higher than that in a non-pregnant woman, clearing the airway and resorting to early intubation, protection of the airway, satisfactory delivery of oxygen and ventilation are vital. Until help is available, the mouth should be checked for any obstructing material such as blood or vomitus and consequently removed using suction. The airway can be made open by either a head tilt and chin lift, or a jaw thrust. A head tilt and chin lift can be carried out by placing a hand on the forehead and gently tilting it back while lifting the chin with the other hand (Figure 7.2). A head tilt should be avoided in trauma victims suspected to have a cervical spine injury. A jaw thrust is performed by pushing the posterior aspect of the lower jaw upwards (Figure 7.3).

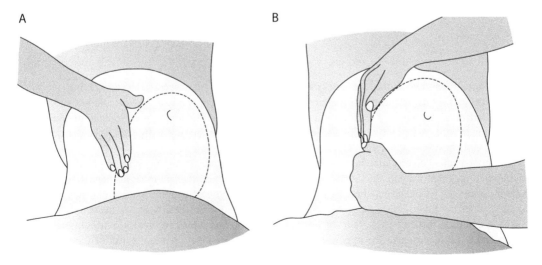

FIGURE 7.1 Manual displacement of the uterus to the left: (A) one-handed technique; (B) two-handed technique.

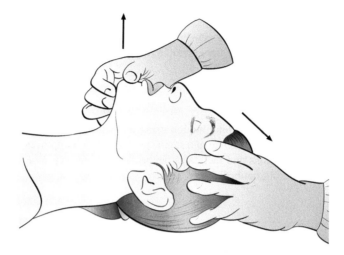

FIGURE 7.2 Head tilt and chin lift.

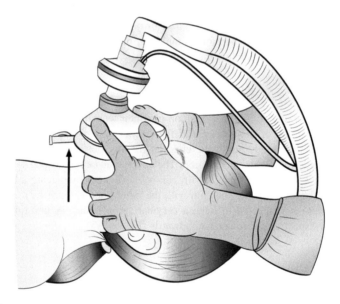

FIGURE 7.3 Jaw thrust.

Afterward, breathing should be assessed for approximately ten seconds by observing for chest movements as well as listening and monitoring for signs of air movement. The circulation should also be simultaneously assessed by feeling for a carotid pulse. Lack of breathing is an indication of a lack of circulation as well. A patient who is unconscious and not breathing normally should be considered as in CRA, and chest compressions should be commenced immediately.

Although a patent airway may be achieved by a laryngeal mask airway in a non-pregnant woman, the airway in a pregnant woman should be secured with a cuffed endotracheal tube, as there is an increased risk of aspiration. As the airway becomes narrower due to laryngeal oedema when pregnancy advances, a slightly narrow tube is necessary. An appropriately skilled anaesthesiologist is needed, because intubation could be difficult as a result of laryngeal oedema and enlarged breasts. Furthermore, hyperaemia and hypersecretion in the upper airway increase the friability of the mucosa of the airway and may possibly result in impaired visualisation and increased bleeding, especially with repeated attempts at intubation. Difficult or failed intubation is a major contributor to poor outcomes in maternal CRA.

The first responders should not try to intubate the woman. They should commence chest compressions, insert an oropharyngeal airway to maintain the airway and gently manually ventilate until an anaesthesiologist arrives. Soft ventilation at a rate of 10–12/minute without the use of excessive pressures or volumes is important.

Supplemental Oxygen

As the demand for oxygen increases during pregnancy, and as the pregnant woman is at an increased risk of developing hypoxia compared to a non-pregnant woman, the addition of high-flow 100% oxygen to whatever method of ventilation is essential.

Chest Compressions

Reduced venous return due to the gravid uterus and skin oedema make chest compressions less effective in a pregnant woman compared to those in a non-pregnant patient. As the heart is pushed upwards due to the splinting of the diaphragm by the gravid uterus, it is recommended that the hands of the resuscitator should be over the centre of the sternum rather than over the lower one-third of the sternum when performing chest compressions. It is important to ensure that the direction of chest compressions is perpendicular to the wall of the chest, and therefore, if a tilt is used, then this factor should be taken into account when performing chest compressions. Chest compressions are more effective when the woman is supine and the uterus displaced manually to the left, rather than when the woman is tilted to the left.

Initially, chest compressions should be performed at a rate of 30 compressions: 2 ventilations until the woman is intubated. Following intubation, chest compressions should be performed at a rate of 100/minute and ventilation at a rate of 10/minute. The beat of the popular song 'Staying Alive' by Bee Gees is a useful guide to the rate of 100/minute at which chest compressions should be performed. The person performing chest compressions should keep their arms straight, and the sternum should be depressed by 4–5 cm allowing for complete chest recoil. In order to avoid getting tired from performing chest compressions, each person in the team should take turns without leaving room for a delay during change over.

Fluid Administration

Haemorrhage is a major cause of CRA, and may also be a consequence of other causes of CRA. In addition, haemorrhage may be concealed as in some cases of placental abruption, uterine rupture and ruptured ectopic pregnancy. Abdominal examination and ultrasound (for free fluid) are helpful in detecting concealed haemorrhage in these cases. Two large-bore intravenous (IV) cannulae with a minimum gauge of 16 should be inserted as soon as possible. If it is difficult to obtain peripheral access, then central venous access or venous cutdown should be considered. Intravenous access should be gained above the femoral vein, because fluids or drugs administered via the femoral veins may not reach the maternal heart until the fetus is delivered due to compression of the inferior vena cava by the gravid uterus. At the time of gaining IV access, blood should be obtained for group and save (at least six units of packed red cells), a full blood count, blood urea, serum electrolytes, liver function tests and a clotting profile.

An aggressive approach to volume replacement should be adopted. However, the pregnant woman is also at heightened risk of developing pulmonary oedema, and there is emerging evidence to support a less aggressive approach to fluid replacement in cases of maternal CRA not resulting from hypovolaemia. Attention to fluid balance is extremely important in cases of pre-eclampsia, in whom the risk of pulmonary oedema is even greater.

Defibrillation

If defibrillation is required, the same settings as for a non-pregnant patient should be used. The shocks from a defibrillator have been shown to have no effect on the fetus. Adhesive defibrillator pads are preferable to defibrillator paddles, and the left defibrillator pad should be placed lateral to the left breast. If fetal monitoring equipment is being used, then these should be removed from the woman before defibrillation is performed. If the uterus is manually displaced to the left or if the left lateral tilt is achieved by a person placing the knees underneath the woman's thorax, then this should be discontinued during defibrillation.

Medication

The types and doses of medication used are the same as the ones for non-pregnant patients. The usual drugs used in resuscitation are identified as safe for both the woman and the fetus.

Perimortem Caesarean Delivery

Rationale

Delivery of the fetus and placenta reduces oxygen consumption, improves venous return, cardiac output and functional residual capacity and also makes chest compressions more effective. This may also facilitate internal chest compressions which are more effective than external chest compressions. Therefore, PMCD should be considered in cases of CRA beyond 20 weeks of gestation, irrespective of the presence of fetal heart activity. The degree of aortocaval compression by the gravid uterus is minimal before 20 weeks of gestation, and the fetus is unlikely to survive even if delivered at this gestation. Therefore, PMCD is not recommended before 20 weeks of gestation.

Time Limits

Perimortem caesarean delivery has been recommended after four minutes of CRA if there is no return of spontaneous circulation, with the aim of delivering the fetus and the placenta within the next minute. The 4-minute rule was proposed, as anoxic brain damage is likely after 4–6 minutes of CRA. However, the pregnant woman is more inclined to develop anoxic brain damage earlier, and resuscitation is prone to be less successful than in a non-pregnant patient. In addition, in a stressful and demanding situation such as maternal CRA, achieving an incision to the delivery time of a minute is unlikely. The shorter the time from arrest to delivery, the better the outcome is for both the woman and the neonate, Therefore, the 4-minute delay is being challenged today in favour of a significantly earlier and even immediate delivery, especially in women with non-shockable rhythms, i.e. pulseless electrical activity and asystole.

Technique

It is imperative that time is not wasted by transferring the woman to the operating room or determining whether the fetus is alive or dead. Perimortem caesarean delivery, which requires only a scalpel and two cord clamps, should be performed at the site of CRA. This could be the labour suite, antenatal or postnatal ward, intensive care unit or at the accident and emergency (A & E) department. Resuscitation should be continued at the time of surgery. There is no need for anaesthesia or analgesia, and with no circulation, blood loss would be minimal.

Traditionally, PMCD has been performed utilising midline incisions on the abdomen and the uterus. However, as delivery can be achieved quickly with a suprapubic transverse incision as well, and, as the majority are unfamiliar with midline uterine incisions today, it is recommended that PMCD is performed using the incisions that the operator is predominantly familiar with.

Once the baby is delivered and if cord clamps are not available, the umbilical cord should be manually compressed to control haemorrhage from the neonate until the cord is clamped or tied later. The baby should be handed over to the neonatal team who should be ready with neonatal resuscitation equipment. Following successful resuscitation and restoration of circulation, the woman may start bleeding, and she should be transferred to the operating room for suturing of the incised layers of the uterus and the abdominal wall while under anaesthesia. If necessary, haemorrhage can be controlled in the short term by compressing the aorta (discussed in Chapter 14). Broad-spectrum intravenous antibiotics, e.g. cefuroxime and metronidazole, should be administered.

Perimortem Caesarean Delivery or 'Resuscitative Hysterotomy'

The procedure of caesarean delivery is thought to have derived its name from 'Lex Caesarea' or 'Law of Caesar' which stated that 'fetuses had to be separated from the mothers who are dying or had died during childbirth'. This was performed in order to try and save the life of the baby, and if this was not possible, this procedure enabled the baby to be buried separately from the mother, as per religious beliefs. Although PMCD has traditionally been performed to save the fetus from a dying mother, today, it is performed to facilitate the resuscitation of the woman and improve her chances of survival, as well as to provide the fetus with an opportunity for survival. Therefore, there are suggestions for the procedure of PMCD to be more appropriately termed 'resuscitative hysterotomy'. It may be required at the most impractical and impossible time to obtain consent from the woman or any other party. Issues with regard to consent are usually circumvented as the procedure is performed in the 'best interests of the mother'.

Place of Instrumental Vaginal Delivery

In rare instances in which delivery can be achieved quickly by a straightforward instrumental vaginal delivery, this should be attempted, provided the necessary criteria are satisfied (discussed in Chapter 9).

Perimortem Hysterectomy

During occasions in which CRA has occurred due to massive obstetric haemorrhage, and in which usual conservative measures have failed to arrest the haemorrhage, it is reasonable to perform hysterectomy at the time of PMCD. The combination of PMCD and hysterectomy not only facilitates effective resuscitation, but this also may be effective in controlling life-threatening haemorrhage.

Fetal Survival

Medication and defibrillation used in the process of maternal resuscitation have been established to have no significant effect on the fetus. Fetal survival depends on the speed and effectiveness of maternal resuscitation, the gestational age, the presence of hypoxia and fetal distress before the event, arrest to the delivery time and the neonatal facilities in the unit.

Continuing Care after Cardiorespiratory Arrest

Continuing care following CRA and successful resuscitation involves seeking and treating the cause. The woman should be transferred to an intensive care setting and managed with multidisciplinary input. Early involvement of experienced personnel, including an intensivist, is essential to ensure a good outcome. There is growing evidence that therapeutic hypothermia following CRA is safe for the woman. However, the concern is the risk of delayed coagulation following the therapy, as most cases of maternal CRA may be complicated by bleeding. If therapeutic hypothermia is not utilised, then efforts should be taken to prevent hyperthermia, at least. If there is no evidence of successful resuscitation, then re-suscitative efforts should be continued until a consensus is reached by the consultant obstetrician, the consultant anaesthesiologist and the cardiac arrest team to discontinue resuscitative efforts.

Documentation, Debriefing, Incident Reporting and Training

Poor documentation can lead to serious medico-legal consequences. Accurate documentation is critical in all cases of maternal CRA irrespective of the outcome. Extensive debriefing of the woman (if she

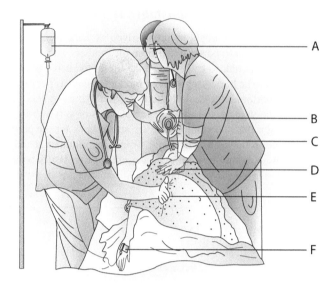

FIGURE 7.4 Cardiopulmonary resuscitation in a pregnant woman; A – rapid administration of intravenous fluids, B – ventilation with 100% oxygen, C – early intubation with a cuffed endotracheal tube, D – chest compressions, E – manual displacement of the uterus to the left, F – venous access above the diaphragm. (Modified from Jeejeebhoy FM, Morrison LJ. Maternal Cardiac Arrest: A Practical and Comprehensive Review. *Emerg Med Int* 2013;2013:274814. doi:10.1155/2013/274814)

survives) and her relatives is mandatory. Maternal CRA is a rare and devastating event, and substandard care is possible. A discussion with the team is important in highlighting the positive as well as negative aspects of management. All cases of maternal CRA should prompt a clinical incident reporting form, and this should be reviewed. Regular drills will ensure optimum management in the face of managing actual cases.

The salient features of CPR in a pregnant woman are shown in Figure 7.4.

Key Points

- Prompt and effective CPR is pivotal to the outcome in maternal CRA.
- Maternal CRA could be due to haemorrhage, but other underlying causes could also result in haemorrhage.
- Early intubation with a cuffed endotracheal tube is important to maintain the airway.
- Manual displacement of the uterus is more advisable over tilting the woman in order to relieve aortocaval compression.
- Perimortem caesarean delivery is required to facilitate resuscitative efforts, if the gestational age is beyond 20 weeks.
- Fetal survival depends on maternal survival.

BIBLIOGRAPHY

1. Chu J, Johnston TA, Geoghegan J, Royal College of Obstetricians and Gynaecologists. Maternal Collapse in Pregnancy and the Puerperium: Green-top Guideline No. 56. *BJOG* 2020;127(5):e14–52. doi:10.1111/1471-0528.15995.
2. Drukker L, Hants Y, Sharon E, Sela HY, Grisaru-Granovsky S. Perimortem cesarean section for maternal and fetal salvage: Concise review and protocol. *Acta Obstet Gynecol Scand* 2014;93:965–72.

3. Eldrige AJ, Ford R. Perimortem caesarean deliveries. *Int J Obstet Anesth* 2016;27:46–54.

4. Jeejeebhoy EM, Zelop CM, Windrim R, Carvalho JCA, Dorian P, Morrison LJ. Management of cardiac arrest in pregnancy: A systematic review. *Resuscitation* 2011;82(7):801–09.

5. Kikuchi J, Deering S. Cardiac arrest in pregnancy. *Semin Perinatol* 2018;42(1):33–38.

6. Lipman S, Cohen S, Einav S, Jeejeebhoy F, Mhyre JM, Morrison LJ, Katz V, Tsen LC, Daniels K, Halamek LP, Suresh MS, Arafeh J, Gauthier D, Carvalho JC, Druzin M, Carvalho B, Society for Obstetric Anesthesia and Perinatology, The Society for Obstetric Anesthesia and Perinatology consensus statement on the management of cardiac arrest in pregnancy. *Anesth Analg* 2014 May;118(5): 1003–16.

7. Monsieurs KG, Nolan JP, Bossaert LL, et al. European Resuscitation Council Guidelines for Resuscitation 2015: Section 1. Executive summary. *Resuscitation* 2015;95:1–80. doi:10.1016/j.resuscitation.2015.07.038

8. Ouzounian J.G., Elkayam U. Physiologic changes during normal pregnancy and delivery. *Cardiol Clin* 2012;30:317–29.

9. Rose CH, Faksh A, Traynor KD, Cabrera D, Arendt KW, Brost BC. Challenging the 4- to 5-minute rule: From perimortem cesarean to resuscitative hysterotomy. *Am J Obstet Gynecol* 2015;213:653–56.

8

Abnormal Labour

Sanjeewa Padumadasa and Malik Goonewardene

The journey through the maternal pelvis is the shortest trip a human being would ever possibly embark upon, but it is probably also the most hazardous. Evolution has led to fetuses with larger heads being born through smaller maternal pelves, and this has made natural childbirth increasingly difficult. Dystocia, dysfunctional labour and poor progress are terms used to describe an abnormal labour pattern that deviates from what is observed in the majority of women who undergo normal deliveries. The diagnosis and optimal management of abnormal labour require a blend of science and the art of obstetrics. The situation is compounded by numerous demands of the woman in the background of malpractice litigation. Acute fetal distress, which could occur consequent to abnormal labour, is also discussed in Chapter 29.

Types of Abnormal Labour

- Poor progress in the first stage, i.e. up to 10 cm dilatation
- Prolonged second stage, i.e. after full dilatation to delivery of the fetus
- Precipitate labour

Poor Progress in the First Stage

The following patterns of poor progress in the first stage have been described.

- Slower than average progress from the onset of labour (prolonged latent phase and primary dysfunctional labour)
- Decrease in progress after initial satisfactory progress (secondary dysfunctional labour)
- Complete cessation of progress (arrest) after initial satisfactory or slow progress

Although a definitive diagnosis of labour is crucial for the further management of a woman, sometimes this is not easy. This is because the onset of labour is not a well defined specific event, but rather it is a dynamic continuum from pregnancy, commencing with effacement of the cervix, especially in nullipara. The diagnosis of labour is actually retrospective. A woman may be assumed to be in the latent phase when actually she is not, and therefore, a definitive diagnosis of a prolonged latent phase is not possible. The duration of labour depends on a woman's unique physiological reproductive process and pregnancy characteristics. Furthermore, a prolonged latent phase of the first stage of labour is generally a benign disorder compared to abnormalities in the active phase of the first stage and the second stage. However, it is still important to provide analgesia and to monitor both fetal and maternal conditions. Interventions should not be based solely on time durations. In a woman with a spontaneous onset of labour, if the maternal and fetal conditions are satisfactory and there is reasonable progressive cervical dilatation, then interventions should not be enforced, and the augmentation of labour with amniotomy and intravenous oxytocin infusion or caesarean delivery would usually be indicated only when she is in the active phase.

Until recently, Friedman's labour curve, dating back to the middle of the 20th century, which suggested that the cervix dilates at a slow rate until 3–4 cm (the latent phase) and more rapidly at approximately 1 cm per hour thereafter (the active phase), has been used as a guide to diagnosing abnormal labour. Friedman also described a deceleration phase at 9 cm. Poor progress was diagnosed by comparing a woman's labour pattern in relation to the expected nomogram which had an 'alert line' drawn at 1 cm per hour from 4 cm. An 'action line' was drawn four hours to the right of the alert line to aid in determining when to intervene, because too soon or inappropriate interventions in labour could be harmful to the woman, the fetus or both.

Recently in a large study, it has been reported that the latent phase of normal labour: continues until about 5–6 cm dilatation; is very much slower than previously reported; and its duration varies considerably from one woman to the other. For example, labour may take more than six hours to progress from 4 to 5 cm and more than three hours to progress from 5 to 6 cm of dilatation, with no adverse maternal or neonatal outcomes. It has also been observed that the median time necessary to progress from a centimetre to the next becomes shorter as labour advances, and that after 6 cm, labour accelerates much faster in multiparous than in nulliparous women. In addition, there is apparently no deceleration phase near 10 cm. Contemporary labour curves have thus been proposed based on these findings (Figure 8.1). It has been suggested that allowing labour to continue for a longer period before 6 cm of cervical dilatation may reduce the rate of intrapartum and subsequent repeat caesarean deliveries.

The methodological validity of these contemporary curves and their safety for use in clinical practice have been questioned by some. On the other hand, the original concept of applying a mean rate of 1 cm per hour for the total duration of the active phase of labour does not take into consideration individual variations in women and the fact that frequently, labour does not progress in a linear fashion. Therefore, use of an alert line at a rate of 1cm per hour and an action line four hour to its right, commencing from the start of the active first stage of labour, is currently not advised. Defining and managing abnormal labour based on time durations only, is also not supported. A new WHO Labour Care Guide has been developed recently, and its main differences from the previous WHO partograph are described below.

- The active phase of the first stage of labour is defined as commencing from 5 cm of cervical dilatation.
- Evidence based time limits of cervical dilatation are used for each centimetre of cervical dilatation, and these are dynamic and vary from up to 6 hours at 5 cm and up to 2 hours at 9 cm. Alert and action lines are not drawn.
- Fetal heart rate monitoring is intensified during the second stage of labour.
- The availability of a labour companion, pain relief, oral fluid intake and the position of the mother are recorded.
- The frequency and the duration of uterine contractions are recorded and no attempt is made to quantify the strength of uterine contractions.

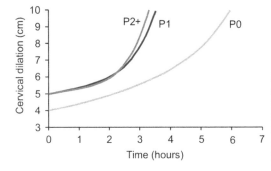

FIGURE 8.1 Contemporary labour curves for women in spontaneous labour, stratified by parity; reproduced with permission from wolters kluwer. P0 = nulliparous, P1 = parity of 1, P2+ = parity of 2 or more. (Zhang J, Landy HJ, Branch DW, et al. Contemporary Patterns of Spontaneous Labour with Normal Neonatal Outcomes. *Obstet Gynecol* 2010;116(6):1283)

- An 'alert column', describing the expected norms, has been included. When any parameter is detected to vary from the expected norms, it needs to be 'flagged', and the response must be recorded.

The new WHO Labour Care Guide includes not only a graphical representation of the progress of labour but also other attributes that contribute to a positive childbirth experience and satisfactory outcomes. In addition, the monitoring during the second stage which was previously not emphasized, has been strengthened. The inclusion of references for the expected norms for the parameters that are documented facilitates the recognition and documentation of an abnormality. This is expected to trigger a response similar to that in the Modified Obstetric Early Warning Score (MOEWS) chart (discussed in Chapter 7). Furthermore, the plan of action is recorded. However, whether the longer durations allowed for cervical dilatation, especially from 5–7 cm, are acceptable to all healthcare practitioners and are applicable in all settings, is yet to be seen.

Causes of Poor Progress of Labour

Labour is a complex interaction of the three Ps; **P**ower, **P**assage and the **P**assenger. Abnormalities in any of these factors may account for poor progress of labour, but frequently, it is a combination of factors that results in poor progress of labour.

Power

The power for labour to progress is provided by uterine contractions, with maternal expulsive efforts contributing during the active phase of second stage. The uterine smooth muscle has the ability not only to contract and relax, but also to retract, a unique feature that is essential to provide the power for labour to progress. Uterine contractions are assessed by clinical examination, external uterine tocography and intrauterine pressure catheters. Uterine contractions may be weak, infrequent or both, making these ineffective (hypotonic uterine dysfunction/uterine inertia), and this is the predominant cause of poor progress of labour. Strong and uncoordinated uterine contractions occurring at an increased frequency (hypertonic pattern) are also associated with dysfunctional labour.

Passage

As far as the passage is concerned, there may be abnormalities in the bony components as well as the soft tissues of the pelvis. Gynaecoid is the normal type, while anthropoid, android and platy-pelloid are abnormally shaped pelves which are sometimes found in women (Figure 8.2). Abnormal labour could also be due to bony irregularities, but is seldom encountered today as a result of the rarity of diseases (e.g. rickets) affecting the pelvic bones and the carrying out of antepartum cae-sarean delivery in women who are suspected to have pelvic abnormalities – for example, after pelvic fractures.

As labour is a dynamic process and involves many changes that take place within the maternal pelvis (e.g. stretching of pelvic ligaments) and the fetus (e.g. flexion, rotation and moulding), clinical pelvi-metry prior to the onset of labour has not been considered useful in predicting the possibility of feto-pelvic disproportion, i.e. the mismatch between the size or shape of the fetus and those of the maternal pelvis, leading to abnormal labour. However, it may be a useful tool during labour in special situations such as assisted vaginal breech delivery or trial of labour after a previous caesarean delivery. An experienced obstetrician should be able to recognise obvious bony abnormalities in the female pelvis during a routine vaginal examination.

A full bladder may hinder the progress of labour, and emptying the bladder may be all that is ne-cessary for labour to progress in this case. Other soft-tissue abnormalities in the passage such as fibroids,

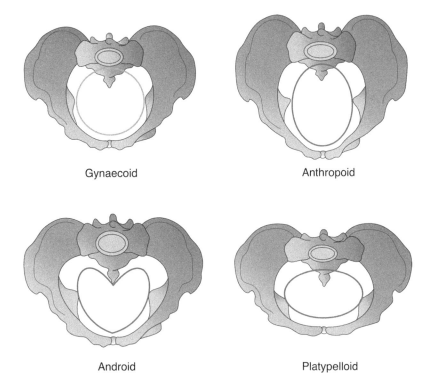

Gynaecoid

Anthropoid

Android

Platypelloid

FIGURE 8.2 Types of female pelves.

cervical dystocia, vaginal septum, tumours and atresia may be diagnosed at vaginal examination during labour. Vaginal delivery may be achieved in case of a vaginal septum, but haemorrhage resulting from tears in the septum should be anticipated. Ovarian tumours tend to lie alongside the upper part of the uterus towards the latter part of pregnancy and are usually not a cause of abnormal labour.

Passenger

The presenting part may be too large (e.g. macrosomia due to maternal diabetes mellitus or post dates or hydrocephalus), or more commonly, the relative diameters of the presenting part may be increased due to a malposition of the vertex, its attitude, or asynclitism, or a malpresentation. Figure 8.3 shows the relevant diameters of the fetal head. The disparity in the relationship between the fetal head and the maternal pelvis is referred to as cephalopelvic disproportion (CPD), a diagnosis that should be made only during labour.

Malpositions of the Vertex

In a vertex presentation, when the fetal occiput is in a posterior or transverse position, it is referred to as a malposition. It is important to identify malpostions of the vertex in early labour before a caput forms.

The fetal occiput presents posteriorly in approximately 25% of early and 10%–15% of active labours. The anthropoid pelvis predisposes to this condition. Majority rotate spontaneously to direct occipitoanterior (DOA) position and deliver. A few may persist as occipitoposterior (OP) position, arrest in occipitotransverse position (deep transverse arrest) or deliver in direct occipitoposterior position (face to pubes) (Figure 8.4). Epidural anaesthesia may hinder rotation of the fetal head, as a result of loss of pelvic floor muscle tone and loss of antero-medial sloping nature of the pelvic floor, and this may lead to persistent OP position.

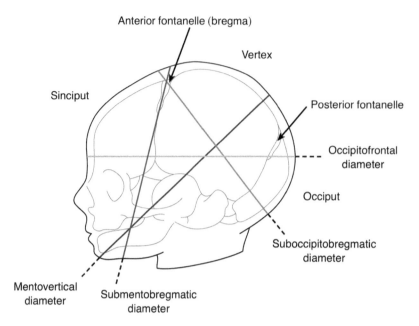

FIGURE 8.3 The diameters of the fetal head.

In OP positions, spontaneous rotation to the DOA position and a normal delivery should be anticipated. This should occur in approximately 80% of cases. If a normal delivery does not happen, then the mode of delivery will depend on a multitude of factors such as the progress of labour, the position and station of the vertex and the clinical skills and experience of the operator. The available options are a vacuum delivery, a face to pubes delivery with or without the application of a long-bladed forceps, rotational forceps delivery using Kielland forceps, digital or manual rotation to occipitoanterior (OA) position followed by a normal or instrumental vaginal delivery (IVD) or a caesarean delivery. Currently, manual rotation has been virtually abandoned and digital rotation is also not easily possible. Delivery with Kielland forceps, long-bladed forceps and vacuum extraction are discussed in Chapter 9. It is essential that a proper evaluation of the position of the vertex, its station within the pelvis and exclusion of CPD is carried out prior to attempting an IVD. It has been observed that, sometimes, a diagnosis of 'Deep Transverse Arrest' is erroneously made when the vertex is neither deep (station +1) nor has the labour been arrested. Attempting an IVD in such a situation is contraindicated.

Fetal Attitude

The attitude of the fetal head refers to the degree of flexion or extension at the upper cervical spine. Different longitudinal diameters are presented to the pelvis depending on the fetal attitude. In a well-flexed head, the anterior fontanelle is not easily felt, and the presenting diameter is the suboccipito-bregmatic, which measures about 9.5 cm at term (Figure 8.5A). In OP and occipitotransverse (OT) positions, which are often associated with deflexion of the fetal head, the anterior fontanelle is felt at a lower plane and assumes a more medial position compared to the posterior fontanelle, and the presenting diameter is the occipito-frontal which measures about 10.5 cm at term (Figure 8.5B). The extension of the fetal head leads to brow and face presentations (Figures 8.5C and D).

Asynclitism

Asynclitism (lateral flexion of the head), which is a physiological phenomenon that can occur during labour when the head enters the sacral hollow with its anteroposterior diameter in the

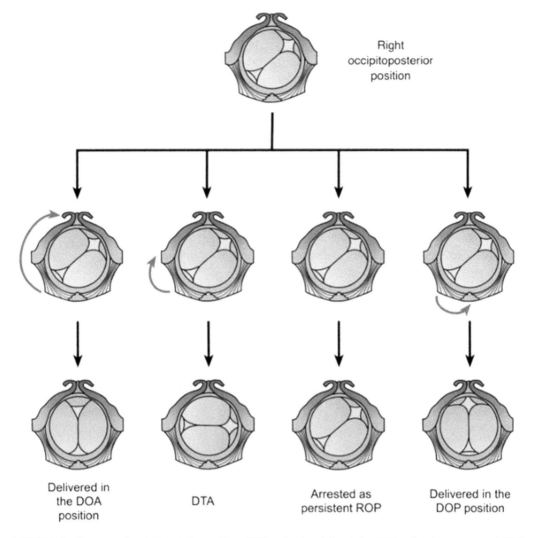

FIGURE 8.4 Outcomes of occipitoposterior positions. DOA = direct occipitoanterior, DTA = deep transverse arrest, ROP = right occipitoposterior, DOP = direct occipitoposterior.

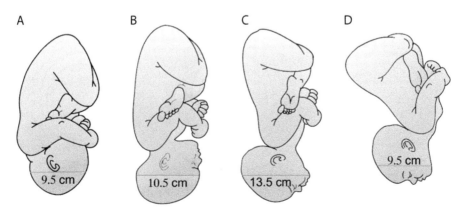

FIGURE 8.5 The changing diameters of the fetal head with deflexion and extension. A = well-flexed vertex, B = deflexed vertex, C = brow, D = face presentation.

transverse plane of the pelvic inlet (Figure 8.6), leads to dysfunctional labour if it is not spontaneously corrected in the mid-cavity of the pelvis. In anterior asynclitism, the anterior parietal bone is more prominently felt than the posterior one and the sagittal suture is felt towards the posterior half of the pelvis, while in posterior asynclitism, the posterior parietal bone is more prominently felt than the anterior one and the sagittal suture is felt towards the anterior half of the pelvis (Figure 8.7).

Malpresentations

When the presenting part is not the vertex of the fetus, it is referred to as a malpresentation. Breech is the most common malpresentation (discussed in Chapter 25).

The following are the other malpresentations.

- Face
- Brow
- Shoulder, dorsal or arm presentation when the lie is transverse or oblique
- Compound presentations

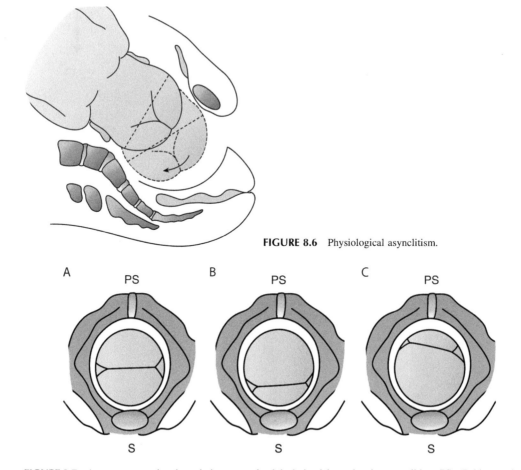

FIGURE 8.6 Physiological asynclitism.

FIGURE 8.7 A transverse section through the maternal pelvis during labour showing asynclitism. PS = Pubic symphysis, S = sacrum, A = synclitism, B = anterior asynclitism, C = posterior asynclitism.

Face and Brow Presentations

Usually, a secondary brow presentation occurs during internal rotation of a vertex presentation from an OP position to an OA position in labour, due to the extension of the fetal head. Similarly, a secondary face presentation may occur by extension of the fetal head at the onset of labour. Rarely, these mal-presentations could persist from the onset of labour, in which case they are referred to as a primary face or brow presentation. Causes of a primary face or brow presentation are given in Table 8.1.

Face Presentation

In face presentation, the fetal head is fully extended and almost at a right angle to the spine. Face presentation may be suspected on abdominal examination if there is a marked depression between the fetal back and occiput. It is diagnosed when the supraorbital ridges, eyes, nose, mouth and chin are felt on vaginal examination once the cervix has sufficiently dilated. The palpation of the chin (mentum) is crucial for the differentiation of a face presentation from a brow presentation, because in a brow presentation, which is incompatible with vaginal delivery, the chin is not palpable. The development of significant facial oedema may make it difficult to distinguish between the mouth and anus. In this case, inserting a finger into the orifice will enable the palpation of the alveolar ridges in the mouth and the detection of the anal sphincter tone in the anus. The presenting diameter in a face presentation is the submento-bregmatic, which is also approximately 9.5 cm in a full-term fetus and is the same as the suboccipito-bregmatic diameter of a favourable and fully flexed vertex presentation. However, the ill-fitting presenting part is a poor dilator of the cervix, and in addition, the base of the skull does not undergo moulding as in the case of the cranial vault. In direct mentoanterior position of a face presentation, and with internal rotation of left and right mentoanterior positions to a direct mentoanterior position, vaginal delivery is possible. Once the chin escapes under the pubic symphysis, the head is born by flexion (Figure 8.8).

Forceps may be applied if there is a need to assist delivery (discussed in Chapter 9), but vacuum delivery is contraindicated in face presentation. In left or right mentoposterior and mentotransverse positions vaginal delivery is possible only if spontaneous rotation to the direct mentoanterior position occurs. Vaginal delivery is not possible in direct mentoposterior position, as the extended fetal neck cannot extend further to accommodate the pelvic curve (Figure 8.9). In this case, caesarean delivery must be performed. In left or right mentoposterior and mentotransverse positions, Kielland forceps can be used to rotate a fetus to a direct mentoanterior position and deliver (described in Chapter 9).

TABLE 8.1

Causes of a primary face or brow presentation

Fetal anomalies
   Major CNS abnormalities
   Anencephaly
   Iniencephaly
   Meningomyelocoele
   Conditions that cause permanent extension of the fetal head
   Cervical spine deformities
   Goitre
   Cystic hygroma
   Brachial cysts
Prematurity
Excessive tone in the extensor muscles of the fetus
Multiparity
Idiopathic (Majority)

A   B

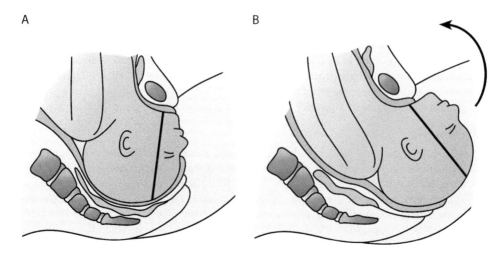

FIGURE 8.8   Face presentation. A = mentoanterior position, B = mechanism of delivery.

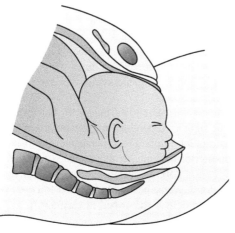

FIGURE 8.9   Face presentation – mentoposterior position.

Brow Presentation

Brow presentation occurs when the fetal head is extended and is midway between a vertex (well flexed) and a face presentation (fully extended). It is diagnosed by easily palpating the anterior fontanelle, and also palpating the supraorbital ridges and nose, vaginally. As mentioned earlier, the chin is not palpable in a brow presentation, differentiating it from a face presentation. The mento-vertical diameter (approximately 13.5 cm), is the largest and the most unfavourable of the anteroposterior diameters of an average-sized fetal skull which presents at the maternal pelvis (Figure 8.10). Persistent brow presentation during labour, with an average-sized fetus, requires a caesarean delivery, as vaginal delivery is not possible. Vaginal delivery has been reported in a very small number of cases with a small fetus in a capacious pelvis. Up to two-thirds of antepartum brow presentations may spontaneously convert during the early stages of labour to either a face presentation (by further extension) or a vertex presentation (by flexion).

Shoulder, Dorsal or Arm Presentation When the Lie is Transverse or Oblique

When the fetus lies with its longitudinal axis perpendicular to the longitudinal axis of the pelvis (transverse lie), the shoulder, back or arm is the presenting part. These presentations may also occur when the lie is oblique. The causes of these presentations are given in Table 8.2.

The complications of shoulder presentation are cord prolapse, arm prolapse (Figure 8.11) and neglected shoulder presentation which can lead to obstructed labour and uterine rupture. When the cause is lax

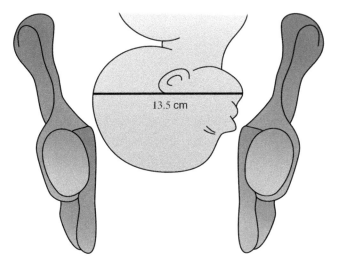

13.5 cm

FIGURE 8.10   Brow presentation.

TABLE 8.2

Causes of shoulder, dorsal or arm presentation

Maternal causes
    Multiparity
    Lax abdominal and uterine muscles
    Uterine abnormality, e.g. septate or subseptate uterus
    Contracted pelvis
    Placenta praevia
    Fibroids in the lower segment
    Full bladder (abnormal lie usually resolves after the bladder is emptied)
Fetal causes
    Prematurity
    Multiple pregnancy
    Polyhydramnios
    Fetal anomalies
    Intrauterine fetal death

uterine musculature associated with multiparity, then the lie is likely to convert to longitudinal in early labour with the increase in uterine tone. If the lie does not convert to longitudinal, a caesarean delivery is necessary in cases of shoulder presentation. However, if shoulder presentation is diagnosed during early labour, the obstetrician may perform external cephalic version followed by stabilising induction, in the presence of adequate liquor. These procedures are discussed in Chapters 27 and 2 respectively.

Compound Presentations

A compound presentation is when one or more of the limbs present with the head or the breech. The most frequent combination is the hand with the head (Figure 8.12), and the next common is a hand with the breech. In the majority of cases, the diagnosis may not be made until labour is advanced. Usually, the head or the breech will descend below the hand, and the outcome is generally good unless it is associated with cord prolapse. If the descent of the head or the breech appears to be hampered by a limb, then the limb should be pushed up, and the woman should be instructed to bear down if the cervix is fully dilated.

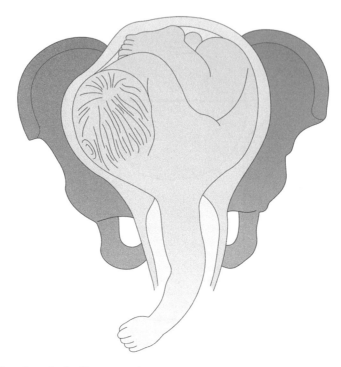

FIGURE 8.11   Prolapsed arm in shoulder presentation.

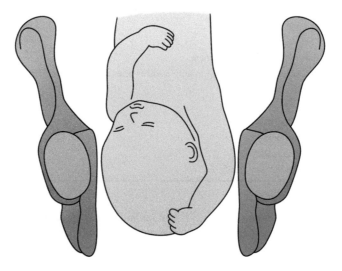

FIGURE 8.12   Compound presentation (hand and head).

Provider and Patient Factors

In addition to the three **P**s mentioned above, **P**rovider and **P**atient factors also play a role in determining the outcome of labour. The provider of intrapartum care may be influenced by personal training and experience, time of day, facilities within the unit and medicolegal climate, while patient factors such as pre-existing medical conditions, previous obstetric history, anxiety and pain, among others should be taken into account when managing dysfunctional labour.

Identification and Management of an Abnormal First Stage of Labour

Each woman with abnormal labour should be considered unique, and her management should consequently be individualised. The methods of identification and management of abnormal labour vary vastly among obstetric units in the world. Although the maintenance of a partograph has been widely recommended, and several designs of partographs are available, the graphic labour pattern should never be used in isolation. Partographs are often not used properly. Furthermore, robust evidence is currently lacking in terms of their effectiveness in improving birth outcomes. Evidence for the acceptability and applicability of the new WHO Labour Care Guide in all settings, and its effectiveness in enhancing a positive childbirth experience in a woman and improving maternal and fetal outcomes, is awaited. Clinical parameters are of paramount importance in intrapartum decision-making. In the management of women with poor progress of the first stage of labour, the following steps are indicated.

- Identify the cause
- Provide continuous support to the labouring woman
- Correct the cause of poor progress, e.g. augmentation of labour with amniotomy and/ or oxytocin infusion after excluding a malpresentation and fetopelvic disproportion
- Carry out continuous electronic fetal monitoring
- Reassess

Identify the Cause

The station of the presenting part is the relationship of the foremost bony part of the fetal head to the ischial spines of the maternal pelvis. When this is at the level of the ischial spines, then the station is zero, and the levels above and below the ischial spines are designated from −3 to +3. Abdominally, the head is divided into five equal parts, and when the entire head is palpable abdominally (described as a head level of 5/5), then the corresponding station of the head vaginally is −3. At station 0, the level of the head, when palpable abdominally, is 2/5. When the entire head has entered the pelvis, and it is not palpable abdominally (i.e. 0/5), the corresponding station of the head is +2 vaginally (Figure 8.13). When the head is crowning, the corresponding station of the head vaginally is +3. Abdominally, overestimations of the descent of the head could occur due to difficulties in palpating the fetal head on account of maternal obesity or the OP position of the vertex where the face of the

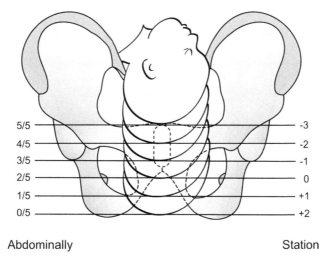

FIGURE 8.13 The relationship of abdominal descent and vaginal station.

fetus is angled upwards and is difficult to be determined. Vaginally, overestimations are possible when there are a caput and moulding (Figure 8.14).

The fetal position should be checked by palpating the entire length of the sagittal suture, as if going along a road, to identify a 'Y' junction, the posterior fontanelle, where three bones meet, and the anterior fontanelle, where four bones intersect. The fontanelles themselves may not be palpable due to significant moulding. In the presence of a large caput, a fetal ear should be identified and the direction of the pinna will point to the posterior fontanelle. The ear canal must also be identified, because rarely, the pinna could be folded forward, therefore giving a false impression of the position. The ear also acts as an important landmark in assessing the station of the head as it is very close to the biparietal diameter. Furthermore, if the ear is easily palpable, then significant CPD is unlikely.

Moulding is defined as the extent of overlapping of fetal skull bones which occurs as the fetal head adapts to the birth canal during labour. The parietal bones overlap the occipital bone, each other and in severe cases, the frontal bone. Moulding is graded from 0 to +3 according to severity (Figure 8.15).

- 0 moulding – bones are separated
- +1 moulding – bones touching, but not overlapping
- +2 moulding – bones overlapping, but easily reducible with digital pressure
- +3 moulding – bones overlapping, and not reducible with digital pressure

Up to +2 moulding is normal and occurs in order to reduce the diameters of the fetal head, thus making it easy for the fetal head to traverse the maternal pelvis during labour. Moulding of +3 is abnormal and is a feature of CPD.

Provide Continuous Support to the Labouring Woman

The woman should be advised to assume whatever position she feels is comfortable other than the supine position which could cause hypotension and even fetal distress as a result of reduced venous return due to compression of the inferior vena cava by the gravid uterus. Continuous support by a professional as well as a companion reduces operative interventions, shortens labour and leads to a better outcome in the neonate as well as the woman, as compared to cases when women are left alone during labour.

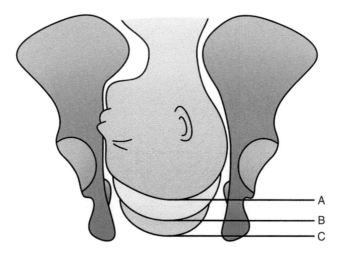

FIGURE 8.14 The effect of the caput and moulding on the assessment of fetal station. A - fetal station, B = effect of moulding, C = effect of caput.

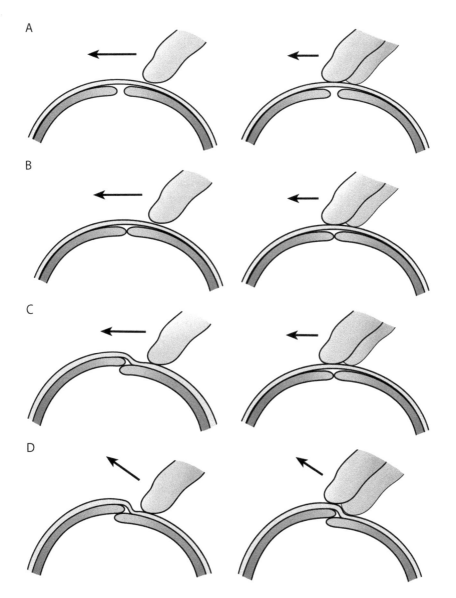

FIGURE 8.15 Degrees of moulding. A = 0 moulding, B = +1 moulding, C = +2 moulding, D = +3 moulding.

Pain activates the sympathetic pathways in the body which leads to inhibition of uterine contractions and results in poor progress of labour. Therefore, pain relief constitutes a vital part of management. Epidural analgesia is an effective method of pain relief during labour and does not interfere with the progress during the first stage, but it prolongs the second stage of labour due to the abolition of the Ferguson reflex and hindering maternal bearing-down efforts during the expulsive phase. However, it has been shown that there is no increase in the rates of instrumental vaginal delivery or caesarean delivery with epidural analgesia. Narcotic analgesics, usually pethidine, are also used to provide effective pain relief during labour. The main side effect of narcotic analgesics is a respiratory depression in the newborn, which can be managed with the antagonist, naloxone and assisted ventilation. Inhalational analgesia, usually a combination of 50% nitrous oxide and 50% oxygen, can be useful during the late first stage and second stage of labour. Overdosage with this method is unlikely to happen. This is because when the medication achieves maximum effect, the woman would feel drowsy and her hand which is holding the inhaler will fall away from her face. As there is a latent period between the commencement of inhalation and the onset of effective analgesia, the woman should start inhaling before the onset of uterine contractions for this method to be effective. Dehydration, if present, should be corrected with intravenous fluids.

Amniotomy

Following amniotomy, the fetal head descends and directly presses on the cervix, and prostaglandins, which increase the sensitivity of oxytocin receptors, are released. Therefore, amniotomy is commonly used to augment labour in case of poor progress in the first stage. Amniotomy shortens the first stage of labour and slightly reduce the rate of caesarean deliveries in cases of an abnormal first stage of labour with no difference in adverse maternal or neonatal outcomes. However, amniotomy is associated with intrauterine infection and, in the presence of a high presenting part, cord prolapse.

Oxytocin

Augmentation with an intravenous oxytocin infusion is usually combined with amniotomy, to manage abnormal progress in the first stage of labour. In this case, the principle of using oxytocin is to mimic natural uterine activity. Although various regimens of oxytocin are used, what is more important than the initial, incremental as well as maximum doses are its effects, both desired and adverse. Common regimens have initial doses varying from 1–5 mU/minute, and increments of 1–5 mU/minute at intervals of 30–40 minutes until an adequate pattern of contractions (at least three contractions per 10 minutes, each lasting at least 30 seconds) is achieved. The recommended maximum dose is 20 mU/minute. Augmentation with oxytocin is expected to cause flexion of the fetal head and rotation to a favourable OA from an OP or OT position, leading to a relatively smaller diameter of the fetal head presenting at the pelvis, with the end result being progressive cervical dilatation and the descent of the fetal head. The fetus should be observed using continuous electronic fetal monitoring following administration of oxytocin.

Oxytocin is not usually associated with significant maternal or neonatal complications. However, it may lead to tachysystole (more than five contractions in 10 minutes), and hypertonus (each contraction lasting ≥2 minutes or within 60 seconds of each other). When either of these results in fetal distress, then it is referred to as hyperstimulation. Although individual definitions vary, all of these terms refer to excessive uterine activity. It is advisable to be cautious and to reduce the oxytocin dose if a contraction lasts >60 seconds or if the interval between contractions is <30 seconds, even in the absence of fetal distress. If a reduction of the oxytocin dose fails to achieve a normal pattern of uterine contractions and a satisfactory fetal condition, then uterine relaxation (e.g. with terbutaline 0.25 mg subcutaneously) is necessary. Oxytocin has also been associated with uterine rupture, water intoxication, cardiac arrhythmias and amniotic fluid embolism. If there is no progress of labour after four hours of administering oxytocin in adequate doses, then caesarean delivery is recommended.

The natural response of a uterus in the case of CPD in a primigravida is to cease contracting. On the other hand, a uterus in a multiparous woman would usually amplify contractions in the presence of CPD. Therefore, augmenting labour with oxytocin in the presence of poor progress of labour in a multiparous woman should only be done after assessing uterine contractions and excluding signs of CPD, as inappropriate use of oxytocin may heighten the risk of uterine rupture.

It is recommended to utilise internal tocodynamometry in order to measure the frequency, duration and magnitude of uterine contractions in special circumstances such as the case for obese women and poor progress of labour despite augmentation with oxytocin.

Carry Out Continuous Electronic Fetal Monitoring

Continuous electronic fetal monitoring is critical in every case of abnormal labour. While external cardiotocography is usually adequate, placement of a fetal scalp electrode is an option in the late part of the first stage.

Reassess the Progress of Labour Following Intervention

It is vital to reassess the progress of labour with uterine contractions, cervical dilatation and the descent of the presenting part after intervening in abnormal labour. The interval between assessments is usually four hours, but it may have to be reduced according to the clinical circumstances, presumed fetal compromise and expected progress. For example, a repeat assessment after four hours may be appropriate in a primigravida with a cervical os of 8 cm, the fetus in OP position and no fetal distress, while a repeat determination after three hours would be more suitable in a multiparous woman with the same findings.

Caesarean Delivery

The most appropriate intervention for abnormal labour in the first stage, in the presence of adequate uterine contractions, is caesarean delivery. Dysfunctional labour is a major contributor to caesarean deliveries worldwide.

Prolonged Second Stage

The second stage of labour consists of two phases, a passive (pelvic) phase, during which the presenting part descends with the aid of uterine contractions, and an active (perineal) phase during which the fetal head rotates to a more favourable position and maternal expulsive efforts aid in delivery of the fetus.

Time Limits of the Second Stage

A prolonged second stage has been defined as more than two hours without epidural and three hours with epidural in nulliparous women, and more than one hour without and two hours with epidural analgesia in multiparous women. Recent studies on the duration of the second stage have shown that approximately 15% of the contemporary obstetric population are identified as having a prolonged second stage as per the above criteria. Furthermore, in a large study, the 95th percentiles of the second stage of labour in nulliparous women with and without epidural analgesia were recently reported to be 3.6 and 2.8 hours, respectively. The length of the second stage has a negligible effect on the overall maternal and neonatal outcome, provided that the fetal and maternal conditions are satisfactory and that there is adequate progress as far as the descent of the presenting part is concerned. This raises the question of whether the criteria for a diagnosis of a prolonged second stage are too stringent and unsuitable for a contemporary obstetric population and whether there is a need for a redefinition.

Factors Affecting the Duration of the Second Stage

Many maternal factors such as age, parity, height, weight, obesity, size and shape of pelvis, uterine contractile forces, soft tissue resistance, expulsion effort, epidural analgesia as well as fetal factors such as size, position, degree of flexion and station at full dilatation have an effect on the progress of the second stage of labour.

Epidural analgesia lengthens the second stage due to sensory blockade, which diminishes a woman's urge to push. It also has an effect on the Ferguson reflex, which leads to a reduction of oxytocin release. Delayed spontaneous pushing during the active phase of the second stage (i.e. the woman pushes with an open glottis, three to four times during the contraction only when she has a strong urge to push or when the head is visible at the vaginal introitus) reduces the duration of active pushing but may not increase the likelihood of a vaginal delivery. Although delayed pushing can lead to a longer second stage as well as a possible higher incidence of intraamniotic infection and low umbilical cord pH, there is no significant advantage in directed early pushing during the passive phase of the second stage (i.e. the woman is advised to take a deep breath at the beginning of each contraction and to bear down with a closed glottis throughout each contraction when she is found to be fully dilated on vaginal examination). This latter practice could also possibly lead to further medical intervention. Evidence for reduction or discontinuation of the epidural while late in labour in order to facilitate full maternal bearing down efforts having beneficial effects on the mode of delivery or neonatal outcome is also rather equivocal. Therefore, in the absence of robust evidence, the woman's preference and comfort and the clinical context should be considered when deciding on the timing (i.e. early or delayed) and method of pushing (i.e. intermittently or continuously during the contraction and with an open or closed glottis), and whether the epidural analgesia should be reduced or discontinued.

Interventions for a Prolonged Second Stage

Although a prolonged second stage is associated with increased perinatal morbidity, this association may mostly stem from the increased rate of interventions, such as operative delivery. However, each case should be handled on an individual basis and there must be a balance between an intervention that happens too early, which may be unnecessary and may possibly even end up in a traumatic delivery, and an intervention that happens too late, which may result in birth asphyxia. Furthermore, in the presence of fetal distress, it is essential that the operator selects the most suitable intervention. If uterine contractions are considered as inadequate, and malpresentations, malpositions and CPD have been excluded, then augmentation with an intravenous oxytocin infusion may be considered by an experienced obstetrician. Instrumental vaginal delivery (discussed in Chapter 9) may be performed by an experienced operator at the correct time, place and under proper analgesia after careful selection of suitable cases and instruments. Caesarean delivery (discussed in Chapter 11) should be performed if any of the abovementioned criteria are unmet. It is imperative that an experienced obstetrician is involved in both the decision-making process and the procedure itself, as both instrumental vaginal delivery and caesarean delivery when the fetal head is impacted in the pelvis are associated with significant maternal and neonatal morbidity.

Use of Ultrasound in Dysfunctional Labour

A combination of transabdominal and transperineal ultrasound using a two-dimensional ultrasound machine and a convex probe can be used to complement clinical examination in assessing position, station, attitude and asynclitism, especially in the presence of dysfunctional labour. Ultrasound in labour is not only useful in differentiating between women who are suited for normal delivery and those who require operative delivery but also in predicting the success rate of IVD.

Assessment of Fetal Position

The position of the fetal spine is determined using the transabdominal approach and at low stations, the transperineal approach. The landmarks are the cervical spine for OA position on a sagittal plane (Figure 8.16A), midline cerebral echo for OT position on a transverse plane (Figure 8.16B), and the two fetal orbits for OP position (Figure 8.16C).

Assessment of Fetal Station

Fetal station is assessed transperineally instead of transabdominally. The sonographic parameters used to assess fetal station are described below.

- Angle of progression - the angle between the long axis of the pubic bone and a line drawn from the lowermost part of the pubic symphysis to the lowermost bony part of the fetal skull (Figure 8.17)
- Fetal head direction - the angle between the longest axis of the fetal head and the long axis of the pubic symphysis

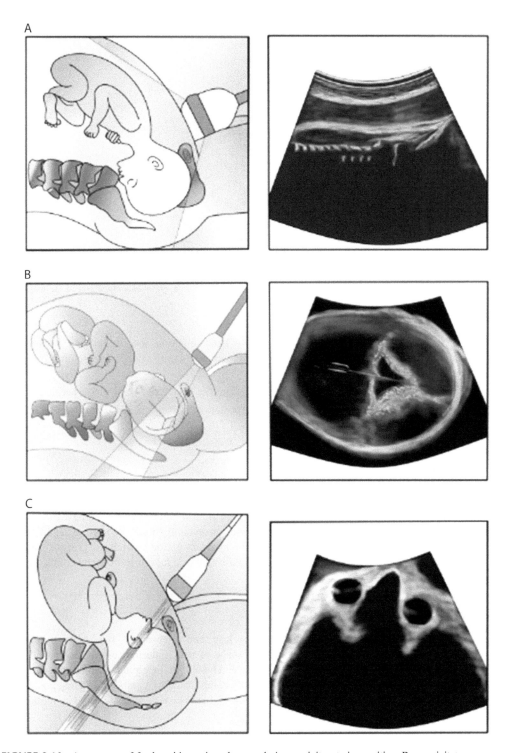

FIGURE 8.16 Assessment of fetal position using ultrasound. A = occipitoanterior position, B = occipitotransverse position, C = occipitoposterior position.

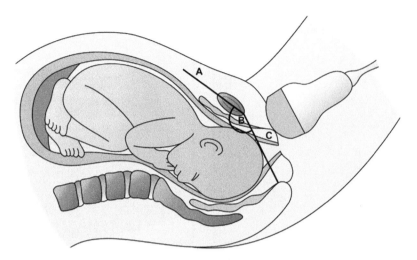

FIGURE 8.17 Assessment of fetal station using the angle of progression. A = line through the long axis of the pubic symphysis, B = angle of progression, C = line from the distal point of pubic symphysis tangential to the fetal skull.

- Sonographic head station - incorporation of the head direction and the distance between the infrapubic plane (which is 3 cm above the ischial spines) and the deepest presenting bony part along the line of head direction
- Head-perineum distance – the shortest distance from the bony fetal skull to the perineum
- Midline angle - the angle between the anteroposterior axis of the fetal skull and the anteroposterior axis of the maternal pelvis

Assessment of Fetal Attitude

Ultrasound has proved to be useful in assessing the degree of flexion/ extension of the fetal head in relation to the spine and in the diagnosis of malpresentation.

Currently, there is no consensus as to when ultrasound should be performed and how the findings should be integrated into clinical practice. In any case, ultrasound should be used as an adjunct to clinical examination and not as a substitute to clinical examination, which, at present times, is probably irreplaceable as the most reliable means of assessment in labour in the hands of the skilled.

Precipitate Labour

Precipitate (rapid) labour is defined as labour lasting less than three hours. It is more common in multiparous than in nulliparous women and in the presence of strong uterine contractions, small-sized fetus, roomy pelvis and minimal soft tissue resistance. History of precipitate labour in a previous pregnancy is also a risk factor. Precipitate labour can be complicated by genital tract tears, postpartum haemorrhage and acute inversion of the uterus. In addition, there is a risk of fetal asphyxia, intracranial haemorrhage, trauma and birth in unsterile conditions.

Complications of Abnormal Labour

Complications of abnormal labour are listed in Table 8.3.

TABLE 8.3

Complications of abnormal labour

Maternal complications
    Postpartum haemorrhage
    Genital tract lacerations
    Intrauterine infection
    Increased rate of operative delivery
    Uterine rupture
    Psychological effects of a traumatic experience
Fetal Complications
    Low apgar score
    Birth asphyxia
    Birth trauma
    Shoulder dystocia
    Increased rate of perinatal morbidity and mortality

Key Points

- The duration of normal labour in a healthy woman is highly variable, dependent on the individual, physiological reproductive process and pregnancy characteristics, and possibly longer than previously described.

- Meticulous assessment of power, passage, passenger and the interactions among these is important for a woman in labour.

- The use of the WHO Labour Care Guide or an appropriately modified version, depending on the setting, could facilitate monitoring of labour, while providing evidence-based, respectful care to the woman, and improve outcomes. However, intrapartum decisions should be guided primarily by clinical criteria rather than on cervicographs and time durations.

- The early identification of abnormal labour (prior to the development of fetal distress) and the ability to determine the cause of the abnormality is pivotal in choosing the most appropriate intervention.

- Management of abnormal labour should be individualised and based on current guidelines.

- Augmentation of labour with amniotomy and oxytocin often corrects ineffective uterine contractions and helps to resolve poor progress. However, oxytocin can be dangerous in high parity women and in the presence of cephalopelvic disproportion.

- Instrumental vaginal delivery should comply with current guidelines.

- Caesarean delivery has an important role to play, but is not a panacea for all abnormal labours.

BIBLIOGRAPHY

1. Zhang J, Landy HJ, Branch DW, et al. Contemporary patterns of spontaneous labor with normal neonatal outcomes. *Obstet Gynecol* 2010;116(6):1283.
2. American College of Obstetricians and Gynecologists. Approaches to limit intervention during labor and birth. ACOG committee opinion No. 766. American College of Obstetricians and Gynecologists. *Obstet Gynecol* 2019;133(2):e164–173.
3. Cohen WR, Friedman EA. Perils of the new labor management guidelines. *Am J Obstet Gynecol* 2015;212(4):420–27.
4. Di Mascio D, Saccone G, Bellussi F, Al-Kouatly HB, Brunelli R, Benedetti Panici P, Liberati M, D'Antonio F, Berghella V. Delayed versus immediate pushing in the second stage of labor in women

with neuraxial analgesia: a systematic review and meta-analysis of randomized controlled trials. *Am J Obstet Gynecol* 2020 Aug;223(2):189–203. doi: 10.1016/j.ajog.2020.02.002. Epub 2020 Feb 15. PMID: 32067972.

5. Ghi T, Eggebo T, Lees C, Kalache K, Rozenberg P, Youssef A, Salomon LJ, Tutschek B. ISUOG Practice Guidelines: intrapartum ultrasound. *Ultrasound Obstet Gynecol* 2018;52:128–39.

6. National Institute for Health and Care Excellence. Intrapartum care for healthy women and babies. Clinical Guideline CG190. London (UK): NICE; 2017.

7. The Royal Australian and New Zealand College of Obstetricians and Gynaecologists. Intrapartum fetal surveillance. Clinical guideline third edition, 2014.

8. WHO recommendations. Intrapartum care for a positive childbirth experience World Health Organisation, Geneva, Switzerland, 2018.

9. Lemos A, Amorim MM, Dornelas de Andrade A, de Souza AI, Cabral Filho JE, Correia JB. Pushing/ bearing down methods for the second stage of labour. *Cochrane Database Syst Rev* 2017;3(3): CD009124. Published 2017 Mar 26. doi:10.1002/14651858.CD009124.pub3

10. Lavender T, Cuthbert A, Smyth RM. Effect of partograph use on outcomes for women in spontaneous labour at term and their babies. *Cochrane Database Syst Rev* 2018;8(8):CD005461. Published 2018 Aug 6. doi:10.1002/14651858.CD005461.pub5

11. WHO recommendation on progress of the first stage of labour: diagnostic test accuracy of a 1–cm/hour cervical dilatation rate threshold. WHO-RHL, World Health Organisation, Geneva, Switzerland 2018.

12. Hofmeyr GJ, Bernitz S, Bonet M, Bucargu M, et al. WHO next generation partograph: revolutionary steps towards individualised labour care. *BJOG*, Epub. 08 March 2021, https://doi:org/10.1111/1471-0528.16694.

9

Instrumental Vaginal Delivery

Malik Goonewardene and Sanjeewa Padumadasa

Early Sanskrit manuscripts (circa 1500 BC) describe the use of single and paired instruments by ancient ayurvedic practitioners in India for 'difficult labour' with a dead fetus, and there is evidence of similar instruments being subsequently used by Egyptians, Greeks and Arabs for delivery. In England, the use of forceps in live childbirth is credited to Peter Chamberlen the Elder. Moreover, this 'secret instrument' was used exclusively by his male descendants for more than a century (circa 16th Century) in order to manage difficult deliveries. This allowed physicians, referred to as 'man-midwives', access to the birthing chambers which were, at that time, solely under the command of the midwives in England. Saving the woman's life took precedence over causing possible harm to the fetus, and these instruments were initially used to extract fetuses from labouring women who were at high risk of death due to prolonged or obstructed labour. The focus has drastically changed over the years, and today, the goal is to assist delivery in favor of both fetal and maternal indications with minimal or no harm to either.

While the concept of using a 'cupping glass fixed to the scalp with an air pump' for delivering a baby has been first described by Yong in 1694, it is Simpson, better known for the introduction of chloroform anaesthesia, who is credited with having invented the first vacuum extractor in 1847 and designing the long curved forceps which are named after him as well, later on. Malstrom, Bird and Vacca have pioneered significant changes to the design of vacuum extractors used in obstetric practice during the last 17 decades.

In 1829, although Arnott described vacuum extraction as a 'substitute for steel forceps in the hands of men who are deficient in manual dexterity, whether from inexperience or natural ineptitude', this is certainly not the case. Instrumental vaginal delivery (IVD), whether it is delivery by forceps or vacuum extraction, requires a perfect blend of the science and the art of obstetrics and should be carried out by the correct person on the correct patient at the correct time at the correct place and using the correct instrument. If not, IVD can be disastrous for the baby, the mother or both. Although IVD has been referred to as 'operative vaginal delivery' and, more recently, as 'assisted vaginal birth', the term IVD will be used in this chapter. Although 'operative vaginal delivery' is acceptable, the authors are of the opinion that, because all normal deliveries should be assisted, preferably by a skilled birth attendant, and no woman should be allowed to deliver spontaneously by herself, 'assisted vaginal birth' appears to be inappropriate for IVD.

Rates of IVD vary from country to country and from hospital to hospital within the same geographical location, but the numbers have dwindled at a steady rate during the past few decades. However, the ability to carry out IVD remains an essential skill that all obstetricians should possess.

Indications for Instrumental Vaginal Delivery

Maternal

Conditions such as cerebrovascular disease, severe pre-eclampsia/eclampsia or cardiac disease in which maternal effort during the second stage could aggravate the condition may require IVD. Exhaustion leading to a poor maternal effort in the expulsive phase of the second stage and conditions in which the woman is unable to effectively bear down, such as neurological or neuromuscular disorders, may also necessitate IVD.

Fetal

Fetal compromise during the second stage as evidenced by the presence of meconium, non-reassuring heart rate pattern or abnormal scalp blood sampling are common indications for IVD, as this is usually quicker than a caesarean delivery. Furthermore, performing a caesarean delivery when the fetal head is impacted within the pelvis could be more dangerous than performing an IVD (discussed in Chapter 11). However, it should be emphasised that the delivery must be straightforward, because the combination of hypoxia and trauma could prove detrimental to the fetus.

Non-Progressive Second Stage of Labour

A non-progressive, prolonged second stage is an indication for IVD. The unfavourable dynamic relationships in labour, such as deflexion and occipitoposterior (OP) positions, can be overcome by skillfully performed IVD. Epidural anaesthesia, which abolishes the Ferguson's reflex and the maternal urge to push during the expulsive phase and results in a prolonged second stage, may also be an indication for IVD.

The time limits that are usually accepted in the second stage of labour, at which point an IVD may be considered, are given below.

- Nullipara – two hours without regional anaesthesia, and three hours with regional anaesthesia
- Multipara – one hour without regional anaesthesia, and two hours with regional anaesthesia

However, it must be emphasised that there are no rigid time limits for the second stage of labour when IVD should be resorted to. A decision to perform IVD should be taken after considering the fetal and maternal factors as well as the progress of labour.

Conditions that Need to be Fulfilled for a Safe Instrumental Vaginal Delivery

Operator and Setting

An experienced operator who is skilled with the use of forceps and vacuum and management of any complications which could arise following the procedure, such as shoulder dystocia, postpartum haemorrhage (PPH) and failure of IVD which requires a second stage caesarean delivery, has the capacity to perform IVD. Additional personnel, including midwives and neonatal staff, should be present. Finally, there should also be immediate access to an operating room.

Indication

There should be a valid indication to perform IVD, which carries considerable fetal and maternal morbidity. Alternatives such as expectant management or second-stage caesarean delivery need to be considered.

Consent

Informed consent must be obtained before IVD. The late second stage, which may be a stressful time for the woman as well as the healthcare provider, is not the ideal time to procure genuine consent. Therefore, it may be prudent to discuss with the woman prior to labour about the option of IVD in case the necessity arises.

Uterine Contractions and Maternal Pushing

Propulsive forces in the form of uterine contractions and maternal pushing which are safer and more effective than traction with either forceps or vacuum extractor should be utilised whenever possible during IVD.

Abdominal and Vaginal Examination

It is mandatory to perform both abdominal and vaginal examinations to assess how far the head has descended into the pelvis. Abdominally, the level of the head is described as 5/5 to 0/5, while the station of the head is described vaginally as −3 to +3 (described in Chapter 8). Before embarking on an IVD, the fetal head should ideally be not palpable abdominally (0/5). A vaginal examination should confirm full dilatation of the cervix and ascertain the position, attitude and asynclitism of the fetus. The station should ideally be +2, and the presence of a caput and moulding should not result in overestimations of descent, when examined vaginally. The presence of a significant caput and moulding, i.e. greater than ++, indicates the possibility of CPD, in which case a caesarean delivery should be performed. Asynclitism, i.e. the relationship of the sagittal suture of the fetal head to the transverse plane of the pelvic cavity, should be identified. Membranes must be ruptured before IVD. Transperineal ultrasonography can be used to complement clinical examination in ascertaining fetal position, station, attitude, asynclitism and evidence of CPD in case of doubt (discussed in Chapter 8).

Maternal Position and Analgesia

The woman must be in the lithotomy position, and epidural or spinal anaesthesia or local anaesthetic infiltration of the perineum should be provided, depending on the station of the presenting part of the fetus and feasibility.

Empty Bladder

Catheterisation relieves the hindrance caused by a full bladder. However, if an indwelling catheter is in place (e.g. in the case of pre-eclampsia), then it should be removed in order to reduce the risk of bladder or urethral damage.

Types of Instrumental Vaginal Delivery

- Non-rotational forceps delivery
- Rotational forceps delivery
- Vacuum delivery

Non-Rotational Forceps Delivery

In addition to a cephalic curve (Figure 9.1A) used to accommodate the fetal head, non-rotational forceps have a pelvic curve (Figure 9.1B) effective to help negotiate the pelvic curve, and therefore, should be applied only for direct occipitoanterior (DOA) and direct occipitoposterior (DOP) positions of the vertex, which do not require rotation of the vertex prior to delivery. However, it is permissible to apply these forceps in the left and right occipitoanterior and occipitoposterior positions (LOA, ROA, LOP, ROP) of the vertex. Alternatively, the vertex could be rotated to the DOA or DOP position digitally or manually, as described later in this chapter.

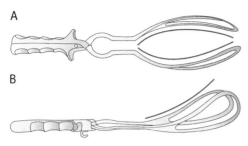

FIGURE 9.1   Non-rotational forceps; A – cephalic curve, B – pelvic curve.

Assemble the Forceps

Before application, the blades of the forceps should be assembled, confirmed as belonging to one set, and orientated in such a way that they would be applied in the pelvis. This also helps to identify the left and right blades, because the left needs to be applied first. The blades and the operator's gloves should then be lubricated with antiseptic cream in order to reduce friction between the blades and maternal tissues.

Application of the Blades of the Forceps in Occipitoanterior Positions of the Vertex

The forceps must be applied directly to the sides of the head along the mentovertical axis of the skull and should cover the area between the orbits and the ears. This is referred to as a biparietal-bimalar application and offers a uniform grip on the two sides where the pressure is evenly distributed to the least vulnerable areas of the fetal head.

The operator should stand in front of the woman, and, between uterine contractions, the left blade should be inserted to the left side of the pelvis, in the following manner: two or more fingers of the right hand should be lubricated and introduced into the posterior aspect of the left side of vagina beside the fetal head. The handle of the left blade should be held in the left hand, using the thumb on one side and the index and middle fingers on the other side, parallel to the right inguinal ligament of the woman and close to her body (Figure 9.2A), and the tip of the blade should be gently passed into the vagina between the fetal head and the palmar surface of the fingers of the right hand, which serves as a guide. It is vital not to use force, but rather to gently guide the blade into the vagina assisted by the thumb of the right hand. As the blade adapts itself to the fetal head, its handle is depressed in a wide arc (Figure 9.2B), and eventually into a horizontal position. An incorrect application would be met with resistance during insertion of the blades, and if this happens, the blade should be withdrawn and reapplied in the correct manner. The closer the blade is to the fetal head, the easier the application is. Once the left blade has been inserted, the guiding fingers should be withdrawn, and the blade should be supported by an assistant. A mirror image of the procedure is performed with the right blade (Figure 9.3).

Ideally, the handle of the right blade should find its way automatically and fit into the handle of the left blade without the need to exert any force and subsequently lock. If there are malalignment and difficulty in locking the handles, then usually this is due to the blades being applied horizontally rather than in the axis of the pelvis, and the handles are pointing upwards. In this situation, the handles should be pushed down towards the floor, which will facilitate the blades to go further into the pelvis along its axis and onto the sides of the fetal head. If this too is unsuccessful, then the blades must be withdrawn, and all relevant factors (size of head, position, station, moulding and the type of forceps being used) should be reassessed.

A reapplication of blades may be attempted after careful consideration of all relevant factors, if no contraindication is detected. For example, Simpson forceps instead of Wrigley forceps should be used for a head that is elongated as a result of moulding in the OP position. If in doubt, the procedure should be abandoned and an emergency caesarean delivery must be carried out.

A

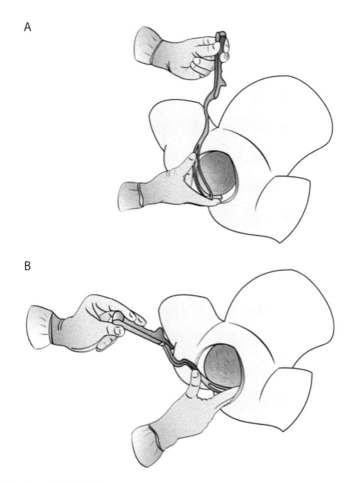

B

FIGURE 9.2   Application of the left blade.

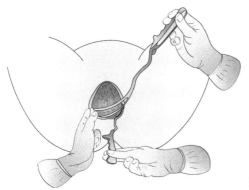

FIGURE 9.3   Application of the right blade.

Confirm Correct Application of Forceps – Occipitoanterior Positions

Figure 9.4 summarises the checks that should be made to confirm the correct application of forceps.

   1. The sagittal suture should be perpendicular to the plane of the shanks (A).

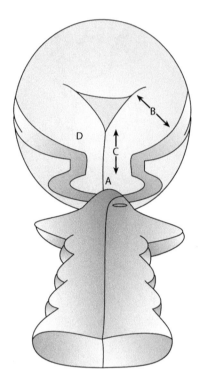

FIGURE 9.4   Checks for correct application of forceps.

2. The blades should be equidistant from the sagittal suture and the lambdoid sutures (B).
3. The posterior fontanelle should be one fingerbreadth above the plane of the shanks (C). This will ensure that the line of traction is through the flexion point of the fetal skull, which is 3 cm anterior to the posterior fontanelle, resulting in flexion of the vertex, and the presentation of the shortest anteroposterior diameter. If the posterior fontanelle is more than one fingerbreadth above this plane, then it will tend to deflex the fetal head during traction, thus presenting a larger diameter at the maternal pelvis.
4. A small and equal amount of space (not more than one fingerbreadth) should be felt between the fetal head and the heel of the blade (D). The presence of a larger space suggests a short application of the blades on the head, which increases the risk of facial nerve injury and the blades slipping off.

If any one of these criteria is not fulfilled, then the blades need to be withdrawn and reapplied, after a careful reassessment of the situation.

The shanks of the forceps will be parallel to the floor only in DOA or DOP positions. In case the fetal head is in a left or right occipitoanterior or occipitoposterior position (LOA, ROA, LOP, ROP) (Figure 9.5A), the fetal head should be gradually and gently rotated between two contractions to DOA or DOP position using forceps, prior to application of traction. Before rotation, the handles should be slightly elevated (Figure 9.5B). This would move the tips of the blades towards the centre of the pelvic cavity, thereby avoiding trauma to the vaginal walls during rotation (Figure 9.5C). Excessive elevation of the handles may cause extension of the fetal head in occipitoanterior (OA) positions, resulting in an increased anteroposterior diameter presenting at the pelvis. Once the rotation has been completed, the handles should be lowered to the horizontal plane (Figure 9.5D). It is important to recheck the position of the fetus to ensure that the blades have not slipped during this rotation. The alternative is to digitally or manually rotate the fetal head from LOA or ROA to DOA, and LOP or ROP to DOP and then apply the blades of the forceps.

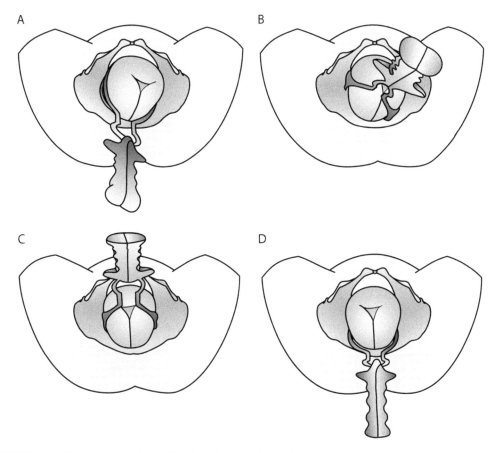

FIGURE 9.5 Slight rotation of the fetal head to direct occipitoanterior position.

Applying Traction

The operator should be comfortably seated in front of the woman. The index and middle fingers of the operator's non-dominant hand should be on the finger guards and in an underhand grip, and the dominant hand should be used to exert downward traction on the shanks (i.e. Pajot's manoeuvre) to ensure that traction is in the axis of the pelvic curve and not against the pubic arch (Figure 9.6). Pajot's manoeuvre replaces the axis traction devices which were previously attached to forceps and ensures that traction is applied downwards in the axis of the pelvic curve, although the handles of the forceps are maintained in a horizontal position. The handles of the forceps should not be lowered, as this will cause elevation of the tips of the blades and increase the risk of vaginal wall tears as well as third and fourth-degree perineal tears.

Traction should be coordinated with uterine contractions and voluntary expulsive efforts by the woman in order to complement the natural process. Mild to moderate traction, only adequate to cause progressive descent of the fetal head, should be applied. The seated position and the use of the non-dominant hand for traction are recommended to ensure that excessive traction is not applied.

The critical head diameter which must be moved is the biparietal diameter. Initially, traction should be directed downwards. Once the occiput emerges from underneath the pubic symphysis, maternal pushing should be discouraged in order to control delivery. Horizontal traction should be applied until the head begins to crown, at which point an episiotomy should be performed if necessary. Primigravidae will usually need an episiotomy, while a policy of selective episiotomy could be adopted in multi-gravidae. Finally, the handles are gradually elevated and the direction of pull arches upwards, and the head is delivered by extension while the perineum is protected manually (Figure 9.7). Lowering the bed

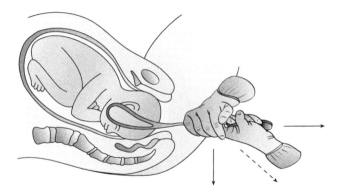

FIGURE 9.6   Pajot's manoeuvre.

A   B   C

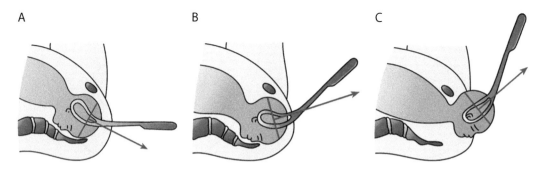

FIGURE 9.7   Direction of traction in the axis of the pelvic curvature.

or rising from the chair during the final stages of delivery of the head aids in applying traction in the desired direction.

Once the head has been delivered, the blades of the forceps should be removed by reversing the sequence used during the application of forceps. The right blade should be removed first, followed by the left.

Forceps Delivery in Occipitoposterior Positions

The application of forceps in OP positions is similar to that in OA positions. However, when checking for correct application, the posterior fontanelle should be one fingerbreadth below instead of above the shanks. A mediolateral episiotomy is generally required, because the fetal head is usually deflexed and presents an increased anteroposterior diameter compared to a flexed OA position, and the occiput would distend the perineum more than the sinciput does in an OA position. There should be no downward traction at this stage, as this would tend to deflex the fetal head further, leading to a greater increase of the anteroposterior diameter to the perineum. Downward traction may be initially necessary to assist the descent of the fetal head along the pelvic curvature if the station is +1 instead of +2. Horizontal traction should be applied until the base of the nose is under the pubic symphysis (Figure 9.8). The handles should then be slowly elevated until the occiput gradually emerges over the anterior margin of the perineum. Then, by performing a downward motion with the instrument, the nose and chin should be successively delivered.

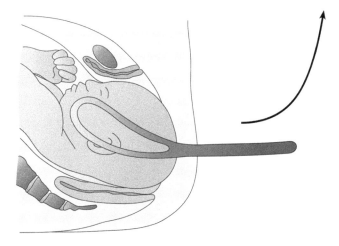

FIGURE 9.8   The direction of traction in OP position.

Digital Rotation of the Vertex to a Direct Occipitoanterior Position

In LOA and ROA positions, it would often be possible to digitally rotate the vertex to the DOA position. In the left and right occipitotransverse positions of the vertex (LOT and ROT) as well, it may be possible to digitally rotate the vertex to a DOA position, while digital rotation of an ROP or LOP position of the vertex to the DOA position is difficult and virtually impossible. For a ROA or ROT position, the tips of the index and middle fingers of the left hand should be used to apply pressure on the edge of the anterior (left) parietal bone along the lambdoid suture in a clockwise direction (Figure 9.9). For an LOA or LOT position, the right hand should be used to apply pressure on the edge of the anterior (right) parietal bone along the lambdoid suture in an anticlockwise direction. These rotations could be aided by the fingers of the free hand which are also being used to apply pressure in a complementary direction from the contralateral side of the fetal head. If digital rotation is successful, then non-rotational forceps should be used to complete the delivery. In LOA or LOT positions, any tendency of the fetal head to rotate back to the original position could be prevented by steadying the head with the fingers used in the rotation during the application of the blades. If digital rotation is not successful, then rotational forceps or vacuum delivery will be necessary.

Manual Rotation of the Vertex to a Direct Occipitoanterior Position

Epidural or spinal anaesthesia provides adequate pain relief for the procedure of manual rotation, but tocolysis may be needed to relax the uterus in case the uterus is firmly contracted around the fetus. In ROT and ROP positions, the left hand is inserted into the vagina, and the thumb is placed over the anterior parietal bone, while the index and middle fingers are placed over the two parietal bones on either side of the sagittal suture and at the edge of the lambdoid sutures with the other fingers supporting the fetal head from below (Figure 9.10A). Next, the fetal head is rotated in a clockwise direction to the DOA position (Figure 9.10B). It is important to ensure that the rotation of the fetal head is accompanied by concomitant rotation of the fetal shoulders in order to avoid damage to the cervical spine. This is achieved by placing the right hand on the maternal abdomen behind the fetal shoulder and pulling the shoulder towards the midline. If possible, applying rotational pressure on the posterior shoulder of the fetus as well while using the vaginal hand (i.e. Pomeroy's manoeuvre) aided by the external hand on the anterior shoulder via the maternal abdomen may be attempted. When manual rotation is successful, the fetus will be in the DOA position. A forceps delivery would be the more ideal option, although commencement of an intravenous oxytocin infusion has also been done in carefully selected cases. In a LOT or LOP position, the right hand is used vaginally and the

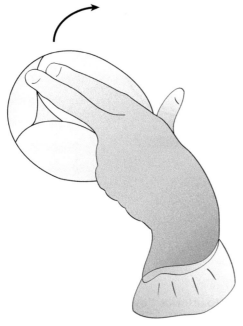

FIGURE 9.9 Digital rotation from right occipitoanterior to direct occipitoanterior position.

left hand abdominally in a similar fashion, and the fetal head is rotated in an anticlockwise direction and into the DOA position. If the manual rotation is unsuccessful, rotational forceps or vacuum delivery will be essential. Historically, a manual rotation was carried out by gripping the fetal head with the entire palmar surface of one hand, dislodging it upwards and then rotating it. At present, this is not advisable.

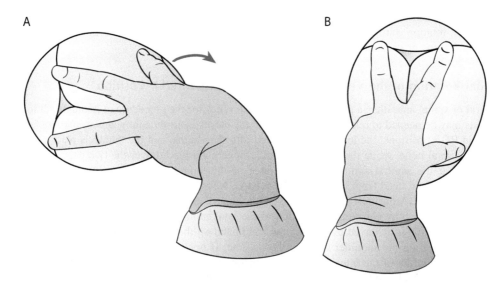

FIGURE 9.10   Manual rotation from right occipitotransverse position to direct occipitoanterior position.

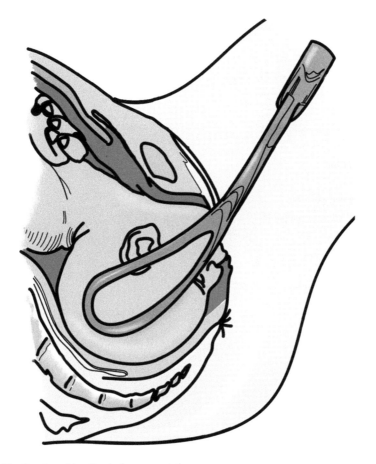

FIGURE 9.11 The direction of traction in face presentation.

Forceps Delivery in a Mentoanterior Position of a Face Presentation

Forceps can be applied to expedite the delivery of a fetus in a mentoanterior position of a face presentation. Slight downward traction should be applied until the chin is delivered beneath the pubic symphysis. Delivery is completed by gradually elevating the handles at up to about 45° above horizontal level (Figure 9.11).

Forceps for Aftercoming Head of the Breech

The technique for the application of forceps for delivery of the aftercoming head of a breech is described in detail in Chapter 25.

Completion of Delivery

Once the head is delivered, the shoulders and the rest of the body should be delivered in the usual manner. Shoulder dystocia and postpartum haemorrhage must be anticipated, and the genital tract should be carefully examined for tears. Accurate documentation is vital. A delivery with forceps can be a traumatic experience for the woman. She may request elective caesarean delivery during subsequent pregnancies or may even plan to not conceive. Therefore, it is imperative that she and her partner are debriefed adequately.

Checklist for Application of Forceps

Maternal factors
Uterine contractions
Maternal pushing
Abdominal examination
Estimated fetal size
Fetal presentation and position
Fetal head abdominally not palpable
Fetal heart rate
Vaginal examination
Cervical dilatation
Fetal presentation and position
Station of the fetal head
Fetal attitude
Asynclitism
Caput, moulding
Prerequisites
Valid indication
Verbal consent
Patient in the lithotomy position
Informed paediatric team
Cleaning and draping
Empty bladder
Anaesthesia

PROCEDURE – APPLICATION OF FORCEPS

Application of Blades

1. Assemble the forceps and lubricate the blades and the gloves of the operator.
2. Hold the handle of the left blade parallel to the right inguinal ligament with the left hand.
3. Insert the middle and index fingers of the right hand into the vagina.
4. Guide the handle in a wide arc until the blade is in place and assisted by the thumb of the right hand.
5. Request assistant to hold the blade in place.
6. Repeat the procedure with the right blade.
7. Lock the handles.
8. If the handles do not lock, push them downwards towards the floor. If this is not successful, then withdraw the blades, reassess the situation and reapply the blades. If this too fails, abandon IVD and perform an emergency caesarean delivery.

Check for Accurate Application

1. Are the shanks of the forceps perpendicular to the sagittal suture?
2. Are the shanks equidistant from the sagittal suture and the blades equidistant from the lambdoidal suture lines?
3. Is the posterior fontanelle one fingerbreadth above or below the plane of the shanks of the forceps?
4. Is there equal space, about one fingerbreadth, between the fetal head and the heel of the forceps?

If any one of these criteria is not fulfilled, withdraw the blades and reapply after a careful reassessment of the situation. If this too fails to fulfil any of these criteria, then abandon IVD and perform an emergency caesarean delivery.

Apply Traction

1. The operator should be seated.
2. Perform the Pajot's manoeuver to aid traction along the axis of the pelvis.
3. Synchronise with uterine contractions and maternal pushing.
4. Carry out a maximum of three attempts over 10 minutes, and abandon if unsuccessful and perform an emergency caesarean delivery.

Selective Episiotomy

- Remove the right blade, followed by the left
- Look out for shoulder dystocia, perineal tears and postpartum haemorrhage
- Documentation

Rotational Forceps Delivery

Rotational forceps delivery with Kielland forceps is an option for the delivery of a fetal head when the sagittal suture is not in the anteroposterior diameter of the pelvis. Therefore, it could be used in the left and right occipitotransverse or occipitoposterior positions of the vertex (LOT, ROT, LOP, ROP). It could also be applied in women with left and right mentotransverse or mentoposterior positions of a face presentation. The lack of a pelvic curve in the Kielland forceps enables its application and the rotation of the fetal head within the pelvis. The Kielland forceps also have overlapping blades with a sliding lock that enables the correction of asynctilism prior to the rotational delivery. However, the rotation of the fetal head within the pelvis using the Kielland forceps carries a high risk of genital tract trauma and must be carried out only by an obstetrician who is skilled in the use of the instrument, after confirming the suitability of its use in the index patient. The prerequisites and the preliminaries for a Kielland forceps delivery are essentially the same as for a nonrotational forceps delivery, except for the fact that the sagittal suture of the fetus need not be in the anteroposterior diameter of the maternal pelvis. It is vital to obtain informed written consent prior to carrying out a trial of rotational forceps delivery, which may lead to an emergency caesarean delivery in case of failure. Although rotational forceps could be carried out in the labour ward under bilateral pudendal block and perineal infiltration, carrying it out in the operation room under spinal or epidural anaesthesia is preferable. In experienced hands, the likelihood of achieving vaginal delivery is higher in rotational forceps compared to rotational vacuum delivery, while there are no significant differences in maternal and neonatal outcomes between the two methods of delivery. When assembling the blades of the Kielland forceps, these should be orientated so that the directional knobs on the shanks face the fetal occiput. Therefore, in OT positions, there will be an anterior blade and a posterior blade instead of left and right blades, with directional knobs pointing towards the fetal occiput and indicating the direction in which it should be rotated. Furthermore, the anterior blade must be applied first.

Rotational Forceps Delivery for Right Occipitotransverse Position

Application of the Blades of the Forceps

Three or more fingers of the right hand should be lubricated and introduced into the posterior aspect of the vagina beside the fetal head. The handle of the anterior blade should be held in the left hand using the thumb on one side and the index and middle fingers on the other side, perpendicular to the floor (Figure 9.12A), and the tip of the blade is gently passed into the vagina between the fetal head and the palmar surface of the fingers of the right hand, and guided with the thumb of the right hand to lie on the right parietal bone of the fetal head (Figure 9.12B). Next, this blade is guided in an anticlockwise direction around the sinciput and face of the fetus with the fingers of the right hand (Figure 9.12C) to

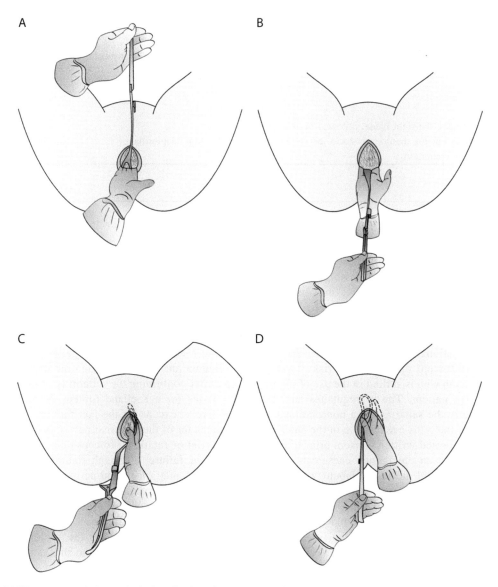

FIGURE 9.12 Wandering method of application of anterior blade for a rotational forceps delivery.

its final position on the left parietal bone of the fetal head, underneath the pubic symphysis (Figure 9.12D), while the left hand rotates the handle in a downward arc. This is referred to as the 'wandering method' of application. After withdrawing the guiding fingers, an assistant should be instructed to support the blade in situ. If there is difficulty in the wandering of the anterior blade, then the procedure should be abandoned, and an emergency caesarean delivery must be carried out. If the application of the anterior blade is successful, then three or more fingers of the lubricated left hand should be inserted into the posterior part of the woman's vagina. The posterior blade of the forceps should be held in the right hand with the handle upwards and perpendicular to the woman's perineum (Figure 9.13), inserted into the posterior aspect of the vagina and guided with the thumb of the left hand to lie on the right parietal bone of the fetal head. The right hand should depress the handle during this process. Usually, the application of the posterior blade is not demanding. The application of blades in LOT, LOP and ROP positions of the vertex is similar except for the prior orientation of the blades with the directional knobs pointing to 3, 5 and 7 o'clock positions respectively, and the wandering of the anterior blade in a clockwise direction with the fingers of the left hand for LOT and LOP positions.

Other Methods of Application of the Blades of the Forceps

The 'direct method' of application may be used if the fetal head is low, particularly in the presence of anterior asynclitism. The four fingers of the left hand are inserted with the palmar surface facing downwards, between the anterior parietal bone of the fetus and the maternal pubic symphysis, and the right hand holds the anterior blade with the handle downwards and perpendicular to the woman's perineum, and guides the anterior blade, assisted by the thumb of the left hand beneath the maternal pubic symphysis, directly over the parietal bone until the cephalic curve accommodates the parietal bone (Figure 9.14). For this procedure, the operating table must be elevated sufficiently to enable the application of the anterior blade from below the maternal perineum. The posterior blade of the forceps is inserted directly, as described earlier, in the 'wandering method'.

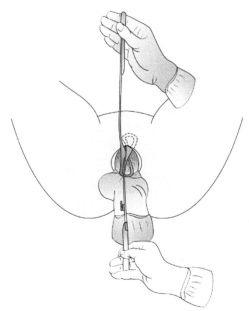

FIGURE 9.13 Application of the posterior blade of Kielland forceps.

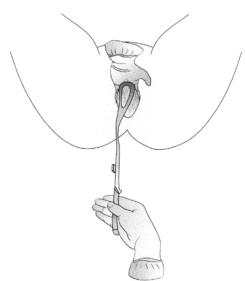

FIGURE 9.14 Direct method of application of anterior blade for a rotational forceps delivery.

The classical method, described by Christian Kielland (1871–1941 AD), the inventor of the instrument, was originally used when the fetal head was higher in the pelvis than what would be acceptable for a forceps delivery today. It was associated with a high risk of uterine perforation and entanglement of the umbilical cord and is described here for historical interest only. The four fingers of the left hand are inserted under the pubic symphysis with the palmar surface facing upwards. The anterior blade with its cephalic curve facing the woman's pubic symphysis is held in the right hand, with its handle facing upwards and almost perpendicular to the perineum and guided along with the fingers of the left hand, while the handle is pressed down until it occupies the space between the anterior shoulder and the fetal head. The blade is then rotated by 180° and adjusted so that the cephalic curve is placed over the anterior parietal bone.

Check for Correct Application

If the blades have been correctly applied, then they should be parallel to the sagittal suture. The handles should be 30°–45° below the horizontal, in line with the axis of the pelvic mid-cavity, and it should be possible to lock the blades. If the blades are not parallel to the sagittal suture, or if these are malaligned and cannot be locked, then the blades need to be withdrawn and reapplied after a careful reassessment of the situation. If this too fails to solve the problem, then IVD must be abandoned and an emergency caesarean delivery should be performed.

Correction of Asynclitism

Once the blades are locked, the malalignment of the sliding lock indicates asynclitism. Asynclitism is at least partially corrected by aligning the sliding lock. This is achieved by pulling the finger guard which is closer to the perineum towards the operator while simultaneously pushing on the other finger guard (Figure 9.15).

Rotation Using Forceps

After the confirmation of the correct application of blades and at least partial correction of asynclitism, rotation should be performed when the uterus is relaxed between contractions. The handles of the forceps should be held in the left hand and in an underhand grip, with the index and middle fingers on the finger guards and the thumb and other fingers resting on the handles. The right hand should be placed on top of the handles for support. The delivery bed should be sufficiently elevated, and kneeling on one knee (with a pillow underneath) will help. Before rotation, the fetal head may need to be, slightly rather than excessively, disengaged upwards. Rotation is achieved by pronation of the left hand while an assistant rotates the fetal shoulder in the same direction as that of the fetal head (Figure 9.16). It is extremely important that no force is used during rotation. Some advise that the right hand should be used to retract the vaginal walls and not placed on the handles for support, so that rotation can be observed directly. After rotation, it should be checked and confirmed that the fetal head, rather than just the blades of the forceps, has rotated around the surface of the fetal head. This is done by examining the position of the vertex after rotation. If the vertex is not in the DOA position, then the IVD should be abandoned and an emergency caesarean delivery should be performed. The rotation in LOT and LOP positions of the vertex are similar except for holding the handles of the forceps in the right hand, supporting the handles (or retracting the vaginal walls) with the left hand and carrying out the rotation by pronating the right hand. Rotation in the ROP position is similar to that in a ROT position other than the fact that it involves a larger rotation.

Applying Traction

After confirming that the vertex is in the DOA position, traction is applied along the pelvic axis, initially downwards with the handles angled 30°–45° below the horizontal. Traction is continued with a gradual

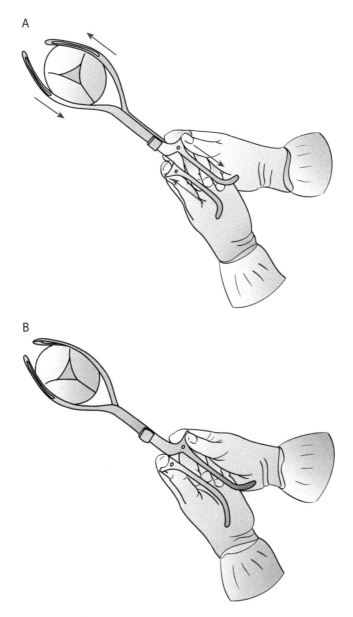

FIGURE 9.15 Correction of asynclitism.

elevation of the handles in an arc to the horizontal position as soon as the occiput appears below the pubic symphysis, and to about 45° above the horizontal level to complete the delivery of the head. Although a routine episiotomy is needed for a primigravida, a policy of selective episiotomy may be adopted in a multigravida. It is essential that an assistant provides perineal support to prevent excessive perineal trauma and damage to the anal sphincter.

An alternative method of applying traction is also used by some operators. This method mimics and aids the natural process of internal rotation, similar to a vacuum delivery as described later in this chapter. The operator leans with his body towards the direction of the desired rotation and a form of 'rotatory traction' is applied. The fetal head will then undergo spontaneous internal rotation and descent,

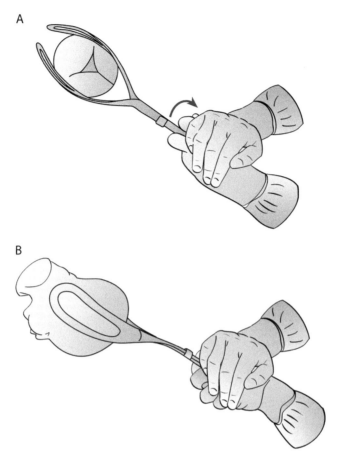

FIGURE 9.16   Rotation of fetal head using forceps.

as in the case of a vacuum delivery. However, if spontaneous internal rotation and descent does not occur, then the previously mentioned method of slight disengagement upwards and rotation followed by traction needs to be completed.

After Completion of Delivery

The fetal shoulders and the rest of the body should be delivered in the usual manner. The possibility of shoulder dystocia and postpartum haemorrhage must also be anticipated. Rotational forceps delivery is associated with the occurence of extensive genital tract tears that involve the vagina and cervix which may even extend into the bladder. There is a risk of circular or 'bucket handle' tears, especially in the cervix with rotation and subsequent traction and spiral tears involving the cervix and vagina with 'rotatory traction'. Therefore, not only should the operator be highly skilled and experienced in the application of rotational forceps, but proper selection of cases is also crucial.

Vacuum Delivery

The basic premise of a vacuum extractor is that a suction cup is connected, via tubing to a vacuum source. Direct traction can then be applied to the presenting part, either directly through the tubing or via a connecting chain. Recently introduced devices have incorporated the vacuum mechanism into handheld cups. Although the risk of maternal genital tract injuries is less in this procedure rather than with a forceps delivery, the risk of fetal injury is akin to that of a forceps delivery. The clinical assessment before vacuum delivery should be just as stringent as for rotational forceps, and the same prerequisites should be fulfilled for a vacuum delivery. Vacuum delivery is best avoided if a fetal bleeding disorder is suspected or at gestations less than 34 weeks due to the risk of haemorrhage in the fetus.

There are rigid as well as soft vacuum cups. Soft cups were developed in an attempt to reduce scalp trauma which is associated with rigid cups, but these have a higher failure-to-deliver rate than rigid cups.

Equipment Check

Before insertion of the cup, it is important to check whether the equipment is complete and functioning. Lubricant gel should be applied to the exterior of the cup.

Application of Vacuum Cup

The vacuum cup should be applied between contractions, and over the flexion point on the fetal skull, which is 3 cm anterior to the posterior fontanelle. As the diameter of a vacuum cup as well as the distance between the anterior fontanelle and the flexion point is about 6 cm, the application of the cup with one of its edges at the posterior fontanelle and the other edge about 3 cm away from the anterior fontanelle will ensure its correct application (Figure 9.17). Proper application of the vacuum cup over the flexion point ensures that the narrowest anteroposterior diameter of the fetal skull, i.e. suboccipito-bregmatic, presents at the maternal pelvis. It is important to note that the flexion point may be located more posteriorly along the sagittal suture than it appears, especially in deflexed OT and OP positions of a vertex presentation.

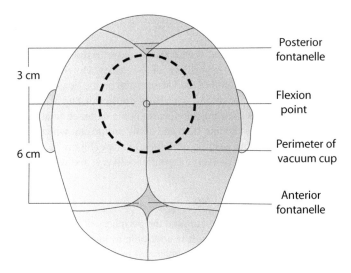

FIGURE 9.17   Application of vacuum cup over the flexion point on the fetal skull.

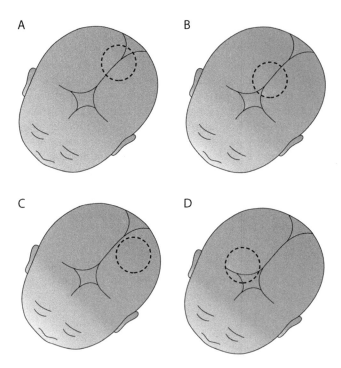

FIGURE 9.18 Correct and incorrect placement of vacuum cup on the fetal head. A - Correct placement: Flexing median B, C, D - Incorrect placement (B - Deflexing median, C - flexing paramedian, D - deflexing paramedian).

A vacuum cup placed more anteriorly causes deflexion of the fetal head and increases the anteroposterior diameter of the fetal head presenting at the maternal pelvis. Similarly, a vacuum cup placed favoring one side of the sagittal suture presents a larger diameter of the fetal head at the maternal pelvis due to asynclitism (Figure 9.18). If the centre of the cup is more than 1 cm from the sagittal suture, then the application is referred to as paramedian.

Anterior and Posterior Cups

Vacuum cups that have both the suction and traction ports close to the midline are known as anterior cups. These are effective in well-flexed OA positions of the vertex. However, the suction port situated centrally may hinder the accurate application of the vacuum cup on the flexion point when the fetal head is deflexed, as present in OT and OP positions. The Bird's posterior cup with its suction port placed peripherally on the vacuum cup allows accurate application on a deflexed fetal skull (Figure 9.19). The currently popular Kiwi Omnicup has a flexible stem and a low profile cup which facilitates its placement over the flexion point irrespective of the position of the fetal vertex (Figure 9.20). Several modifications of this are available: for use in caesarean delivery; for outlet delivery; and with a traction force indicator.

Creation of the Vacuum within the Cup

After ensuring that no maternal tissue is caught around the periphery of the cup, the vacuum is created to a maximum of about 600 mmHg (0.8 kg/cm^2). It is advisable to initially increase suction to about 150 mmHg (0.2 kg/cm^2) and recheck to ensure that no maternal tissue is caught under the edge of the cup. Next is to increase suction to the desired level. There is no advantage in creating a vacuum gradually or reducing the vacuum between episodes of traction.

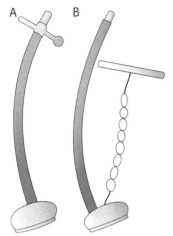

FIGURE 9.19 Anterior and posterior vacuum cups; A – anterior cup, B – posterior cup.

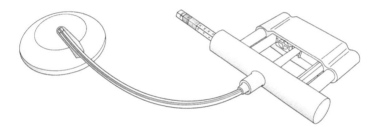

FIGURE 9.20 Kiwi omnicup.

Traction Application with the Vacuum Cup

Traction should be applied with the index and middle fingers of the dominant hand on the traction bar. The thumb of the non-dominant hand should be placed on the vacuum cup and the index and middle fingers on the fetal scalp. The thumb provides countertraction to prevent detachment of the cup while the fingers assess whether it is the bony part of the fetal skull or just the scalp that is descending (Figure 9.21). As the case in forceps delivery, traction should coincide with uterine contractions and maternal effort and should be in line with the axis of the pelvis. Traction should be perpendicular to the plane of the cup to avoid detachment, and the best guide for this is to secure that the direction of pull is not outside the circumference of the cup (Figure 9.22).

Provided that the cup has been placed in the correct flexing median application, the fetal head will undergo autorotation to OA position during traction at the most suitable level in the pelvis. In some cases of OP position, especially in a woman with an anthropoid pelvis where the anteroposterior diameter is larger than the transverse, which predisposes to OP position, the head does not undergo rotation to OA position but will instead be delivered as face-to-pubes.

Complete Delivery

With adequate flexion of the fetal head and perineal support, the need for a selective episiotomy in a vacuum delivery is usually less than that in a forceps delivery. Once the fetal head has been delivered, the vacuum should be released and the cup eased off the scalp. Shoulder dystocia and postpartum

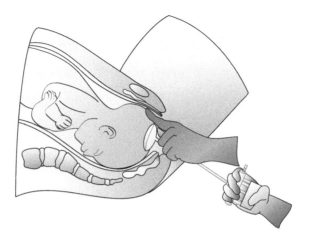

FIGURE 9.21   Technique of vacuum delivery.

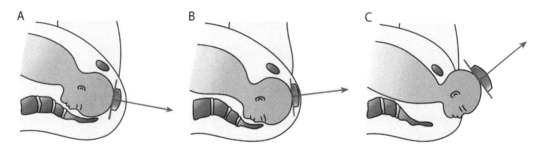

FIGURE 9.22   Direction of traction with vacuum cup.

haemorrhage must be anticipated. Although trauma to the genital tract is less likely compared to a forceps delivery, the cervix, vagina and perineum should still be meticulously inspected.

A chignon is a temporary swelling left on the infant's head following vacuum delivery. The parents should be reassured that the chignon would disappear within 48 hours and is not indicative of any long-term harm.

When to Abandon the Procedure

Traction should be synchronised with uterine contractions and maternal straining. Delivery should be completed at the end of three pulls or earlier and ideally within 10 minutes. If there is no descent with each pull, it is best to abandon the procedure and proceed to caesarean delivery.

If the vacuum cup detaches during traction, then a careful appraisal should be done as to whether it is due to CPD or technical issues with the vacuum extractor. Excessive caput, which can prevent the formation of an adequate chignon, may also cause the vacuum cup susceptible to being detached easily. A decision has to be taken as to whether the cup should be reapplied and vacuum delivery reattempted, forceps delivery performed or caesarean delivery should be resorted to instead. If vacuum delivery is not feasible due to technical issues or the presence of significant caput, then a forceps delivery may be attempted, provided that there is no CPD. Sequential use of instruments (e.g. forceps after failed vacuum delivery) to complete delivery of the fetus, especially in the presence of CPD, has been shown to lead to a worse neonatal as well as maternal outcome, compared to the use of just one instrument. At the same time, performing a caesarean delivery at this stage, with the fetal head deeply impacted within the maternal pelvis, can be technically problematic and can cause considerable maternal morbidity due to extension of the uterine incision, haemorrhage and sepsis. Therefore, fine clinical judgement is essential if an attempted vacuum delivery fails. The involvement of a skilled and experienced obstetrician is mandatory in such cases.

PROCEDURE – VACUUM DELIVERY

- Confirm the indication.
- Exclude contraindications.
- Ensure that prerequisites for an IVD are satisfied.
- Apply the vacuum cup over the flexion point on the fetal head.
- Establish that no maternal tissue is caught around the periphery of the cup.
- Place the thumb on the vacuum cup and the fingers on the fetal scalp.
- Create a vacuum inside the cup.
- Apply traction that is perpendicular to the cup while coinciding with uterine contractions and maternal pushing.
- Accomplish a maximum of three attempts over 10 minutes and abandon if unsuccessful, and perform an emergency caesarean delivery.

Trial of Instrumental Vaginal Delivery

If an IVD is not deemed straightforward, then it may be prudent to conduct a trial of IVD. This entails obtaining informed written consent, moving the woman to the operating room and attempting IVD with preparations made for an emergency caesarean delivery. This alleviates any pressure on the operator to persist with repeated attempts at IVD. In addition, caesarean delivery can be done immediately in case the procedure fails. This long-established procedure avoids an unnecessary caesarean delivery in some and a potentially agonising IVD in others.

Main Differences Between Forceps and Vacuum Delivery

The main differences between forceps and vacuum deliveries are summarised in Table 9.1.

BD Odon device

The BD Odon device, a low-cost tool used to assist delivery during the second stage, has been recently invented by Jorge Odon, a car mechanic from Argentina. The use of an air chamber in applying traction on the fetal head prevents the greater pressures applied on the fetal head by the metal blades of forceps as well as the negative pressures by the vacuum devices which predispose to the formation of haematomas. A double layer of plastic is inserted via the birth canal to surround the fetal head. A minimal amount of air, only adequate to grip the head, is then pumped between the two plastic layers. Finally, the fetus is pulled out through the birth canal.

How the BD Odon device, which requires no formal training for its application and is applied without considering the natural birth mechanisms, will compete with long-established forceps and vacuum, which are applied after careful consideration of the delicate relationships of the fetus and the birth

TABLE 9.1

The main differences between forceps and vacuum delivery

	Forceps	**Vacuum**
Indications		
Prematurity <34 weeks	Preferred	Contraindicated
Face presentation	Used	Contraindicated
Aftercoming head of breech	Used	Contraindicated
Prerequisites		
Requirement for analgesia	More	Less
Amount of time for delivery	Less	More
Traction force on the head	More	Less
Failure rate	Less	More
Maternal complications		
Post-operative pain	More	Less
Perineal tears	More	Less
Anal sphincter dysfunction	More	Less
Voiding dysfunction	More	Less
Neonatal complications		
Scalp trauma	Less	More
Intracranial haemorrhage	Less	More
Subgaleal haemorrhage	Less	More
Retinal haemorrhage	Less	More
Cephalhaematoma	Less	More
Neonatal jaundice	Less	More
Forceps marks on the face	Yes	No
Chignon	No	Yes
Maternal worries about the baby	Less	More

passage in order to correct the unfavourable dynamic factors characteristic of prolonged second stage of labour, is yet to be discovered.

Key Points

- Instrumental vaginal delivery, also referred to as operative vaginal delivery, is a surgical procedure and requires strict adherence to surgical principles.
- A thorough assessment of the delicate relationship of the fetus to the passage, which includes cervical dilatation, station, position, attitude, asynclitism and the absence of CPD such as an excessive caput and moulding, is the key to a safe and successful IVD.
- Vacuum delivery can be just as dangerous as a forceps delivery.
- A maximum of three attempts of IVD over ten minutes can be accomplished, and this must be abandoned if unsuccessful and an emergency caesarean delivery should be performed.
- In the vast majority of cases of IVD, normal delivery will occur in subsequent pregnancies.
- An obstetrician who has mastered the management of labour can master IVD as well.
- It is up to the present generation of obstetricians to impart the skill of safe IVD to future generations. This should remain indispensable in the armamentarium of an obstetrician.

BIBLIOGRAPHY

1. Murphy DJ, Strachan BK, Bahl R, on behalf of the Royal College of Obstetricians and Gynaecologists. Assisted vaginal birth: Green-top Guideline No. 26. *BJOG* 2020;127(9):e70–112. doi:10.1111/1471-0528.16092.
2. Tempest N, Hart A, Walkinshaw S, Hapangama DK. A re-evaluation of the role of rotational forceps: retrospective comparison of maternal and perinatal outcomes following different methods of birth for malposition in the second stage of labour. *BJOG* 2013;120:1277–84.
3. Bird GC. The importance of flexion in vacuum extraction delivery. *BJOG* 1976;83:194–200.
4. Baskett TF, Fanning CA, Young DC. A prospective observational study of 1000 vacuum assisted deliveries with the OmniCup device. *J Obstet Gynaecol Can* 2008;30:573–80.
5. Vacca A. Trials and tribulations of operative vaginal delivery. *BJOG* 2007;114:519–21.
6. O'Brien S, Hotton EJ, Lenguerrand E, et al. The ASSIST Study - The BD Odon Device for assisted vaginal birth: a safety and feasibility study. *Trials*. 2019;20(1):159. Published 2019 Mar 5. doi:10.1186/s13063-019-3249-z

10

Shoulder Dystocia

Sanjeewa Padumadasa and Malik Goonewardene

Shoulder dystocia, which occurs in approximately 1% of vaginal deliveries, is due to the anterior shoulder of the fetus being impacted above the maternal pubic symphysis (PS), while the posterior shoulder has descended below the maternal sacral promontory. There is a failure of the fetal shoulders to deliver spontaneously or with mild downward traction on the fetal head, as these have failed to rotate to the wider oblique diameter of the maternal pelvis. The fetal chin will be tightly pressed against the perineum (turtle sign). Sometimes, restitution may occur, but an external rotation of the fetus will not happen following the delivery of the head. Bilateral shoulder dystocia, where both shoulders are arrested above the pelvic brim, is a theoretical possibility that could only arise as a result of excessive traction and gross elongation of the fetal neck during a forceps delivery.

Factors Associated with Shoulder Dystocia

The factors given in Table 10.1 should alert the clinician of the possibility of shoulder dystocia. However, it should be borne in mind that some of these factors are quite common and may not necessarily be associated with shoulder dystocia in individual cases and that the vast majority of shoulder dystocia cases develop in women with no associated factors. Therefore, shoulder dystocia is largely unpredictable and unpreventable, and it is imperative that every birth attendant is mindful of the possibility of shoulder dystocia with any vaginal delivery.

Prevention of Shoulder Dystocia

Two strategies that have been recommended to prevent shoulder dystocia are: elective caesarean delivery if the estimated fetal weight is greater than the 95th centile at term for a given population and induction of labour after 38 weeks of gestation in women with hyperglycaemia in pregnancy. Recent evidence suggests that the induction of labour at or near term in non-diabetic women with suspected fetal macrosomia also reduces shoulder dystocia without increasing the rates of instrumental vaginal delivery or caesarean delivery, although perineal injuries appear to be heightened. However, there is inadequate evidence in guiding the optimum gestation for inducing labour, as delivery after 38 weeks of gestation with no hyperglycaemia does not significantly reduce the birth weight, while delivery at 37 weeks of gestation has a slightly higher risk of prematurity related complications.

The majority of brachial plexus injuries (BPI) following shoulder dystocia are not permanent. A history of shoulder dystocia in a previous pregnancy which has given rise to a permanent BPI is an indication for caesarean delivery in a subsequent pregnancy. An experienced obstetrician should attend the delivery of women with predisposing factors for shoulder dystocia. Simulation-based training forms an important part of preparing to manage shoulder dystocia.

TABLE 10.1

Factors associated with shoulder dystocia

Maternal characteristics
　　Maternal obesity
　　Excessive maternal weight gain during pregnancy
Previous obstetric history
　　Previous shoulder dystocia
Antepartum
　　Fetal macrosomia
　　Maternal diabetes mellitus
　　Post-term pregnancy
Intrapartum
　　Augmented labour
　　Prolonged first stage of labour
　　Prolonged second stage of labour
　　Instrumental vaginal delivery

Complications

Fetal Complications

Asphyxia

When shoulder dystocia occurs, the fetus is prone to developing hypoxia as a result of reduced blood flow to the intervillous space due to uterine contractions and the inability of the fetal chest to expand due to compression within the maternal pelvis. There are around four minutes before permanent hypoxic damage to the fetal brain occurs, provided that the fetus is not already hypoxic before the event. However, in the presence of hypoxia before the delivery of the head, serious asphyxia may ensue in a very short period of time. The triad of hypoxia, trauma and reduced cerebral venous return may aggravate damage to the fetal brain.

Brachial Plexus Injury

Brachial plexus injury is a serious complication, occurring in 5%–15% of deliveries complicated by shoulder dystocia. Excessive traction on the fetal head, which leads to an aggravation of the impact of the anterior shoulder against the maternal PS is the most common cause of BPI (Figure 10.1).

The majority of injuries occur as a result of neuropraxia and resolve spontaneously with no residual effects. However, one in ten such injuries may be permanent, and this is a major cause of litigation in the field of global obstetrics. The most common type of BPI is Erb's palsy involving nerve roots C5 and C6. Involvement of the whole brachial plexus or Klumpke's palsy involving nerve roots C8 and T1 could also occur.

In Erb's palsy, the affected arm hangs down and is internally rotated and pronated. If the C7 nerve root is also involved, the wrist will be flexed and the fingers will be curled up. The appearance is classically known as the 'porter's tip position' (Figure 10.2). Total BPI results in a paralysed arm with no sensation. There may be respiratory distress and feeding difficulties resulting from hemiparalysis of the diaphragm if the phrenic nerve is damaged, as well as contraction of the pupil and ptosis (i.e. Horner's syndrome) if the sympathetic nerves are damaged. In Klumpke's palsy, there is partial or total paralysis and loss of sensation in the forearm, wrist and hand.

It is important to note which shoulder is impacted anteriorly in the maternal pelvis, as this may have medico-legal implications. When BPI is associated with shoulder dystocia, it is the anterior shoulder that is likely to be affected. Brachial plexus injury of the posterior shoulder could happen even before

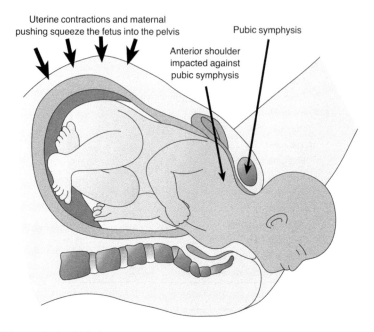

FIGURE 10.1 Injury to the brachial plexus.

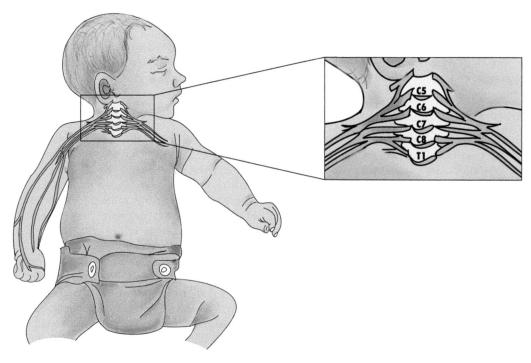

FIGURE 10.2 Erb's palsy.

the head is delivered as a result of maternal forces (which are greater than the forces applied by the clinician) associated with an ultrashort second stage of labour, and is unlikely to result from shoulder dystocia or any manoeuvres used by the clinician.

Fractures

Fractures of the clavicle may occur in about 15% of cases of shoulder dystocia. Rarely, fractures of the humerus may also happen. Even more seldom, fractures of the cervical spine have also been reported.

Maternal Complications

Genital Tract Lacerations

There is an increased incidence of genital tract lacerations, including obstetric anal sphincter injuries (OASIS), as a result of internal manoeuvres used to manage shoulder dystocia. Infrequently, uterine rupture has been reported.

Postpartum Haemorrhage

Shoulder dystocia is associated with postpartum haemorrhage (PPH), as a result of bleeding from genital tract lacerations as well as uterine atony as a result of prolonged labour.

Other Rare Maternal Complications

Rarely, bladder rupture, uterine rupture, separation of PS, sacroiliac joint dislocation and lateral femoral cutaneous neuropathy have been reported following management of shoulder dystocia.

Management

When shoulder dystocia is encountered, additional personnel must be summoned immediately. This includes the most experienced obstetrician, neonatologist and staff to help place the woman in positions that might be necessary to aid delivery. An anaesthesiologist should be called if the shoulder dystocia does not get resolved with initial measures and surgical measures are consequently anticipated.

Persisting with the application of downward traction on the fetal head is one of the main reasons for BPI, and this should be avoided. Fundal pressure should not be applied as this could aggravate the impaction of the anterior fetal shoulder against the maternal PS, as well as increase the risk of uterine rupture. Maternal pushing should also be discouraged, as this also aggravates the condition (Figure 10.3). Shoulder dystocia should be managed using one or a set of manoeuvres given in Table 10.2.

First-Line Measures

Shifting the Woman to the Lower Edge of the Bed and Placing Her in McRobert's Position

If there is evidence of shoulder dystocia, then it is essential to call for help immediately. The woman should be taken to the lower edge of the bed, and two assistants should be instructed to take the woman's knees to her chest (McRobert's position with hyperflexion of maternal thighs) with a jerking movement. Synchronised with the jerk, mild axial traction should be applied on the anterior shoulder (Figure 10.4). The McRobert's position may result in a slightly increased anteroposterior diameter of the pelvis, but more importantly, it leads to the rotation of the PS superiorly and the straightening of the lumbosacral angle. This brings the longitudinal axis of the pelvis in line with the direction of the forces required for delivery, thereby making these forces more effective (Figure 10.5). Taking the woman to

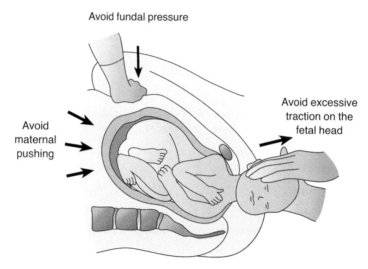

Avoid fundal pressure

Avoid excessive
traction on the
fetal head

Avoid
maternal
pushing

FIGURE 10.3   Avoid excessive traction on fetal head, fundal pressure and maternal pushing when managing shoulder dystocia.

TABLE 10.2

Manoeuvres used in shoulder dystocia

First-line measures
  Call for help
  Shift woman to the lower edge of the bed
  Assume McRobert's position
  Apply suprapubic pressure
Second-line measures
  Perform episiotomy
  Use internal manoeuvres involving rotation
  Apply internal manoeuvres involving the delivery of the posterior arm
  Administer all-fours manoeuvre
Third-line measures
  Carry out cleidotomy
  Render symphysiotomy
  Perform the zavanelli manoeuvre or abdominal rescue

the lower edge of the bed enables the application of mild downward traction on the fetal head in line with the longitudinal axis of the maternal pelvis, without the bed getting in the way.

Application of Suprapubic Pressure

If the anterior shoulder cannot be delivered by placing the woman in McRobert's position, then the woman's knees should be slightly abducted to allow the application of suprapubic pressure. The aim of applying suprapubic pressure is to cause adduction of the fetal shoulders in order to reduce the bia-cromial diameter and to dislodge these from the anteroposterior diameter of the maternal pelvic inlet thereby pushing these to the wider oblique diameter. A third assistant should apply suprapubic pressure with the heels of both hands, one on top of the other, continuously or by rocking movements, from the posterior to the anterior side of the fetal anterior shoulder (Figure 10.6). If a third assistant is not available, the assistant who is on the same side as the baby's back will have to apply suprapubic pressure using one hand. If restitution has occurred, then the direction of the fetal face will help in

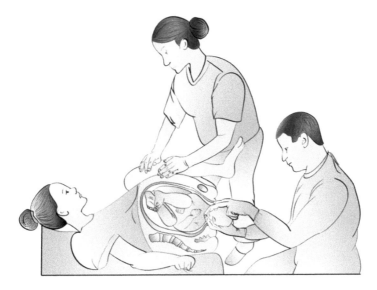

FIGURE 10.4 McRobert's position.

identifying the posterior side of the shoulders. If restitution has not occurred and the posterior side of the shoulders is not known by previous abdominal and vaginal examinations, then the anterior shoulder should be pushed in one direction. Next, the operator should place himself / herself between the woman's thighs, apply routine, mild, axial traction on the fetal head and attempt to deliver the anterior shoulder. If this fails, suprapubic pressure should be applied in the opposite direction and mild, axial traction applied again on the fetal head.

FIRST-LINE MEASURES

- Call for help.
- Position the woman to the lower edge of the bed.
- Instruct two assistants, "take the woman's knees to her chest" (McRobert's position).
- Instruct a third assistant to apply suprapubic pressure from the posterior side of the fetal anterior shoulder towards the anterior side. If this fails, change the direction and reapply pressure.
- Apply routine, mild, axial traction on the fetal head.

A vast majority of cases of shoulder dystocia can be successfully dealt with by these first-line measures. However, if the fetal shoulders are not delivered within 30 seconds, then second-line measures are indicated.

Second-Line measures

Episiotomy

Shoulder dystocia is an emergency concerning the maternal bony pelvis instead of a soft tissue problem. However, an episiotomy may be necessary after external measures have failed to resolve the shoulder dystocia in order to gain more access within the vagina to be able to perform internal manoeuvres.

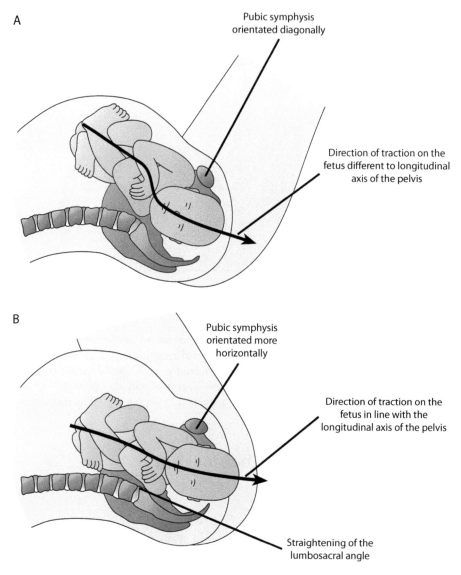

FIGURE 10.5 The mechanism of McRobert's manoeuvre; A – before McRobert's manoeuvre, B – after McRobert's manoeuvre.

Internal Manoeuvres

The decision as to which of the internal manoeuvres (rotational or delivery of posterior shoulder) should be attempted first lies at the discretion of the operator. After performing any of these manoeuvres, mild, axial traction should be applied in order to deliver the shoulders. If any resistance is encountered during the use of mild traction, then this indicates that the shoulder dystocia still exists, and traction must be immediately discontinued and new manoeuvres must be employed to free the shoulder. If one manoeuvre does not work within the 30-second timeframe, then it is essential to proceed to the next, rather than choosing to persist with the same ineffective manoeuvre for much longer, as the fetus can become hypoxic within a few minutes.

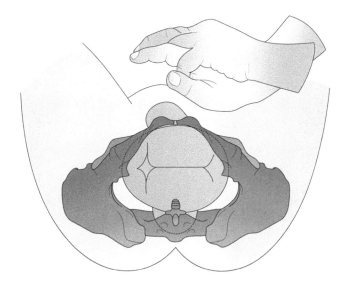

FIGURE 10.6   Application of suprapubic pressure.

Manoeuvres Involving Internal Rotation

The most spacious part of the maternal pelvis is the sacral hollow. In addition, the posterior shoulder is usually accessible, as it would have already descended below the sacral promontory. The assistant in charge of applying suprapubic pressure and the operator performing internal rotational manoeuvres should ensure that pressure is applied in complementary directions to each other. Suprapubic pressure should not be applied when the hand is being inserted into the vagina. The principle behind the initial internal rotational manoeuvres is to dislodge the biacromial diameter of the fetus away from the anteroposterior diameter of the maternal pelvic inlet and push it to a larger, oblique diameter. The following description is for cases when the posterior side of the shoulders is towards the woman's left. A hand should be inserted, with the fingers held together in the shape of a cone (Figure 10.7), posteriorly into the vagina, in front of the fetal posterior shoulder, and that shoulder should be pushed off the midline towards the woman's left (Figure 10.8). If performing this manoeuvre is challenging with the right hand, then the left hand should be used. This manoeuvre should be combined with suprapubic pressure on the anterior shoulder in a complementary opposite direction, i.e. from the left to the right of the woman, and this will also promote adduction of the fetal shoulders (Figure 10.9). If the shoulder dystocia is not resolved with this manoeuvre, then the right hand should be reinserted behind the posterior shoulder of the fetus, and it should be pushed towards the right of the maternal pelvis, promoting adduction of the shoulders, while the assistant pushes the anterior shoulder in a complementary, opposite direction, i.e. from the right to the left of the woman (Figure 10.10). If this too fails to resolve the shoulder dystocia, then the operator should reach up to the anterior shoulder from behind the

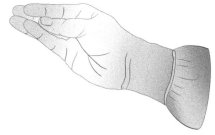

FIGURE 10.7   Correct method of vaginal access.

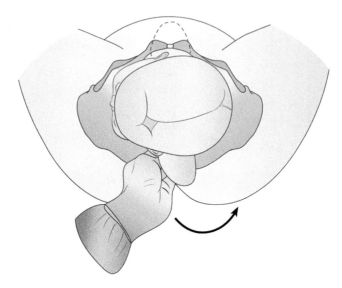

FIGURE 10.8   Application of pressure from the anterior aspect of the posterior shoulder.

posterior shoulder and apply pressure on the back of the anterior shoulder from the left to the right of the woman's pelvis, while the assistant applies suprapubic pressure in the same direction, left to right (Figure 10.11). It is more effective if pressure is applied anterior to the posterior shoulder with the operator's left hand simultaneously (Figure 10.12).

   If it is still not possible to deliver the anterior shoulder, then pressure should be continued in the same direction and rotation of the shoulders by 180° attempted, assisted if possible, with the left hand inserted in front of the posterior shoulder (Figure 10.13). If this is successful, the original anterior shoulder which was arrested behind the PS will now enter the sacral hollow and the original

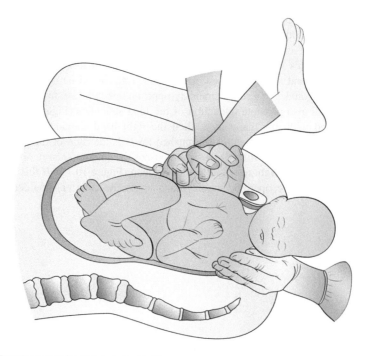

FIGURE 10.9   Complementary internal and suprapubic pressure.

posterior shoulder which was in the sacral hollow will now come to lie anteriorly and below the level of the PS, enabling the delivery of the shoulders. If this manoeuvre fails to rotate the shoulders by 180°, then the directions of pressure should be reversed, i.e. from the back of posterior shoulder and front of anterior shoulder, and rotation of the shoulders by 180° in the opposite direction attempted (Figure 10.14). The objective is the same, i.e. to bring the original anterior shoulder which was arrested behind the PS into the sacral hollow and the original posterior shoulder which was in the sacral hollow to lie anteriorly and below the level of the PS, thus enabling the delivery of the shoulders. If the posterior side of the shoulders is towards the woman's right, then the same manoeuvres should be employed with corresponding changes in the directions of the application of pressure.

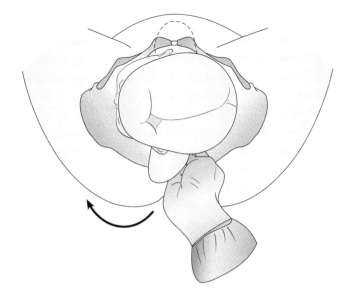

FIGURE 10.10   Application of pressure from the posterior aspect of the posterior shoulder.

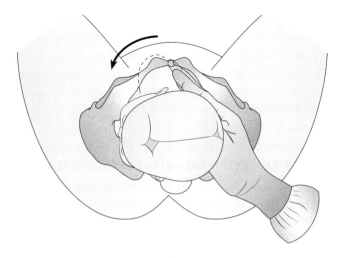

FIGURE 10.11   Application of pressure from the posterior aspect of the anterior shoulder.

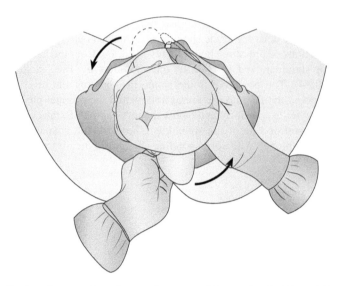

FIGURE 10.12   Application of pressure from the posterior aspect of the anterior shoulder and the anterior aspect of the posterior shoulder.

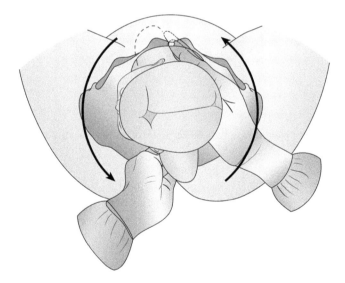

FIGURE 10.13   Rotation of the shoulders by 180° in an anticlockwise direction.

PROCEDURE – INTERNAL ROTATIONAL MANOEUVRES

When inserting a hand into the vagina, it should be in the shape of a cone with the fingers held together, and suprapubic pressure should not be applied. Instruct the assistant to apply synchronous suprapubic pressure in a complementary direction when performing internal rotational manoeuvres. After performing any of these manoeuvres, apply mild traction on the anterior shoulder.

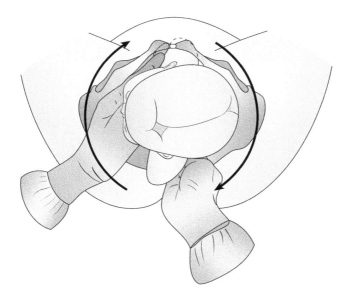

FIGURE 10.14 Rotation of the shoulders by 180° in a clockwise direction.

1. Insert one hand into the posterior aspect of the vagina and anterior to the fetal posterior shoulder, and push that shoulder off the midline to the wider oblique diameter of the pelvis.
2. If the shoulder dystocia is not resolved with the first step above, then insert the hand into the vagina, posterior to the posterior shoulder, and push that shoulder off the midline to the wider oblique diameter.
3. If the shoulder dystocia is still not resolved with the second step above, then insert the hand into the vagina, posterior to the posterior shoulder, move it up and place it behind the anterior shoulder and push that shoulder off the midline to the wider oblique diameter. If possible, insert the left hand anterior to the posterior shoulder and push it to the oblique diameter simultaneously.
4. If delivery of the shoulders is not possible with the first, second and third steps above, then continue to push the anterior shoulder and attempt to rotate the shoulders by 180°, assisted if possible, by the other hand inserted anterior to the fetal posterior shoulder.
5. If rotation of the shoulders by 180° is not possible with the fourth step above, then reverse the direction of pressure and attempt to rotate the shoulders by 180° in the opposite direction.

Manoeuvres Involving the Delivery of the Posterior Arm

- Delivery of the posterior arm across the fetal chest
- Delivery of posterior arm using traction on the posterior axilla
- Delivery of posterior arm and rotation of the fetal trunk by 180°

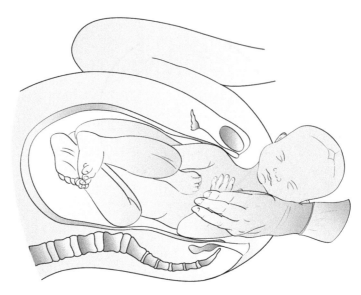

FIGURE 10.15 Delivery of the flexed posterior arm.

Delivery of the Posterior Arm Across the Fetal Chest

Suprapubic pressure should not be applied when attempting to deliver the posterior arm. A hand, with the fingers held together in the shape of a cone, should be inserted posteriorly into the vagina, in front of the fetal posterior shoulder, and then passed upwards, while slightly elevating the posterior shoulder with the other hand in order to increase the space available for manipulations. If the fetal arms are flexed, and the posterior hand and forearm are palpable, the posterior wrist should be grasped between the fingers and the thumb of the operator, and traction must be applied in a straight line downwards in line with the forearm and across the fetal head in order to extend the arm and deliver (Figure 10.15). Traction applied in a perpendicular direction to the forearm may result in fracture of the radius and/or ulnar bones. If the posterior hand and forearm are not palpable, then the posterior upper arm should be followed up to its elbow and by placing the thumb on the antecubital fossa and applying pressure posteriorly on the forearm just below the elbow, the forearm should be flexed (Figure 10.16). Next, the posterior wrist should become accessible for traction. Direct traction on the upper arm to reach the elbow is not recommended, as this could result in fracture of the humerus.

Delivery of the Posterior Arm Using Traction on the Posterior Axilla

Application of traction on the fetal posterior axilla, with the index and middle fingers of the operator anterior to the posterior shoulder along the sacral curve of the maternal pelvis, may be effective in severe cases (Figure 10.17). In this manoeuvre, the presenting diameter at this stage which is biacromial is converted to the axillo-acromial diameter, which is approximately 3 cm shorter, thereby facilitating delivery of the fetal shoulders. Traction may also be applied using a sling (Figure 10.18).

Delivery of Posterior Arm and Rotation of the Fetal Trunk by 180°

If the anterior shoulder is not accessible after the delivery of the posterior arm, then the fetal head should be supported while the trunk is rotated by 180° by applying pressure on the anterior part of the posterior shoulder. This brings the former posterior shoulder anteriorly and below the level of the pubic

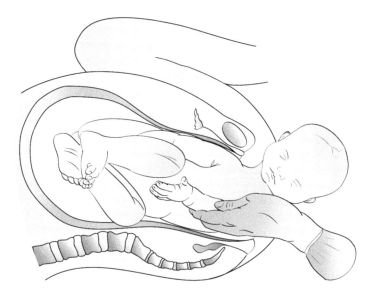

FIGURE 10.16   Flexion of the forearm to make the wrist accessible.

symphysis, and the former anterior shoulder into the sacral hollow, enabling the delivery of the shoulders (Figure 10.19).

PROCEDURE – DELIVERY OF THE POSTERIOR ARM

1. Insert the hand posteriorly into the vagina and anterior to the fetal posterior shoulder while slightly elevating the posterior shoulder with the other hand.
2. Identify the posterior forearm and hand.
3. Grasp the posterior wrist and apply traction in a straight line downwards and across the fetal chest.
4. If the arm is extended, flex the forearm at the elbow to make the wrist accessible, and continue as indicated in the third step above. Alternatively, apply traction on the posterior axilla, with the index and middle fingers or a sling anterior to the fetal posterior shoulder along the maternal pelvic curve, especially in severe cases. If the anterior shoulder is still not delivered following the emergence of the posterior arm, then support the baby's head and rotate the trunk by 180°.

All-Fours Manoeuvre

Placing the woman in the all-fours position may cause a 1–2 cm increase in the anteroposterior diameter of the pelvic inlet due to the effects of the fetal weight and gravity on the sacroiliac joints which become relatively flexible due to pregnancy. However, it may not be practical to place the woman in an all-fours position if she is obese or is on epidural analgesia. In this position, it is the fetal posterior shoulder that is delivered first. If the shoulders fail to deliver following gentle traction on the fetal head, then internal manoeuvres must be adopted (Figure 10.20).

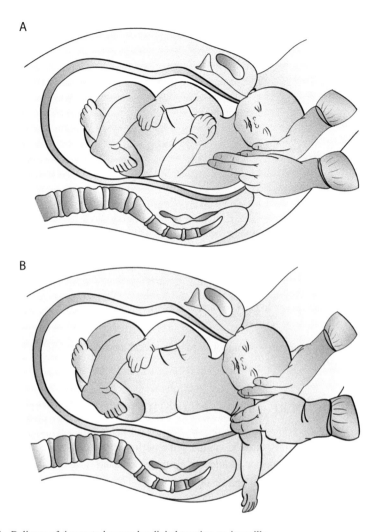

FIGURE 10.17   Delivery of the posterior arm by digital traction on its axilla.

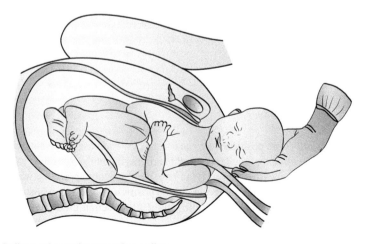

FIGURE 10.18   Delivery of posterior arm using a sling.

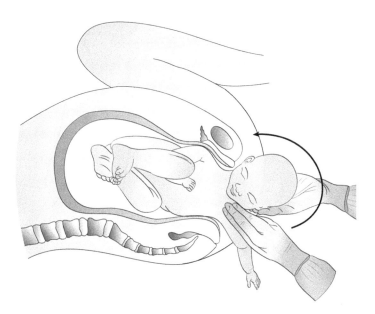

FIGURE 10.19 Following delivery of the posterior arm, the fetus could be rotated by 180°.

Third-Line Manoeuvres

If even second-line measures fail, then this would be a case of severe shoulder dystocia. The third-line manoeuvres available for these severe cases of shoulder dystocia are; cleidotomy, symphysiotomy, the Zavanelli manoeuvre and abdominal rescue. These are associated with considerable neonatal and maternal morbidity.

Cleidotomy

Cleidotomy is the surgical division or fracturing of one or both clavicles, thereby reducing shoulder girth (Figure 10.21). Fracturing or cutting the clavicle is not easy in a term fetus, and in addition, this could damage the subclavian vessels and the brachial plexus. Cleidotomy may be applicable in the case of a dead fetus or one with a lethal anomaly. Specially designed 'cleidotomy scissors' have been developed and used in the past for this purpose.

Symphysiotomy

The woman is placed in the lithotomy position with an angle of abduction of 60°–70° in order to prevent excessive separation of the PS, and this angle must be maintained especially after the symphysiotomy is completed. Adopting sterile procedures, the skin overlying the PS, subcutaneous tissue and the fibrocartilage joint space of the PS should be infiltrated with a local anaesthetic and the syringe removed, leaving the needle in situ to help identify the joint space. A silastic urinary catheter should be inserted, and the left index and middle finger should be inserted into the vagina alongside the catheter. The urethra must be displaced laterally, and the middle finger is placed under the PS joint space. The catheter would be felt between the left index finger in the vagina and the thumb placed over the PS. Next, a small incision is made about 2–3 cm below the upper border of the PS, until the tip of the scalpel is felt by the middle finger in the vagina. Thereafter, the incision is carefully extended from superficial to deep, first downwards and then upwards, and the left thumb should be able to detect the separation of the PS. The separation should be kept no more than the width of the thumb (approximately 2.5 cm), and as mentioned earlier, it is essential to maintain the angle of abduction of the thighs at 60°–70° (Figure 10.22). A generous mediolateral episiotomy must be

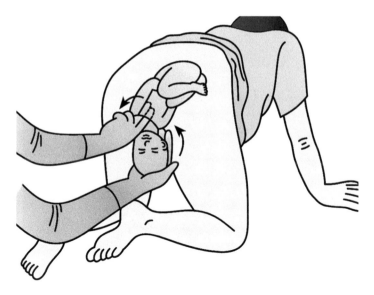

FIGURE 10.20 Use of internal manoeuvres to deliver the shoulders in an all-fours position.

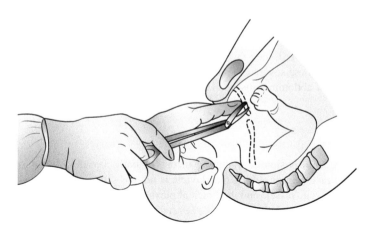

FIGURE 10.21 Cleidotomy.

performed, and the angle of abduction should be reduced to 50°–60° in order to minimise the stretching of the anterior vaginal wall and urethra and to prevent excessive separation of the PS respectively during delivery of the shoulders and the trunk of the baby.

Following the delivery of the baby and the placenta, the PS should be compressed between the thumb on the skin and the index and middle fingers in the vagina for a certain amount of time to achieve haemostasis. Analgesics and antibiotics should be administered. The urinary catheter should be left in situ for five days, and the woman should be nursed on her side as much as possible with her knees strapped for about three days in order to avoid any strain on the PS. Gradual mobilisation must be encouraged afterward.

In skilled hands, symphysiotomy could be a life-saving procedure. It has also been described for the delivery of a trapped aftercoming head of a breech and in obstructed labour at full dilatation when immediate caesarean delivery is not feasible. However, it is associated with considerable maternal morbidity, such as urethral and bladder injury, osteitis pubis, pain and difficulty in walking for about

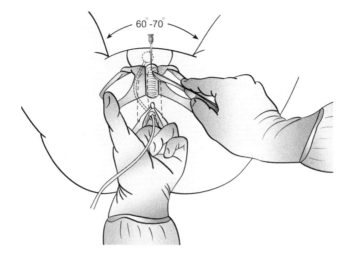

FIGURE 10.22 Symphysiotomy.

three months. Although it would not be applicable in well-resourced settings, it may still have value in under-resourced settings.

PROCEDURE – SYMPHYSIOTOMY

- Achieve strict sterile procedures.
- Insert a silastic catheter into the urethra.
- Infiltrate local anaesthetic agent to the pubic area including the PS joint space.
- Displace the catheter and the urethra laterally using the index finger vaginally, and place middle finger beneath the PS joint space inside the vagina.
- Incise the PS commencing from the anterior fibres, starting 2–3 cm below its upper border, first downwards and then upwards.
- Maintain the angle of abduction of the woman's thighs between 60°–70° and limit the separation of the PS to not more than 2.5 cm.
- Perform a mediolateral episiotomy and reduce the angle of abduction to 50°–60° during the delivery of the shoulders and trunk.

Zavanelli Manoeuvre or Abdominal Rescue

The Zavanelli manoeuvre consists of replacing the fetal head in the vagina and performing caesarean delivery. In order to achieve this, the processes of the delivery of the head have to be reversed. Under regional or general anaesthesia, relaxation of the uterus is achieved by the subcutaneous administration of 0.25 mg of terbutaline. This is followed by a rotation of the fetal head back to occipitoanterior position (reverse restitution) if restitution has occurred, and flexion of the fetal neck (Figure 10.23A). Next, by applying upward, constant, firm pressure on the fetal head, it should be replaced in the vagina (Figure 10.23B). Finally, a caesarean delivery is carried out.

If the fetal head has not been replaced high enough in the vagina to allow for a caesarean delivery, then the fetal anterior shoulder must be directly rotated to the oblique diameter of the maternal pelvis by the abdominal operator, as the fetal anterior shoulder would be easily accessible when the incision is

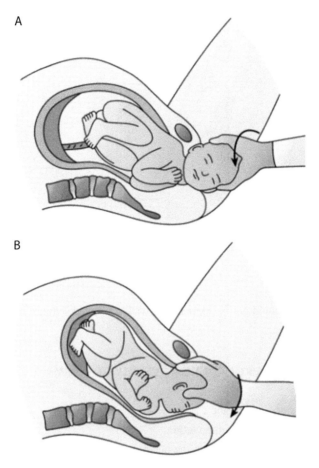

FIGURE 10.23   Zavanelli manoeuvre or abdominal rescue.

made on the uterus following laparotomy. The posterior shoulder would then be easily accessible for internal (vaginal) manoeuvres and the completion of the delivery vaginally by another skilled operator.

PROCEDURE – ZAVANELLI MANOEUVRE ABDOMINAL RESCUE

- Provide regional or general anaesthesia.
- Administer 0.25 mg of terbutaline subcutaneously to cause the uterus to relax.
- Rotate the fetal head back into the occipitoanterior position if it is not in this position.
- Flex the fetal neck.
- Apply pressure to replace the fetal head in the vagina.
- Perform a caesarean delivery.
- In cases in which the fetal head has not been replaced high enough in the vagina; push the fetal anterior shoulder to the oblique diameter of the maternal pelvis directly, and another skilled operator should then carry out vaginal manoeuvres.
- Complete the delivery of the fetus vaginally.

Choice of Manoeuvres in Shoulder Dystocia

The majority of cases of shoulder dystocia can be successfully managed by shifting the woman to the edge of the bed and placing her in McRobert's position, and if necessary, applying suprapubic pressure. In case these first-line measures fail, the next step would be to internally dislodge the anterior shoulder to the wider oblique diameter of the pelvis. If this also fails, then it is reasonable to attempt delivery of the posterior arm if the forearm is flexed or attempt to rotate the fetus by 180° if the forearm is extended. Rotating the fetus by 180° with the application of pressure posterior to the posterior shoulder and anterior to the anterior shoulder is particularly useful in instances where, following instrumental vaginal delivery for occipitoposterior position, the fetal shoulders are stuck in the oblique diameter of the maternal pelvis, with the chest facing either the 2 o'clock or 10 o'clock position. If the shoulder dystocia remains unresolved following internal manoeuvres, then delivery should be attempted after placing the woman in an all-fours position, and if necessary, attempting internal manoeuvres once again in this position.

If the need for third-line manoeuvres arises, then it is worthwhile to resort to symphysiotomy or Zavanelli manoeuvre, which is associated with considerable maternal morbidity, if the fetus is still alive. If the fetus is already dead, cleidotomy is a reasonable option.

Post-Delivery Management

Following delivery, the baby should be handed over to the neonatal team for resuscitation if necessary, and for examination for birth injuries. Umbilical cord blood gases should be performed. The woman should be inspected for genital tract lacerations including OASIS, and PPH should be anticipated (discussed in Chapters 24 and 14). Accurate documentation of the event, including the shoulder involved (whether it was the left or right shoulder that was impacted anteriorly), personnel associated and manoeuvres attempted with an emphasis made on timelines, is imperative. Debriefing of the woman, her partner and the staff forms an important aspect of management. Risk management and regular, in-service simulation-based training in the management of shoulder dystocia is vital.

Key Points

- Shoulder dystocia may occur following any vaginal delivery.
- The vast majority of shoulder dystocia cases can be managed by placing the woman in McRobert's position and applying suprapubic pressure.
- It is mainly the posterior part of the vagina that provides space for performing internal manoeuvres.
- Regular, in-service simulation-based training in shoulder dystocia management is fundamental.

BIBLIOGRAPHY

1. Mehta SH, Sokol RJ. Shoulder dystocia: risk factors, predictability, and preventability. *Semin Perinatol* 2014;38(4):189–93. doi:10.1053/j.semperi.2014.04.003
2. Menticoglou S. Shoulder dystocia: incidence, mechanisms, and management strategies. *Int J Womens Health* 2018;10:723–32. Published 2018 Nov 9. doi:10.2147/IJWH.S175088
3. Boulvain M, Irion O, Dowswell T, Thornton JG. Induction of labour at or near term for suspected fetal macrosomia. *Cochrane Databse Syst Rev* 2016;2016(5):CD000938. doi.org/10.1002/1465185 8.CD000938.pub2
4. Pollack RN, Buchman AS, Yaffe H, Divon MY. Obstetrical brachial palsy: pathogenesis, risk factors, and prevention. *Clin Obstet Gynecol* 2000;43:236–46.
5. Buhimschi CS, Buhimschi IA, Malinow A, Weiner CP. Use of McRoberts' position during delivery and increase in pushing efficiency. *Lancet* 2001;358:470–71.

6. Dahlke JD, Bhalwal A, Chauhan SP. Obstetric emergencies: shoulder dystocia and postpartum hemorrhage. *Obstet Gynecol Clin North Am.* 2017;44(2):231–43. doi:10.1016/j.ogc.2017.02.003

7. Gilstrop M, Hoffman MK. An Update on the Acute Management of Shoulder Dystocia. *Clin Obstet Gynecol* 2016;59(4):813–19. doi:10.1097/GRF.0000000000000240

8. Hofmeyr GJ, Cluver CA. Posterior axilla sling traction for intractable shoulder dystocia. *BJOG* 2009;116:1818–20.

9. Kung J, Swan AV, Arulkumaran S. Delivery of the posterior arm reduces shoulder dystocia dimensions in shoulder dystocia. *Int J Gynaecol Obstet* 2006;93:233–37.

10. Menticoglou SM. A modified technique to deliver the posterior arm in severe shoulder dystocia. *Obstet Gynecol* 2006;108:755–57.

11

Difficult Caesarean Delivery

Sanjeewa Padumadasa and Hemantha Senanayake

Caesarean delivery is increasingly being performed worldwide. However, not all caesarean deliveries are straightforward. Some are complicated, and these are covered under the following sections in this chapter.

- Second stage caesarean delivery
- Difficulties at caesarean delivery (apart from second stage caesarean delivery)
- Extension of the uterine incision

Caesarean delivery for placenta praevia and placenta accreta spectrum (PAS) disorders are discussed in Chapter 13, and perimortem caesarean delivery is discussed in Chapter 7.

Second Stage Caesarean Delivery

Second stage caesarean delivery, the incidence of which has increased over the past few years, carries a higher maternal as well as perinatal morbidity than one that is performed as an elective procedure or during the first stage of labour. Perception of increased safety of caesarean delivery, decreasing rates of mid-cavity instrumental vaginal deliveries as well as possible erosion of skills in instrumental vaginal delivery during recent times have contributed to the increase in second stage caesarean deliveries.

Risk Factors

A deeply impacted fetal head happens in approximately 1.5% of all caesarean deliveries. The incidence can be expected to rise even further, given the increasing trend for caesarean delivery rather than instrumental vaginal delivery in case of a delay or fetal distress during the second stage, and the increasing incidence of fetal macrosomia and maternal obesity. The other risk factors for a deeply impacted fetal head include failed trial of instrumental vaginal delivery and fetal malposition.

Complications

Maternal

Second stage caesarean delivery with the fetal head deeply impacted within the pelvis is associated with increased blood loss, uterine vessels tearing, an extension of the uterine incision into the cervix, vagina, posterior uterine wall ('bucket handle tear') or broad ligament, damage to bladder, ureter and bowel and postpartum infections. The extension of the uterine incision also has implications on the woman's future obstetric performance, as it increases the risk of uterine rupture in a subsequent attempt at vaginal delivery. Therefore, these women are usually subjected to repeat caesarean delivery, which heightens the risk of placenta praevia and placenta accreta spectrum (PAS) disorders. Second stage caesarean delivery is also associated with laparoelytrotomy, i.e. mistaking the upper vagina for the lower uterine segment, thus leading to abdominal delivery through a vaginal incision.

Several factors contribute to the difficulty in delivery of the fetus when the fetal head is deeply impacted within the maternal pelvis. The lower segment of the uterus is thin and distended, which increases the risk of extension of the uterine incision. Only the fetal shoulder may be visible on opening into the uterine cavity ('shoulder sign'), and the fetal head is usually deflexed and elongated with significant caput and moulding. In addition, with the membranes having been ruptured for a long time, the uterus would usually be more or less gripping the fetus. Any attempt at reducing the effective diameter of the fetal head by flexing may be limited by splinting of the fetal spine within the contracted uterus.

Fetal

Second stage caesarean delivery is also associated with significant perinatal morbidity and mortality, including fetal long bone fractures, skull fractures, scalp lacerations, low Apgar scores at birth and admission to the neonatal intensive care unit. Some studies have also found an association between second stage caesarean delivery complicated by extension of the uterine incision, and preterm delivery in subsequent pregnancies.

Management in Case of a Deeply Impacted Fetal Head within the Maternal Pelvis

Preparation

A caesarean delivery with an impacted head must be undertaken by a highly skilled obstetrician, as the complications of the procedure could prove life-threatening for both the woman and baby. This is an important consideration even from the perspective of risk management. Informed written consent should be obtained from the woman. Preparations for an emergency caesarean delivery must be made. This includes prophylaxis against acid aspiration, and crossmatching of blood. Preoperative broad-spectrum intravenous antibiotics (e.g. cefuroxime) should be administered, and the bladder must be emptied. However, catheterising the bladder when the fetal head is impacted within the pelvis could be difficult, and in this case, the fetal head should be pushed slightly upwards.

Arrangements for neonatal resuscitation should be in place. Nitroglycerin or subcutaneous terbutaline may be used to relax the uterus. However, studies have not proven the benefit of uterine relaxants for this purpose. On the other hand, the use of uterine relaxants can impair postpartum uterine contractions and increase the risk of postpartum haemorrhage. Finally, the operating table should be at a lower level than normal in order to facilitate manoeuvres that may be necessary to disengage the fetal head from the maternal pelvis.

Technique

A generous low transverse incision should be made on the skin. It should be at a higher level than normal in order to facilitate proper placement of the uterine incision, because the lower segment of the uterus will be stretched and distended. The anatomical landmarks that help to differentiate between the vagina, cervix and the uterine body are usually obscured. It is also essential to make a generous incision transversely on the uterus at a higher level than normal. This should be curving upwards on both sides to prevent the incision from extending into the uterine vessels.

Once the uterine incision is made, an attempt is made first to deliver the impacted head in a manner similar to that of the standard technique, with the following modifications.

1. The operator waits for the uterus to relax between two contractions.
2. The dominant hand is inserted into the pelvis along the lateral aspect of the fetal head in a manner similar to the insertion of a shoehorn below the heel of the foot (Figure 11.1A). This is because the transverse diameter is the largest at the pelvic inlet, and the impaction of the fetal head would have obliterated the space anteriorly.
3. The fetal head is grasped firmly in the palm of the hand and levered out of the pelvis, by a 'shrugging movement' of the operator's shoulder and elevation of the elbow while avoiding movements at the wrist joint.
4. Grasping the wrist of the dominant hand with the other hand is useful in order to prevent levering movements of the wrist which could lead to tears in the lower segment while elevating the head into the uterine incision (Figure 11.1B).

If the first attempt fails, then the operator has any one of the following options to deliver the impacted fetal head. The choice would depend on the operator's familiarity with the technique.

'Push' Disengagement Technique

A commonly used method for disengagement of the fetal head is the 'push' disengagement technique which is also referred to as the 'head first' technique or 'abdomino-vaginal delivery' (Figure 11.2). The woman is kept in lithotomy position. An assistant inserts a gloved hand into the vagina and gently displaces the fetal head cephalad using the palm of the hand or cupped fingers. This helps spread the force widely across the fetal head. At the same time, the surgeon should apply traction on the fetal shoulders or flex and elevate the fetal head into the uterine incision. Both the surgeon and the assistant should try to flex the fetal head because a flexed head presents the smallest effective diameter.

PROCEDURE – THE 'PUSH' DISENGAGEMENT TECHNIQUE OF DISENGAGING THE IMPACTED HEAD

- Place the woman in lithotomy position.
- An assistant should use the palm of the hand or cupped fingers to push the fetal head into the upper part of the maternal pelvis while flexing the fetal head.
- The surgeon should apply traction on the fetal shoulders and subsequently flex and elevate the fetal head into the uterine incision.
- Complete the delivery of the fetus.

A   B

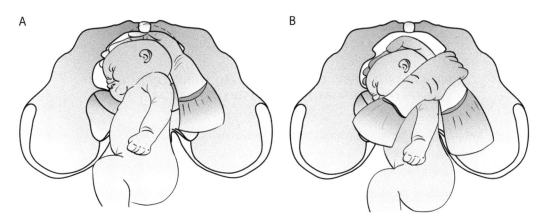

FIGURE 11.1 Levering the head out of the pelvis.

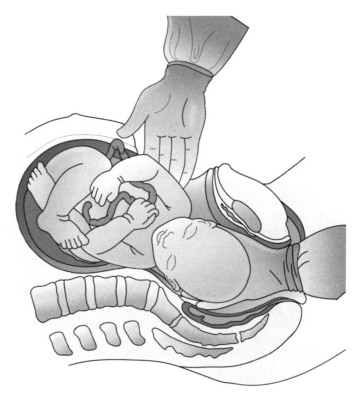

FIGURE 11.2   The 'push' disengagement technique.

'Pull' Disengagement Technique

An alternative to the 'push' technique is the 'pull' disengagement technique, which is also referred to as 'reverse breech extraction' or the 'feet first' technique (Figure 11.3). In this technique, the surgeon reaches towards the upper segment of the uterus, grasps preferably both or at least one foot of the fetus, and applies gentle traction on the fetus as in internal podalic version and breech extraction (discussed in Chapter 28). If one leg is grasped, then one should apply gentle traction on that leg until the other leg appears. Then, the other leg should be delivered. Finally, both legs should be held together, and the fetus is pulled out of the uterus. It is important to apply traction that is parallel to the axis of the fetal legs in order to avoid fracturing the tibia and fibula. Standard breech delivery manoeuvres should be used to deliver the fetal arms and head. These include Lovset's and Mauriceau-Smellie-Veit (MSV) manoeuvres respectively. If the transverse uterine incision has to be extended to maximise space within the uterus, a J-shaped incision, which heals better, is preferred over an inverted T-shaped incision.

PROCEDURE – THE 'PULL' DISENGAGEMENT TECHNIQUE OF DISENGAGING THE IMPACTED HEAD

- Insert the hand towards the upper segment of the uterus.
- Grasp preferably both or at least one foot of the fetus.
- Apply gentle traction on the fetus.
- Pull the fetus out of the uterus using standard manoeuvres as utilised in internal podalic version and breech extraction.

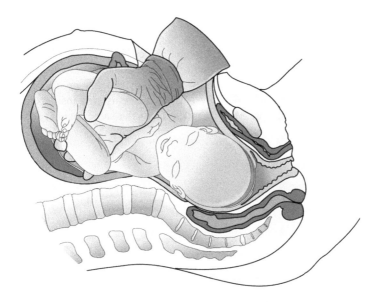

FIGURE 11.3 The 'pull' disengagement technique or reverse breech extraction.

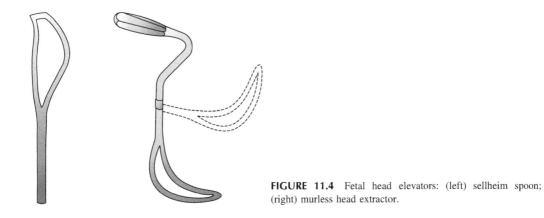

FIGURE 11.4 Fetal head elevators: (left) sellheim spoon; (right) murless head extractor.

Several studies comparing the 'push' and 'pull' disengagement techniques, have reported a nearly 8-fold increased risk of extension of the uterine incision, blood loss, requirement for blood transfusion and longer operating time with the 'push' technique. The rate of fetal injury was reported as similar between the two techniques. Theoretically, the 'push' technique may also be associated with the risk of infection due to contamination from vaginal flora, as well as the risk of fetal scalp trauma.

Use of Fetal Head Elevators

If available, fetal head elevators such as the Sellheim spoon or the Murless head extractor, which take up less space inside the pelvis than the operator's hand, can be used to lift the fetal head into the uterine incision (Figure 11.4).

Patwardhan Technique

The Patwardhan technique, which is also referred to as 'shoulders first' technique, is another method that has been described for the delivery of a fetus at caesarean delivery during the second stage. It was pioneered by Patwardhan and Motashaw as far back as 1957. This technique has been used successfully ever since. In this procedure, an incision is made on the lower uterine segment at the level of the fetal shoulders. When the fetus is in the occipitoanterior position, both fetal shoulders are delivered first. Afterward, the surgeon places his/her hands on the fetal thorax and, with gentle traction on the fetal trunk, the fetal chest, abdomen, buttocks and lower limbs are brought out of the uterus (Figure 11.5). An assistant may aid the process by applying fundal pressure. Finally, the head, which is the only part of the fetus still inside the uterus, is gently delivered out of the pelvis using the MSV manoeuvre in the same manner as in reverse breech extraction.

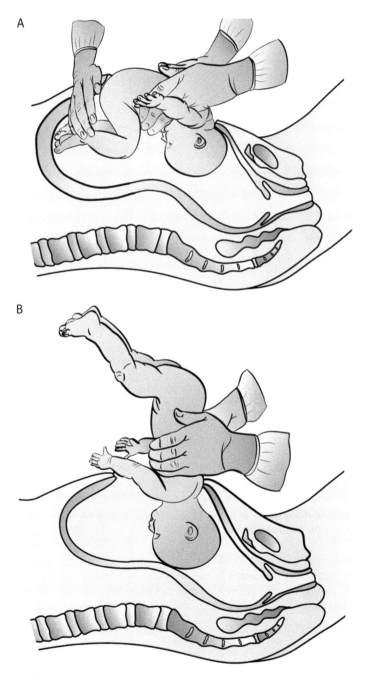

FIGURE 11.5   Patwardhan technique.

PROCEDURE – PATWARDHAN TECHNIQUE (WHEN THE FETUS IS IN OCCIPIT-OANTERIOR POSITION)

- Deliver both arms.
- Apply traction on the fetal thorax.
- Deliver the fetal chest, abdomen, buttocks and lower limbs.
- Gently deliver the fetal head out of the pelvis using the MSV manoeuvre.

When the fetus is in occipitoposterior position and once one shoulder is delivered, the hand of the operator is introduced into the fundus of the uterus and the leg on the same side as the shoulder is grasped and brought out of the uterine incision. This is followed by the delivery of the breech. At this time, an assistant may press on the fundus to help deliver the fetal breech. Afterward, the rest of the fetal body is delivered, finally ending with the fetal head.

Modified Patwardhan Technique

A modification of Patwardhan technique is described for second stage caesarean delivery when the fetus is in the occipitolateral position. In this technique, an incision is made on the lower uterine segment at the level of the anterior shoulder. This is followed by delivery of the anterior shoulder and arm. Then, the fetus is gently rotated and the posterior shoulder and arm are delivered. The rest of the delivery is the same as that of the Patwardhan technique.

Other Methods

Various innovative devices, such as the fetal disimpacting system and the C-snorkel, which help release the vacuum created between the impacted fetal head and the maternal pelvis, have been used to assist the delivery of the fetus at second stage caesarean deliveries. However, there is no data available at the moment regarding the efficacy, safety and cost-effectiveness of these devices.

Post-Delivery Management

Caesarean delivery in the second stage of labour carries the risk of uterine tears that may extend into the adjacent structures and the rest of the uterus. It is of paramount importance that the uterus is inspected carefully for this damage. This may require exteriorising the uterus so that it could be inspected in its entirety, including its posterior wall. As there is a risk of postpartum haemorrhage due to uterine atony as a result of prolonged labour, an oxytocin infusion (20 units in 500 mL of normal saline over four hours) should be commenced. Broad-spectrum intravenous antibiotics (e.g. cefuroxime) should be continued in the immediate postpartum period. If the woman has been in labour for a significant length of time, then it may be wise to leave the indwelling catheter longer than usual, to avoid the formation of vesicovaginal fistula due to ischaemic necrosis of the neck of the bladder.

Reducing the Incidence of Second Stage Caesarean Deliveries

Appropriate management of labour, including the appropriate use and interpretation of the partogram to recognise dysfunctional labour and the judicious use of oxytocin, reduce the need for caesarean delivery during the second stage (discussed in Chapter 8).

It has been suggested that better training in instrumental vaginal deliveries (discussed in Chapter 9), may reduce the incidence of second stage caesarean deliveries. Increasing rates of failed instrumental vaginal delivery and reduced attempts have been implicated in the current increasing trend of second stage caesarean deliveries. Although there may be a reluctance to perform instrumental vaginal delivery due to fear of litigation, recent studies have found that the maternal and perinatal outcomes are similar in cases of failed instrumental vaginal delivery to the ones in which caesarean delivery was performed without a trial. Decisions made by a consultant rather than a clinician with limited experience, are important in determining whether the safer option for the delay in second stage of labour is either caesarean delivery or instrumental vaginal delivery.

Some of the second stage caesarean deliveries are performed to deliver the second twin after the delivery of the first twin vaginally, the indications being non-vertex presentation, fetal distress, cord prolapse and placental abruption. Better training at internal podalic version and breech extraction for delivery of the second twin may have a place in reducing the number of such second stage caesarean deliveries in twin pregnancies (discussed in Chapters 26 and 28).

A reluctance in conducting vaginal breech delivery has resulted in women being subjected to emergency caesarean deliveries even when they present in advanced second stage of labour. Training in the art of assisted vaginal breech delivery will certainly reduce some of these difficult caesarean deliveries (discussed in Chapter 25).

Difficulties at Caesarean Delivery (Apart from Second Stage Caesarean Delivery)

There are causes other than a deeply impacted fetal head, which pose difficulties at caesarean delivery. These causes and their respective management are summarised in Table 11.1. Moreover, management options depend on the cause.

TABLE 11.1

Causes for difficult caesarean delivery (apart from an impacted fetal head) and management thereof

Cause	Management
Scar at the previous surgical site	Excise the scar with an elliptical incision
Possible intra-abdominal adhesions	Consider midline abdominal incision
Inadequate skin incision	Extend the skin incision
Inadequate space between recti muscles	Incise the rectus muscle transversely (Maylard incision) - be cautious about injury to inferior epigastric vessels as these are notorious to retract into tissues.
Inadequate uterine incision	Extend the uterine incision in the shape of J
Poorly formed lower segment	Consider upper segment caesarean delivery
Dense intra-abdominal adhesions	Open the peritoneum as high as possible.
	Take extra care to avoid injury to the bowel and bladder.
	Incise fibrous adhesions close to the uterus with the point of scissors directed towards the uterus. Clamping, cutting and ligating may be necessary.
	Incise the peritoneum on the uterus about 2 cm above the bladder.
	Alternatively, consider upper segment caesarean delivery.
	Consider filling the bladder with a crystalloid solution via the indwelling catheter using an intravenous infusion set. This will delineate the margin of the bladder better.
Deflexed fetal head	Manually flex the fetal head and deliver.
	Apply Wrigley forceps (with the concave pelvic curve towards the fetal occiput) or a handheld ventouse.
Floating fetal head	Confirm the placental location and exclude placenta praevia.
	Anticipate poorly formed and highly vascular lower segment.
	Manipulate the fetus to a longitudinal lie and ask the assistant to maintain the fetal lie by providing lateral support.
	Rupture the membranes, allow liquor to drain and the fetal head to descend, flex the head and deliver.

(*Continued*)

TABLE 11.1 (Continued)
Causes for difficult caesarean delivery (apart from an impacted fetal head) and management thereof

Cause	Management
	Ask the assistant to apply gentle fundal pressure. Excessive force may cause the fetal head to move to one side of the uterus rather than towards the uterine incision.
	Apply Wrigley forceps or hand-held ventouse.
	Alternatively, a combination of external version and internal podalic version and breech extraction may be used.
Breech presentation	Discussed in Chapter 25.
	The aftercoming head of the preterm breech could get entrapped by the retracting uterus.
Transverse lie of the fetus	Combination of external and internal cephalic versions.
	Combination of external and internal podalic versions and breech extraction.
	May have to extend the uterine incision in the shape of a 'J'.
	Consider acute tocolysis with terbutaline 0.25 mg subcutaneously.
Extremely low birth weight fetus	Anticipate poorly formed and highly vascular lower segment.
	There is a possibility of maternal intestines descending and obstructing the operative field. Pack the bowels away if this occurs.
	Incise the deeper layers of the myometrium carefully to prevent scalp injury to the fetus.
Fibroids in the lower segment	Make a transverse incision on the uterus (lower or upper segment) avoiding the fibroid.
	Consider upper segment caesarean delivery.
	Be aware of the abnormal lie of the fetus.
	In exceptional circumstances, a decision may be made by an experienced operator to perform a caesarean myomectomy with preparations to handle blood loss.
Delivery of conjoined twins	Classical incision or extension of a transverse incision on the lower segment to a shape of J may be necessary.
Fetus with hydrocephalus	The mode of delivery depends on the prognosis.
	Where ventriculo-peritoneal shunting is planned, the fetus may be delivered via an upper segment caesarean delivery.
	Where the prognosis is poor, cerebrospinal fluid may be aspirated and the cephalic diameters reduced before accomplishing vaginal delivery.

Extension of the Uterine Incision

A difficult caesarean delivery may result in an extension of the uterine incision. Management of such cases is summarised in Figure 11.6.

Key Points

- The involvement of an experienced obstetrician is essential when making decisions on and when performing second stage caesarean deliveries.
- Both the skin and uterine incisions have to be made at a higher level than normal when performing second stage caesarean deliveries.
- Reverse breech extraction carries less morbidity than 'push' disengagement technique at second stage caesarean deliveries.

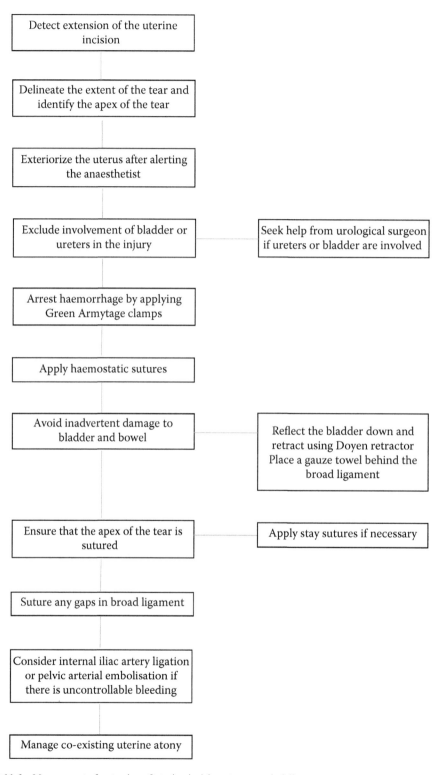

FIGURE 11.6   Management of extension of uterine incision at caesarean delivery.

- Exteriorisation of the uterus helps to reduce blood loss in cases of haemorrhage as well as in identifying the extent of uterine tears and ultimately managing them.

BIBLIOGRAPHY

1. Manning JB, Tolcher MC, Chandraharan E, Rose CH. Delivery of an impacted fetal head during cesarean: a literature review and proposed management algorithm. *Obstet Gynaecol Surv* 2015;70:719–25.
2. Nooh AZ, Abdeldayem H, Ben-Affan O. Reverse breech extraction versus the standard approach of pushing the impacted fetal head up through the vagina in caesarean section for obstructed labour: A randomized controlled trial. *J Obstet Gynaecol* 2017;37:1–5.
3. Schwake D, Petchenkin L, Younis JS. Reverse breech extraction in cases of second stage caesarean section. *J Obstet Gynaecol* 2012;32:548–51.
4. Veisi F, Zangeneh M, Malekkhosravi S, Rezavand N. Comparison of 'push' and 'pull' methods for impacted fetal head extraction during cesarean delivery. *Int J Gynaecol Obstet* 2012;118:4–6.
5. Fong YF, Arulkumaran S. Breech extraction—an alternative method of delivering a deeply engaged head at cesarean section. *Int J Gynecol Obstet* 1997;56:183–4.
6. Saha PK, Gulati R, Goel P, Tandon R, Huria A. Second stage caesarean section: evaluation of Patwardhan technique. *J Clin Diagn Res* 2014;8(1):93–95.
7. Patwardhan BD, Motashaw ND. Caesarean section. *J Obstet Gynaecol India* 1957;8(1):1–15.
8. Vousden N, Cargill Z, Briley A, Tyderman G, Shennan AH. Caesarean section at full dilatation: incidence, impact and current management. *TOG* 2014;16(3):199–205.

12

Complications of Obstetric Anaesthesia

Bhaagya Gunetilleke and Asantha de Silva

Anaesthetic complications contribute to maternal morbidity and mortality. Although recent advances in obstetric anaesthesia have largely mitigated this risk, the potential for anaesthesia related complications should not be underestimated. Pregnant woman may require analgesia or anaesthesia in the following situations.

- Labour
- Elective caesarean delivery
- Emergency caesarean delivery
- Emergency surgery for peripartum complications
- Non-caesarean surgery

The risks associated with anaesthesia develop due to the anatomical and physiological changes associated with pregnancy. These risks can be further exaggerated due to advanced maternal age, hypertensive disorders, cardiac disease and other medical and pregnancy-related conditions. The complications related to general and regional anaesthesia are listed in Table 12.1.

Airway-Related Complications

Physiological changes including oedema of the airway, enlargement of the gravid uterus and the breasts resulting in a shortening of the safe period of apnoea, rapid desaturation, difficulty in face mask ventilation as well as complexity in securing the airway by intubation, heighten the risk of hypoxia and pulmonary aspiration (discussed in Chapter 7). Therefore, it is paramount that an experienced anaesthesiologist is involved in the management of general anaesthesia during pregnancy.

There are two main priorities in the period preceding induction of general anaesthesia.

a. Reduction of the risk of aspiration
b. Prolongment of the safe period of apnoea

Neuraxial anaesthesia in the form of subarachnoid, epidural or combined subarachnoid and epidural anaesthesia is more advisable over general anaesthesia as the lucid patient is able to maintain a patent airway and spontaneous respiration, thus reducing the risk of airway-related complications.

Aspiration

Aspiration of particulate or acidic gastric contents causes obstruction of airways and pneumonitis. Aspiration pneumonitis in pregnancy is associated with a poor outcome.

TABLE 12.1

Complications of obstetric anaesthesia

General anaesthesia
  Aspiration
  Difficult airway
  Failed intubation
  Hypotension
  Uterine hypotonia
  Neonatal depression
  Awareness
  Dental trauma and other oropharyngeal injuries
  Malignant hyperthermia
  Suxamethonium apnoea
Regional (Neuraxial) anaesthesia
  Hypotension
  Bradycardia
  Hypoventilation
  Inadequate, asymmetric analgesia or dense motor block
  Post-dural puncture headache
  Neurological injury
    Transient
    Permanent
  Central nervous system infection
  Epidural haematoma
Others
  Nausea and vomiting
  Pruritus
  Backache
  Anaphylaxis
  Porphyrias
  Anterior spinal artery syndrome

The following measures should be adopted to minimise the risk of aspiration.

i. Ingestion of food during labour and for six hours prior to elective caesarean delivery should be avoided. Clear liquids during labour up to two hours prior to caesarean delivery could be permitted.

ii. Pharmacological prophylaxis with histamine 2 receptor anatagonists, e.g. ranitidine to reduce the acidity and volume of gastric fluid, and a prokinetic such as metoclopramide must be administered. These drugs should be provided eight hours and two hours prior to caesarean delivery. Intravenous (IV) antacid and prokinetic medication should be employed as soon as a decision is made for an emergency caesarean delivery.

iii. In emergencies, 30 mL of 0.3M sodium citrate, a nonparticulate solution, should be administered.

iv. Neuraxial anaesthesia should be used as the default mode of anaesthesia in pregnancy.

v. Rapid sequence induction of general anaesthesia must be carried out while applying cricoid pressure.

vi. Once the woman is conscious, she must be extubated (awake extubation) or placed in left lateral position.

vii. A tiltable surgical bed, a high-volume suction device, and experienced theatre personnel should be readily available.

If the woman vomits during induction of anaesthesia, the cricoid pressure is released in order to prevent oesophageal rupture. The following measures should be applied immediately.

  i. Perform suctioning of the oropharynx.
  ii. Position the woman in a head low, left lateral position.
  iii. Maintain adequate oxygenation via a mask.
  iv. Perform endotracheal intubation and gentle suction of trachea through a catheter inserted via the endotracheal tube, preferably prior to initiating positive pressure ventilation.
  v. Treat bronchospasm with bronchodilators.

Antibiotics are indicated only in women with evidence of pneumonia. Prophylactic antibiotics and steroids are not recommended.

Difficulty in Maintaining a Patent Airway

Difficulty in maintaining the airway in an obtunded pregnant woman is compounded by the anatomical and physiological changes of pregnancy. The triple airway manoeuvre, i.e. jaw thrust, chin lift and extension of the neck, may need to be supplemented with an oropharyngeal airway. It is vital that measures in preventing aspiration are adopted for these women. Maintenance of oxygenation by the use of a face mask and a manual resuscitator (Ambu bag) with a reservoir bag connected to an oxygen source could be supplemented with oxygen administered via nasal prongs (Figure 12.1) or by the use of high-flow humidified oxygen therapy. These women should be nursed in a head-up position. Airway compromise may occur at extubation. Women who are likely to benefit from a period of ventilation prior to extubation should be identified. Awake extubation minimises the risk of airway compromise and aspiration. If there is any doubt about the woman's ability to maintain a patent airway on her own, extubation should be performed after placing her in the left lateral position.

Failure of Endotracheal Intubation

The incidence of difficult intubation and oxygenation is more common among pregnant women than in non-pregnant women. Failure to oxygenate could lead to serious neurological injury or death. Preoxgenation is crucial in order to prolong the safe period of apnoea. A video laryngoscope used by a

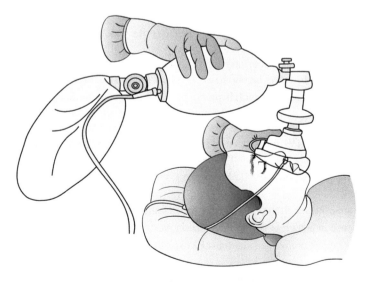

FIGURE 12.1   Simultaneous delivery of oxygen via a face mask and nasal prongs.

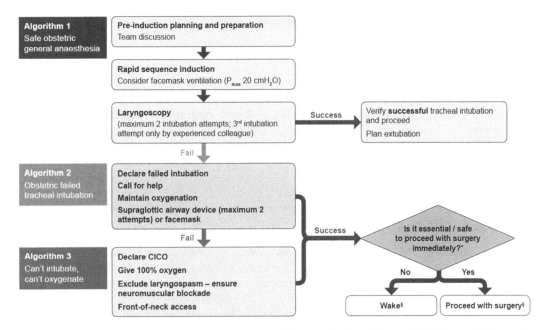

FIGURE 12.2 The failed intubation protocol. (Reproduced with permission from Mushambi MC, Kinsella SM, Popat M, Swales H, Ramaswamy KK, Winton AL, Quinn AC. Obstetric Anaesthetists' Association and Difficult Airway Society guidelines for the management of difficult and failed tracheal intubation in obstetrics. *Anaesthesia* 2015;70:1286–1306)

trained operator improves the chances of successful intubation. Special equipment such as a Magill laryngoscope with a short handle, Polio blade and McCoy blades are useful if a videolaryngoscope is unavailable. Nasal prongs or high-flow humidified oxygen therapy should be used to oxygenate the woman while intubation is attempted. If intubation fails, the succeeding failed intubation protocol in obstetrics should be followed (Figure 12.2). Capnographic confirmation of correct placement of the endotracheal tube is essential. After failed intubation, the immediate situation should be considered in deciding whether to awaken the woman or to proceed with surgery. The woman should be awakened unless it is safe or is essential to proceed. Moreover, the front of neck's airway access should be considered early on.

Hypotension Following Induction of Anaesthesia

Hypotension is multifactorial and results from the impaired venous return due to compression of the inferior vena cava by the gravid uterus, the cardiac depressant effects of anaesthetic drugs and the responses to positive pressure ventilation. Since these factors could exacerbate hypotension due to ongoing haemorrhage or sepsis, extreme caution should be exercised when selecting anaesthetic drugs and corresponding doses in these circumstances. Severe hypotension may contribute to acute fetal distress and even fetal death. Hypotension can be minimised by a left lateral tilt of the woman, re-suscitation with intravenous fluids and vasopressors prior to or soon after induction of anaesthesia. Ventilation with low tidal volumes is recommended until haemodynamic stability is achieved.

Left lateral tilt or manual displacement of the uterus (discussed in Chapter 7) is vital when re-suscitating hypotensive women at more than 20 weeks of gestation. The use of rapid fluid infuser-warmers, balanced salt solutions such as Ringer lactate, maintenance of normothermia, point of care tests of coagulation to guide the use of blood products, clotting factors and tranexamic acid are likely to improve the outcome in haemorrhage-induced hypotension. Efforts at gaining multiple large-bore intravenous access, placement of central venous catheters and hemodynamic monitoring should not delay the resuscitation of the woman.

Uterine Hypotonia

Anaesthetic drugs including inhalational agents, e.g. isoflurane, contribute to uterine hypotonia and can cause postpartum haemorrhage. Volatile anaesthetic agents should be used at a minimum concentration which will prevent awareness. Uterotonic agents (e.g. oxytocin, ergometrine, misoprostol), with or without surgical measures, should be used in its treatment. Management of uterine hypotonia is further described in Chapter 14.

Neonatal Depression

Anaesthetic agents and opioids used for labour analgesia, e.g. intramuscular pethidine, could result in neonatal cardiorespiratory depression. A greater incidence of neonatal respiratory depression is noted when the delivery happens 2–3 hours after administration of opioids. Trained personnel, equipment and drugs (e.g. naloxone) required for the resuscitation of the newborn must be available.

The use of parenteral opioids for labour analgesia could be avoided by the judicious use of epidural analgesia with local anaesthetic drugs in low concentration (0.0625% bupivacaine). The ability to convert a labour epidural to provide anaesthesia for caesarean delivery makes epidurals a versatile option for labour analgesia.

Awareness

General anaesthesia carries a risk of awareness, pain and recall. The use of suboptimal doses for induction and maintenance of anaesthesia to minimise neonatal depression and uterine hypotonia, or in the setting of haemorrhage and hypotension, contributes to awareness. All efforts must be made to use optimal doses after the acute situation which necessitated the use of suboptimal doses is controlled. The psychological effects of awareness are exacerbated in women who are in pain during this period. Hence, optimal analgesia, e.g. with opioids, must be provided at all times. A complaint of awareness must be given serious consideration and should be dealt with empathy and input from psychiatrists when necessary.

Hypotension, Bradycardia and Hypoventilation Following Neuraxial Anaesthesia

A drop in systolic blood pressure exceeding 30 mmHg from the baseline is a common complication of neuraxial anaesthesia. The aetiology is multifactorial. The neuraxial anaesthesia induced sympathetic block is exacerbated by hypovolemia and aortocaval compression. In order to minimise supine hypotension, women greater than 20 weeks of gestation should be placed in a left lateral tilt.

Vasoplegia caused by local anaesthetics is countered by the use of intravenous boluses of ephedrine 5 mg or phenylephrine 50–100 micrograms. fetal acidosis is slightly more prominent with ephedrine than with phenylephrine. Preloading with 10% hydroxyethyl starch is more effective than preloading with a balanced salt solution such as Ringer lactate in minimising hypotension which follows subarachnoid anaesthesia. Bradycardia may evolve rapidly and should be treated with intravenous atropine 0.6 mg boluses.

Impairment of respiration due to paralysis of respiratory muscles by ascending local anaesthetic drugs in neuraxial anaesthesia must be treated with oxygen, assisted respiration with manual respirator (Ambu bag) and, in the presence of hypoxia or a high risk of aspiration, with endotracheal intubation. Minimal doses of sedatives and muscle relaxants, if at all, should be used for intubation in the presence of coexisting hypotension.

Cardiopulmonary resuscitation (CPR) should be commenced in the event of cardiorespiratory arrest (CRA) (discussed in Chapter 7). An intravenous bolus dose of the lipid emulsion Intralipid® (1.2-2 mL/kg), followed by an infusion of 0.5 mL/kg/minute is used for the treatment of CRA which follows an inadvertent intravascular injection of bupivacaine. Intravenous injection of local anaesthetic may precipitate seizures. Management of this includes supplementary oxygen, airway protection with endotracheal intubation if required, control of convulsions with 1–2 mg midazolam or 50–100 mg thiopentone intravenously, and CPR if CRA occurs.

Post-Dural Puncture Headache

Certain side effects follow dural puncture during neuraxial anaesthesia. The incidence could be up to 10%, depending on the gauge of the spinal needle, and with a Tuohy epidural needle it is more than 70%. The symptoms usually appear 24 hours after the dural puncture, and these include photophobia, tinnitus and extreme distress in addition to postural headache. Post-dural puncture headache must be differentiated from other potentially lethal causes of headache, such as impending eclampsia, infections of the central nervous system, intracerebral haemorrhage and cerebral venous thrombosis.

The incidence of this extremely distressing and potentially dangerous complication is reduced by the use of narrow gauge (25, 27 gauge) pencil-point spinal needles. Treatment options include hydration with liberal volumes of oral fluid supplemented with intravenous fluids, progressive escalation of the analgesic regime, caffeine, sedatives, and stool softener. Cerebral imaging is required to exclude intracerebral lesions if the headache does not respond to treatment. An epidural blood patch is used in those with a debilitating headache and not responding to conservative management or those with diplopia or hearing impairment.

Inadequate, Asymmetric Analgesia

Inadequacy and asymmetry could occur with epidural analgesia in labour, and this is evident particularly during instrumental vaginal delivery. A bolus dose of 3–5 mL of 0.125% bupivacaine with fentanyl 50 micrograms would restore the neuraxial analgesia in most instances. Haemodynamic stability should be confirmed prior to administration of the bolus doses of local anaesthetic. In many instances, inadequate analgesia during caesarean delivery under spinal anaesthesia is due to failure to allow adequate time for the onset of action of local anaesthetic. If the level of anaesthesia is below T4, then immediate repositioning of the woman with a head low tilt can achieve an adequate level of anaesthesia, in most cases. Repeating the spinal anaesthetic using lower doses of drugs or conversion to general anaesthesia may be required if pain persists.

Neurological Injury

Major neurological injury that is attributable to neuraxial anaesthesia is rare. The vast majority of neuraxial anaesthetic procedures are carried out using a 'landmark'-based technique. The identification of the site of injection is difficult in women in labour, in the obese and when optimal positioning is not possible. A prolonged neural blockade and bladder dysfunction are common following epidural analgesia, but these resolve completely within 48 hours of stopping the epidural infusion. Injury to nerves is usually transient, lasting for 4–6 weeks.

Permanent neurological injury is extremely rare. The use of neuraxial anaesthesia in the presence of coagulopathy or in those treated with anticoagulants is associated with a greater risk of epidural haematoma, a serious condition that requires immediate diagnosis and decompression within six hours, in order to prevent permanent neurological injury. It is important to ensure a normal coagulation profile and a platelet count of at least 80×10^9/L before administering neuraxial anaesthesia.

Infections of the Central Nervous System

Meningitis is a dreaded complication of neuraxial anaesthesia. Neuraxial blocks are contraindicated in the presence of infection at the site of infection. The use of neuraxial blocks in women with systemic infection should follow a careful risk-benefit assessment and administration of appropriate antibiotics. Adhering to a meticulous, aseptic technique would minimise this complication.

Nausea and Vomiting

These could be multifactorial due to hypotension, traction on the peritoneum or the effect of systemic opioids. Early treatment of hypotension, ensuring adequate analgesia and avoiding exteriorisation of the uterus reduce the prevalence of these problems. The use of antiemetics, e.g. ondansetron, metoclopramide, is helpful in these cases.

Pruritus

Pruritus associated with neuraxial anaesthesia is attributed to the opioids in the solution injected. It is usually self-limiting, but severe pruritus is treated with intravenous chlorpheniramine or naloxone.

Backache

Multiple attempts at neuraxial anaesthesia are associated with localised pain at the site, which is usually self-limiting. Epidural placement does not worsen backache due to preexisting osteoporosis or arthritis. A severe backache with local tenderness and neurological features involving the bladder and lower limbs, following neuraxial anaesthesia, are suggestive of an epidural haematoma and requires immediate neurosurgical review and decompression, as previously discussed.

Anaphylaxis

Anaphylaxis could present with the typical muco-cutaneuos manifestations within seconds of administering a drug intravenously. Progressive obstruction of the airway and hypotension could lead to CRA. Adrenaline 1:1,000, 0.5 mL intramuscularly, or 1:10,000, 0.5 mL intravenous bolus should be administered in the case of cardiovascular collapse, followed by hydrocortisone 200 mg IV and chlorpheniramine 10 mg IV. Furthermore, oxygenation must be maintained. Bronchospasm is treated with nebulization with salbutamol, IV aminophylline and IV magnesium sulphate. Severe hypoxaemia, exhaustion and respiratory failure would require endotracheal intubation and mechanical ventilation. Cardiopulmonary resuscitation should be initiated immediately in the event of CRA.

Key Points

- In pregnancy, neuraxial anaesthesia is safer than general anaesthesia.
- Adhering to fasting guidelines and the use of antacids and prokinetics prior to caesarean delivery, neuraxial anaesthesia, rapid sequence induction of general anaesthesia and awake extubation are employed to reduce the risk of aspiration and its complications.
- Following neuraxial anaesthesia, a persistent headache that is not responding to simple measures needs thorough evaluation in order to exclude sinister pathology in the central nervous system.

- Continued emphasis on education, training and teamwork will facilitate the provision of safe anaesthesia in pregnancy.

BIBLIOGRAPHY

1. Mushambi MC, Kinsella SM, Popat M, et al. Obstetric Anaesthetists' Association and Difficult Airway Society guidelines for the management of difficult and failed tracheal intubation in obstetrics. *Anaesthesia* 2015;70(11):1286–1306. doi:10.1111/anae.13260
2. Clark V, Van de Velde M, Fernando R. Oxford Textbook of Obstetric Anaesthesia. UK: Oxford University Press; 2016.
3. Knight M, Bunch K, Tuffnell D, Shakespeare J, Kotnis R, Kenyon S, Kurinczuk JJ, Eds. on behalf of MBRRACE-UK. Saving Lives, Improving Mothers' Care - Lessons Learned to Inform Maternity Care From the UK and Ireland Confidential Enquiries Into Maternal Deaths and Morbidity 2015-17. Oxford: National Perinatal Epidemiology Unit, University of Oxford; 2019. ISBN: 978-0-9956854-8-2.

13

Antepartum Haemorrhage

Sanjeewa Padumadasa

Antepartum haemorrhage (APH) is defined as bleeding from the genital tract after 20 weeks of gestation and prior to the onset of labour. The cut-off for the period of gestation varies from 20 to 24 weeks among different countries in keeping with national definitions of fetal viability. The causes of APH are listed in Table 13.1.

Placental abruption, placenta praevia and placenta accreta spectrum (PAS) disorders are discussed in detail in this chapter. Although vasa praevia cannot be categorised under APH, it is discussed at the end of this chapter, as it should be considered in any woman who presents with vaginal bleeding during the antenatal period, and it is a serious emergency as far as the fetus is considered.

General Principles of Management

Irrespective of the diagnosis, resuscitation should be the priority if the woman is haemodynamically unstable (discussed in Chapter 14). In contrast to primary postpartum haemorrhage (PPH), bleeding would have started at home in the case of the majority of women with APH, and the estimation of blood loss that is based only on the information given by the woman will be difficult. Therefore, a detailed clinical assessment is necessary for the heamodynamically stable woman. Specific management will depend on the aetiology.

Although placental abruption is generally a clinical diagnosis, there is considerable overlap between the clinical features of placental abruption and those of placenta praevia, especially in regard to the presence or absence of abdominal pain, a malpresentation or high presenting part of the fetus, as well as the amount of bleeding. The placental location should be checked by going through previous antenatal ultrasound reports. However, it is possible that an anomaly scan may not have been performed, and only a first-trimester dating scan may be available. As transvaginal scanning is not part of routine antenatal care, a low-lying placenta could have been missed. Therefore, an abdominal ultrasound scan for placental location is mandatory in all cases of APH. A transvaginal scan should be performed if a low-lying placenta is detected or suspected on abdominal scanning. A digital vaginal examination should not be done until placenta praevia or low lying placenta is excluded by an urgent abdominal ultrasound scan. A speculum examination is required to assess the bleeding and to exclude cervical and vaginal causes which could have given rise to the mentioned bleeding.

It is advisable to palpate through the fornices and exclude a placenta praevia or a low lying placenta before assessing cervical dilatation prior to artificial separation or artificial rupture of membranes, as well as the insertion of a Foley catheter for induction of labour in all pregnant women, due to the possibility of undetected placenta praevia or low lying placenta. On gentle palpation, if the presenting part is not directly palpable through the vaginal fornices, and if a boggy mass is detected between the examining finger and the presenting part, then there is a strong possibility of a placenta praevia or a low lying placenta.

TABLE 13.1

Causes of antepartum haemorrhage

Site	Cause
Uterus	Placental abruption
	Placenta praevia
	Placenta accreta spectrum disorders
	Marginal placental bleeding
	Uterine rupture
Cervix	Cervical ectropion
	Cervical polyp
	Cervical carcinoma
Lower genital tract	Vulvo-vaginal varices
	Vulvo-vaginal infections
	Trauma
Unclassified	Excessive show
	Unexplained

Placental Abruption

Placental abruption is defined as the partial or complete separation of a normally situated placenta before the delivery of the fetus. Although the incidence of placental abruption has decreased over the years to approximately 1 in 100 pregnancies at the present time, it continues to be a major contributor to maternal mortality, severe acute maternal morbidity and perinatal mortality and morbidity. The maternal effects depend primarily on its severity, while the fetal outcome depends on its acuteness as well as the gestational age when it occurs.

Risk Factors for Placental Abruption

- History of placental abruption in the index pregnancy and previous pregnancies
- Hypertensive disorders of pregnancy
- Increased maternal age
- Multiparity
- Maternal smoking and cocaine use
- Prolonged prelabour rupture of membranes
- Multiple pregnancy
- Sudden decompression of an overdistended uterus, e.g. uncontrolled rupture of membranes with polyhydramnios
- Trauma to the abdomen
- Short umbilical cord
- Circumvallate placenta
- Placenta implanted over a uterine septum or submucous fibroid
- Thrombophilia

Types of Placental Abruption

Placental abruption can be classified into revealed, concealed or mixed (Figure 13.1). The most common type is revealed, in which the edge of the placenta separates from the uterine wall, and blood tracks down between the membranes and the uterine wall to escape through the cervix. Sometimes, the bleeding can be concealed between the placenta and the uterine wall. In this case, blood may seep into the myometrium, leading to a 'Couvelaire uterus' which may not contract effectively after delivery and, along with the associated disseminated intravascular coagulation (DIC), leads to PPH. Sometimes, placental abruption can be mixed, with the haemorrhage being simultaneously revealed and concealed.

Clinical features

A high index of suspicion is necessary for the diagnosis of placental abruption. The clinical presentation can vary from mild vaginal bleeding to severe abdominal pain, profound hypovolaemic shock and even fetal death. Abruption of an anteriorly located placenta may be associated with abdominal pain, and that of a posteriorly located placenta may be associated with back pain. The causes of acute abdominal pain during pregnancy are noted in Table 13.2. The changes in location of intra-abdominal organs that take place during pregnancy need to be taken into consideration when looking for a possible cause of abdominal pain. For example, acute appendicitis or torsion of the ovary may present with pain in the upper abdomen during the latter part of pregnancy rather than in the iliac fossa, which is the typical site in a nonpregnant woman.

Following placental abruption, women will usually present in labour as blood traverses the myometrium and generates thrombin as well as prostaglandins locally, which act as powerful contractile agents of the uterus. In addition, the blood clot resulting from abruption creates a barrier between the placental bed and villi, and interferes with the perfusion of the placenta. When the bleeding is concealed, the uterus is usually hard and tender, especially in the case of an anteriorly located placenta, and the fetus may be either dead or severely asphyxiated. Meanwhile, the uterus may be soft in case of abruption of a posteriorly located placenta.

Management

The management depends on the severity of the abruption. The degree of hypovolaemic shock may be out of proportion with the vaginal blood loss in cases of concealed abruption. A quick assessment of vital signs should be performed, and the woman should be resuscitated if deemed haemodynamically unstable. A cardiotocograph may reveal reduced baseline variability or late decelerations and an increased uterine tone with no periods of relaxation. Ultrasound may reveal a retroplacental clot, but more importantly, it

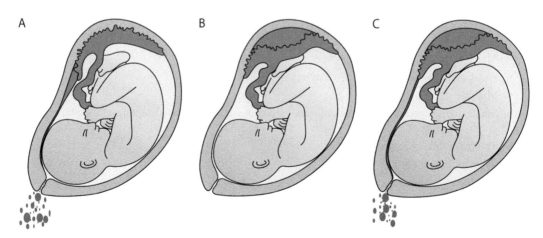

FIGURE 13.1 Types of placental abruption; A – revealed, B – concealed, C – mixed.

TABLE 13.2

Causes of acute abdominal pain during pregnancy

Uterine causes
    Labour
    Placental abruption
    Uterine rupture
    Acute degeneration of fibroid
    Round ligament pain

Ovarian causes
    Torsion of the ovary
    Tubo-ovarian abscess

Gastrointestinal causes
    Acute appendicitis
    Acute cholecystitis
    Small bowel obstruction

Renal causes
    Acute pyelonephritis
    Renal stone
    Ureteral obstruction due to enlarging uterus

Vascular causes
    Rupture of abdominal aortic aneurysm
    Rupture of liver
    Rupture of spleen

Traumatic causes
    Trauma to abdomen

helps to exclude placenta praevia or a low-lying placenta. Immediate caesarean delivery is recommended in case of maternal haemodynamic instability or fetal distress, unless vaginal delivery is imminent.

Most women will present in labour, and usually labour will progress rapidly in these women, thus making vaginal delivery feasible. Vaginal delivery could be assisted with the use of forceps or a vacuum in order to expedite delivery, when the criteria for an instrumental vaginal delivery are fulfilled (discussed in Chapter 9). The associated consumptive coagulopathy that follows placental abruption, as well as uterine atony which occurs as a result of extravasation of maternal blood into the myometrium, may cause severe PPH, and preparations should be in place to manage such an event (discussed in Chapter 14). The placenta should be examined following delivery to confirm abruption. The consumptive coagulopathy should be aggressively managed. Management in the case of a 'Couvelaire uterus' may include hysterectomy, if medical and uterus-conserving measures are not successful in controlling haemorrhage. Anti D immunoglobin should be administered if the woman's blood group is Rhesus negative. A Kleihauer test should also be conducted in order to ensure that an adequate dose of anti D immunoglobulin is given to cover the feto-maternal haemorrhage.

If the woman is at term and not in labour, then labour can be induced with amniotomy and oxytocin, provided that both maternal and fetal conditions are satisfactory.

Minor placental abruption, occurring before term, can be managed expectantly, given that there is no maternal or fetal compromise. Dexamethasone should be considered in pregnancies that are less than 36 weeks in order to improve fetal lung maturity and magnesium sulphate is advised in pregnancies that are less than 32 weeks for neuroprotection of the fetus, but tocolytics should be avoided. However, the possibility of recurrent bleeding should be borne in mind when managing these women. Women with placental abruption who are managed expectantly should be advised on immediate admission to a hospital in case they develop vaginal bleeding or abdominal pain. Repeated episodes of bleeding are associated with fetal growth restriction.

The management of placental abruption is summarised in Figure 13.2.

Recurrence Risk

There is a 25% risk of recurrence of placental abruption in a subsequent pregnancy. Therefore, these women should be closely monitored during successive pregnancies.

Placenta Praevia

In Latin, 'praevia' means 'going before or leading the way'. Therefore, the term 'placenta praevia' is used to describe a placenta that is implanted in the lower uterine segment, over or close to the internal os, thus lying in front of the fetus in the birth canal. The incidence of placenta praevia at term is estimated to be 1 in 200 pregnancies, and can be expected to rise in the future with the increasing rates of caesarean delivery, advanced maternal age and assisted reproductive technology.

Risk Factors for Placenta Praevia

- Previous caesarean delivery (risk increases with the number of caesarean deliveries)
- Other surgeries involving the lower segment of the uterus, e.g. myomectomy, hysteroscopic surgery
- Multiparity
- Assisted reproductive technology
- Multiple pregnancies
- Advanced maternal age
- Maternal smoking
- Previous history of placenta praevia

Placental Localisation

A transvaginal scan is superior to a transabdominal scan in localising the placenta, especially in the case of a posteriorly located placenta. It is safe in experienced hands. Transvaginal scanning allows the precise determination of the distance between the edge of the placenta and the internal os and enables a practical classification of placental location in pregnancies greater than 16 weeks into normal, low-lying or praevia (Figure 13.3). The mid-trimester anomaly scan gives the opportunity to localise the placenta and identify women at risk of a persistent low lying placenta or a persistent placenta praevia. The term 'placenta praevia' is reserved for a placenta lying directly over the internal os. When the placental edge is less than 20 mm from the internal os, then it is referred to as 'low lying', and when it is 20 mm or more from the internal os, it is considered 'normal'.

If the placenta is found to be low-lying or praevia at early gestations, a follow-up ultrasound scan is recommended at 32 weeks and, if necessary, again at 36 weeks of gestation in order to diagnose persistent low-lying placenta or placenta praevia. The dynamic process of formation of the lower segment of the uterus during the latter part of pregnancy, resulting in the apparent 'placental migration', leads to the resolution of about 90% of low-lying placentae diagnosed during the mid-trimester.

Historically, placenta praevia was graded according to the distance between the lower edge of the placenta and the internal os of the cervix, as follows.

- Grade I (lateral or low-lying) - Placenta extends to the lower uterine segment, but not as far as the edge of the internal os
- Grade II (marginal) - The edge of the placenta extends to the internal os, but does not cover it

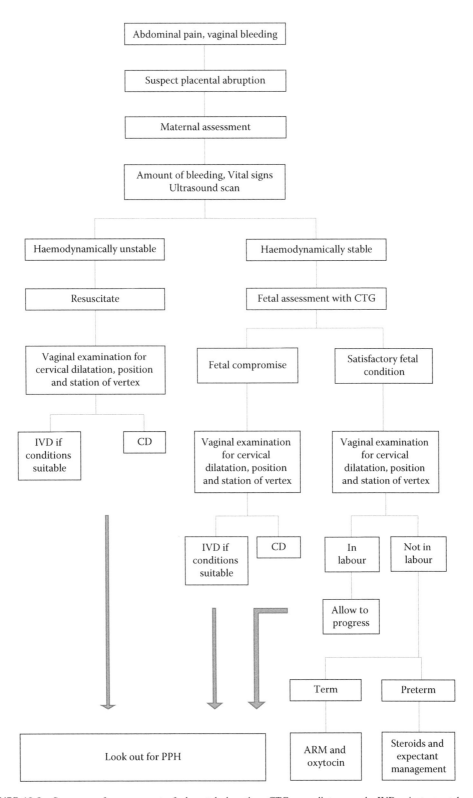

FIGURE 13.2 Summary of management of placental abruption; CTG – cardiotocograph, IVD – instrumental vaginal delivery, CD – caesarean delivery.

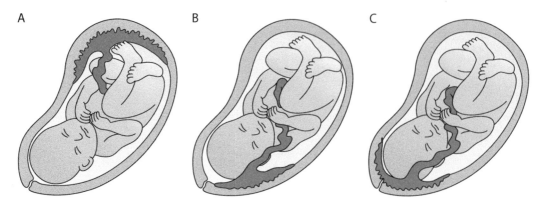

FIGURE 13.3   The classification of placental location; A – normal, B – low lying placenta, C – placenta praevia.

- Grade III (partial) - The edge of the placenta covers the internal os, but only partially when it is dilated
- Grade IV (complete or central) - The placenta completely covers the cervix even at full dilatation

Grades I and II constituted 'minor' placenta praevia, while grades III and IV constituted 'major' placenta praevia.

Clinical Features

Many women with placenta praevia are asymptomatic. However, as the lower segment of the uterus stretches during the latter part of pregnancy and during labour, the placenta implanted in this part of the uterus separates and may cause vaginal bleeding. Usually, the bleeding is painless, because there is little or no extravasation of blood into the uterine muscle, in contrast to a placental abruption. However, the woman could possibly be having labour pains. The initial bleed, known as the 'sentinel bleed', is usually mild and resolves spontaneously, but only to recur later. The uterus is usually soft and nontender unless the woman is in labour. The woman's haemodynamic status is in keeping with the amount of blood loss through the vagina. Coagulopathy is rare in placenta praevia. The presenting part of the fetus is usually high or there may be a malpresentation, as the placenta hinders the head from occupying the lower pole of the uterus and descending into the pelvis. These features should suggest the possibility of a placenta praevia or a low lying placenta even in the absence of bleeding. The fetus is generally not affected in placenta praevia. These features help to clinically differentiate between placenta praevia and placental abruption. However, many cases of placenta praevia may not have these typical features. There could be pain and significant blood loss even leading to maternal haemodynamic instability and fetal death.

Management

Prevention and treatment of anaemia (haemoglobin < 11 g/dl) during the antenatal period is important. The possible need for blood transfusion, midline skin incision, classical caesarean delivery and hysterectomy should be discussed with the woman during the antenatal period, and informed written consent must be obtained. A backup plan should be prepared for women who refuse transfusion of blood or blood products, e.g. Jehovah's Witnesses. Furthermore, digital vaginal examination which could provoke massive bleeding is contraindicated.

The management of placenta praevia or low lying placenta depends on the amount of bleeding, whether the bleeding is ongoing or it has stopped, the health of the woman and the fetus, the gestational age, the position of the placenta and the coexistence of PAS disorder. In case the woman presents with bleeding, a quick assessment should be made and resuscitation must be directed depending on the haemodynamic status of the woman. In case of haemodynamic instability, immediate caesarean delivery or hysterotomy should be performed following resuscitation and stabilisation of the woman. Delivery may be indicated if the woman is at or close to term or is in labour, even in the presence of haemodynamic stability. Anti D immunoglobulin should be administered in Rhesus negative women who present with vaginal bleeding in order to prevent Rhesus isoimmunisation, the dose being guided by the Kleihauer test.

Usually, the fetus is not affected unless the bleeding is severe. Perinatal mortality and morbidity are largely associated with preterm delivery which might be necessary for the management of placenta praevia. Antenatal corticosteroid therapy, used to improve fetal lung maturity, is indicated for women requiring delivery before 36 weeks of gestation. Tocolytics for 48 hours may be considered if the vaginal bleeding is mild in order to facilitate the administration of corticosteroids. However, continued tocolysis is not recommended for ongoing APH. Magnesium sulphate is advised for neuroprotection of the fetus in gestations that are less than 32 weeks.

Most minor bleeds will resolve spontaneously, and the majority of women can be managed expectantly until close to term. However, even the initial minor bleeds should be taken seriously, as there is a risk of a much larger bleed later on. These women may be discharged home after 2–3 days following admission in the absence of further bleeding, provided that there are safety precautions in place, including constant support at home and efficient access to a hospital. They should be advised against penetrative sexual intercourse and strenuous activities and should further be instructed to seek immediate help in case vaginal bleeding occurs/recurs.

Mode of Delivery

As discussed earlier, caesarean delivery should be performed in case of active bleeding. Caesarean delivery is generally recommended if the lower edge of the placenta is less than 20 mm from the internal os during the third trimester. However, the formation of the lower segment of the uterus and the associated placental migration is a dynamic process, and recent evidence suggests that the majority of women with a lower placental edge of more than 10 mm from the internal os can achieve a safe vaginal delivery with minimal bleeding. A practical point is that if the maximum diameter of the presenting part of the fetus is below the leading edge of the placenta, then there is a high success rate for vaginal delivery. In addition, if the placenta is anterior, the presenting part is likely to compress the bleeding placental bed against the pubic symphysis, creating a tamponade effect. However, this tamponade effect is less likely to happen if the placenta is posteriorly located.

As the lower segment continues to form during the third trimester and may allow further placental migration, awaiting spontaneous labour may be the most reasonable option for women in whom vaginal delivery is planned. In case induction of labour is needed, one should palpate through the vaginal fornices and exclude any intervening placenta between the fetal head and the lower segment of the uterus before proceeding to amniotomy. Vaginal prostaglandins may be used if there is a need to ripen the cervix, but an artificial separation of membranes or supracervical Foley catheter insertion should be avoided. Preparations should be in place to manage haemorrhage during labour, and an emergency caesarean delivery should be performed if bleeding ensues.

Caesarean Delivery

Preoperative Preparation

Placenta praevia or low-lying placenta in the presence of a uterine scar should alert the clinician with the possibility of PAS disorder, and this should be excluded by ultrasonography. Placental mapping is important in determining the skin and uterine incisions. The timing of delivery should be based on maternal symptoms, and it is recommended that if a caesarean delivery is planned, asymptomatic women with placenta praevia are delivered between 36 and 37 weeks of gestation, and those with a history of vaginal bleeding or at risk of preterm delivery are delivered between 34 and 37 weeks of gestation, after a course of antenatal corticosteroids. As the risk of massive obstetric haemorrhage is high, delivery should be arranged in a maternity unit with corresponding expertise in managing these cases, on site blood transfusion services as well as access to critical care.

Surgical Technique

Ideally, a consultant obstetrician and a consultant anaesthesiologist should attend the delivery. Regional anaesthesia is considered safer and is associated with a lower risk of haemorrhage compared to general anaesthesia. However, it may be necessary to switch to general anaesthesia if massive bleeding ensues following delivery. Crossmatched blood should be available, preferably in the operating theatre. The majority of cases can be managed with a suprapubic transverse skin incision and a transverse incision on the lower segment of the uterus. However, vertical skin and uterine incisions may be necessary in cases where the placenta extends towards the umbilicus. The possibility of PAS disorder, which may not have been diagnosed during the antenatal period, should be considered at every caesarean delivery for placenta praevia. If there is evidence of PAS disorder after the abdominal cavity has been opened, then surgery should be deferred until resources to manage massive haemorrhage are available.

The bladder should be adequately mobilised, and blood vessels in the line of the incision should be tied before making the incision on the uterus. Diathermy is usually not sufficient in controlling bleeding from these vessels. Malpresentation of the fetus should be prepared for. Incising the placenta must be avoided as much as possible. Once the uterine incision is made, it is advisable to go to the edge of the placenta, rupture the membranes and procure the presenting part through the incision. Oxytocics should be administered to cause contractions of the uterus. A combination of ergometrine 0.5 mg IV and oxytocin 5–10 units IV bolus injections, followed by a slow infusion of 20 units of oxytocin, may be used for this purpose. In the absence of active bleeding, delayed cord clamping should be followed by controlled cord traction to deliver the placenta. The uterus should have contracted by then, often with spontaneous separation of the placenta from its bed. Immediate clamping of the cord and delivery of the placenta by controlled cord traction are needed if there is active bleeding. If the placenta is not separated and delivered in 2–3 minutes, then a manual removal is required. This should be attempted only after uterine contractions have been established. Uterotonic agents should not be administered and manual removal of the placenta must not be attempted if there is suspicion of PAS disorder, as these may provoke uncontrollable bleeding.

Haemorrhage Following Delivery

As the lower segment of the uterus does not contract as well as the upper segment, bleeding from the placental site following delivery is common. Exteriorisation of the uterus and early administration of misoprostol, carboprost and tranexamic acid help to control the haemorrhage until definitive measures are utilised. Cell salvage should be considered, especially in women who refuse transfusion of blood or blood products. Uterine balloon tamponade, application of sutures to the placental bed, uterine compression sutures and devascularization and pelvic arterial embolisation should be used depending on available expertise (discussed in Chapters 14, 17 and 18). Early resort to hysterectomy is recommended if medical and conservative surgical procedures fail to control haemorrhage (discussed in Chapter 19). Total hysterectomy is recommended, as subtotal hysterectomy would not stop the bleeding from the lower segment of the uterus and the cervix.

Compression stockings should be used as prophylaxis against venous thromboembolism (VTE). The decision to administer low molecular weight heparin in the postpartum period after haemostasis has been achieved should be made by a consultant after considering the patient's risk profile for VTE.

Vaginal Delivery in Placenta Praevia in the Presence of Fetal Death or Lethal Fetal Abnormality

Vaginal delivery may sometimes be the most reasonable option to deliver a fetus that is either dead or bearing a lethal abnormality even in the presence of placenta praevia. This is usually done before 24 weeks of gestation after embolisation of internal iliac arteries, foeticide and induction of labour with a high dose vaginal misoprostol regimen. This practice will bypass the need for a hysterotomy, an operation that carries significant maternal morbidity as far as future obstetric performance is concerned. However, hysterotomy may possibly be performed for maternal safety if there is unacceptable bleeding. In countries where fetocide is illegal, women with placenta praevia in the presence of a lethal fetal abnormality are managed similarly as the case of a live viable fetus.

Vaginal Delivery in Cases of Placenta Praevia with Bleeding

In very low resource settings with no immediate access to operating theatre facilities, historical techniques of assisted vaginal delivery may have to be utilised in case of a low-lying placenta with bleeding in the presence of a dead, nonviable fetus or a lethal fetal abnormality, especially before 24 weeks of gestation. These techniques utilise the fetus to provide tamponade on the placenta and the lower segment of the uterus. Depending on the fetal presentation, there are two options available. In a breech presentation or a transverse lie, using one hand on the abdomen and the fingers of the other hand through the cervix, Braxton Hicks bipolar podalic version could be performed and traction may be applied on one foot which is brought out through the cervix, so that the fetal buttocks will not only provide tamponade against the placenta and the bleeding lower segment of the uterus but also act as an effective dilator of the cervix (Figure 13.4). If it is a cephalic presentation, then Willet's technique can be adopted by attaching an Allis tissue forceps or a multitoothed tenaculum to the fetal scalp and applying traction on it, so that the tamponade on the bleeding placental edge is provided by the fetal head itself (Figure 13.5). However, it is important to note that these techniques are unacceptable if the fetus is alive and normal.

The management of placenta praevia and low lying placenta is summarised in Figure 13.6.

Placenta Accreta Spectrum Disorders

'You cannot save the world, but you might save the woman in front of you if you act fast and diligently'.

The above statement is very much appropriate when it comes to the management of placenta accreta spectrum (PAS) disorder, one of the most devastating conditions ever encountered in obstetrics, where skill, speed and diligence on the part of the obstetric team play a pivotal role in the management. Placenta accreta spectrum disorders refer to abnormal invasion of part or all of the placenta into the myometrium or beyond (Figure 13.7). In these cases, any attempt at manual removal of the placenta can lead to massive haemorrhage due to the lack of a plane of cleavage between the placenta and the uterine wall. Furthermore, the most widely adopted treatment method for the condition, which is the caesarean hysterectomy, carries a considerable risk of serious maternal morbidity and mortality. Thankfully, conservative and expectant management options which mitigate hysterectomy-related complications are emerging. Inconsistencies in definition make an accurate estimation of global incidence difficult, but the incidence can be expected to increase in the future due to the escalating rates of caesarean delivery and assisted reproductive technology, as well as advanced maternal age.

Range of Placenta Accreta Spectrum Disorders

Placenta accreta spectrum disorders are subdivided, depending on the degree of trophoblastic invasion into the muscular layer of the uterus, as follows (Figure 13.8);

- Placenta accreta (placenta creta/vera/adherenta) – placenta invades the superficial myometrium without interposing decidual tissue
- Placenta increta – placenta invades the deeper myometrium

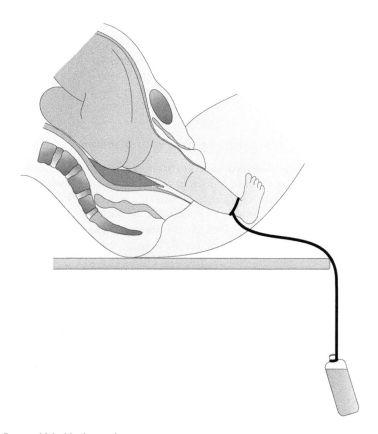

FIGURE 13.4   Braxton hicks bipolar version.

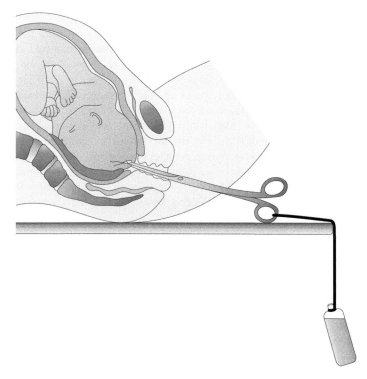

FIGURE 13.5   Willet's technique.

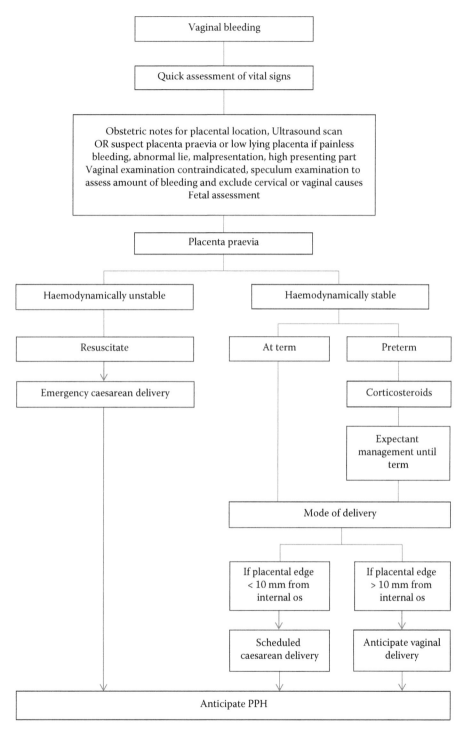

FIGURE 13.6 Summary of management of placenta praevia and low lying placenta.

- Placenta percreta – placenta invades through the serosal layer of the uterus to adjacent organs, most frequently the bladder

These subtypes may coexist in the same placental bed and evolve with advancing gestation.

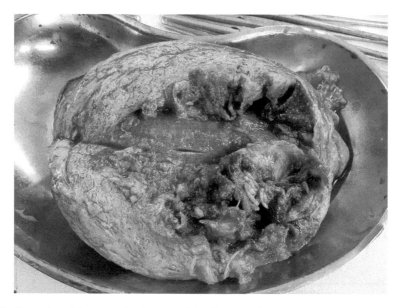

FIGURE 13.7   Cut section of the uterus showing part of the placenta which has invaded the myometrium.

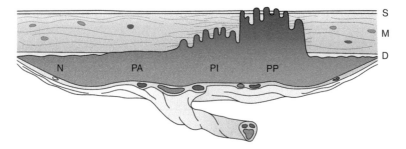

FIGURE 13.8   Types of placenta accreta spectrum disorders; N – Normal, PA – placenta accreta, PIE – placenta increta, PP – placenta percreta, S – serosa, M – myometrium, D - decidua.

Risk Factors for Placenta Accreta Spectrum Disorders

- History of accreta in a previous pregnancy
- Previous caesarean delivery (the risk increases with the number of caesarean deliveries)
- Previous myomectomy
- Previous surgery for correction of uterine anomaly
- Previous surgery for uterine perforation
- Repeated endometrial curettage
- Endometrial ablation
- Manual removal of placenta
- Endometritis

- Pregnancy following treatment of Asherman's syndrome
- Uterine artery embolisation
- Irradiation of the uterus
- Advanced maternal age
- Placenta praevia
- Caesarean scar pregnancy

What is common to all of these risk factors is that there is injury to the endometrium which transforms into the decidua during implantation. The pathogenesis is considered to be placental implantation at a site of defective decidualization caused by preexisting damage to the endometrial-myometrial interface. However, this hypothesis fails to explain the rare occurrence of PAS disorders in nulliparous women with no previous uterine surgery. The cellular changes in trophoblast observed in PAS disorders are probably secondary to the unusual myometrial environment in which it develops rather than a primary defect of trophoblast biology.

Diagnosis of Placenta Accreta Spectrum Disorders

Previous caesarean delivery or any other risk factor mentioned above and the presence of an anterior low lying placenta or placenta praevia should warn the clinician of the possibility of PAS disorder. Antenatal diagnosis is the key to planning management, because delivery in a tertiary level maternity care facility with the expertise and resources to manage PAS disorders considerably improves the outcome for both the woman and the fetus.

Women with PAS disorder may remain asymptomatic throughout pregnancy, even when the placenta has invaded surrounding structures. The invaded placenta does not usually lead to bleeding as long as it does not separate. Haematuria may be present in cases of placental invasion into the bladder. Rarely, uterine rupture has been reported in these cases (discussed in Chapter 16). Ultrasound complemented with colour Doppler studies is the most accurate and cost-effective method of diagnosing PAS disorders. The ultrasound features which are useful in the diagnosis of PAS disorders are;

- Loss of normal hypoechoic zone between the placenta and myometrium (Figure 13.9)
- Extreme thinning of the underlying myometrium (less than 1 mm)
- Multiple vascular lacunae within the placenta (Figure 13.10)
- Hypervascularity of placental bed
- Abnormalities of the uterine serosa-bladder interface
- Extension of placenta into myometrium, serosa or bladder

Once a primary diagnosis of PAS disorder has been made, the next priority is to assess the size and depth of placental invasion. This helps in predicting the difficulty of surgery and also prevents vascular, bladder and ureteric injury during surgery.

It is important to note that pressure from the ultrasound probe, full bladder or a 'uterine window' (defect in myometrium) may lead to an erroneous diagnosis of PAS disorder. At the same time, the absence of ultrasound features does not refute a diagnosis of PAS disorder. Therefore, clinical risk factors are equally as important as ultrasound features in predicting this condition.

Magnetic Resonance Imaging (MRI) scanning is not necessary when ultrasound is performed by an experienced sonographer. However, MRI allows the depth of placental invasion to be determined better when compared with colour Doppler ultrasound and may also have a place in identifying extrauterine placental tissue. It is particularly useful in cases of suspected lateral or posterior placental invasion.

However and as a final note, the definitive diagnosis can only be made clinically at delivery and should be confirmed by histopathology.

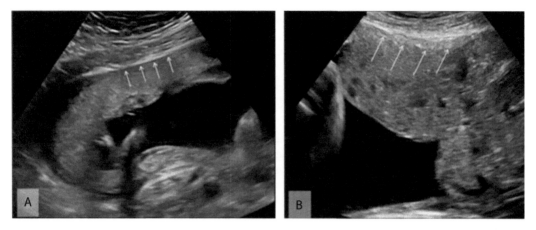

FIGURE 13.9   A – The normal hypoechoic zone between the placenta and the uterine wall, B – absence of retroplacental hypoechoic zone in PAS disorders. (Reproduced with permission from john wiley and sons. Berkley EM, Abuhamad AZ. Prenatal diagnosis of placenta accreta: Is sonography all we need? *J Ultrasound Med* 2013;32:1345–50.)

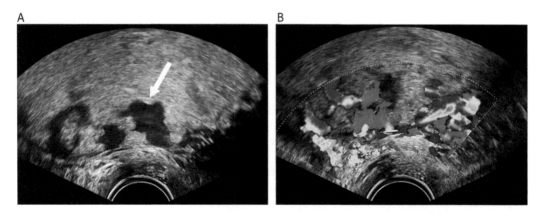

FIGURE 13.10   Ultrasound imaging showing the 'moth-eaten' appearance suggestive of placental lacunae in PAS disorders. A – greyscale imaging, B – colour doppler imaging. (Reproduced with permission from Elsevier. Jauniaux E, Collins S, Burton GJ. Placenta accreta spectrum: pathophysiology and evidence-based anatomy for prenatal ultrasound imaging. *Am J Obstet Gynecol* 2018;218(1):75–87.)

Management of Placenta Accreta Spectrum Disorders

The critical nature of the condition means that recommendations on the management of PAS disorders are not substantiated with well-designed, randomised clinical trials but are based on case series and reports, personal experience, expert opinion and good clinical judgement.

General

Ideally, women diagnosed with PAS disorder should be managed at a centre of excellence with the involvement of a number of clinical specialties. These include an obstetrician, an obstetric anaesthesiologist, a transfusion medicine specialist, a gynaeoncological surgeon, a vascular surgeon, a urological surgeon, a critical care specialist, an interventional radiologist and a neonatologist, depending on the unique demands of the clinical situation. There should be round-the-clock access to a blood bank that is capable of employing massive transfusion protocols (discussed in Chapter 14). Women diagnosed with PAS disorder, a condition that carries a considerable risk of serious morbidity and mortality, need continuous support and reassurance throughout the antenatal period. Haemoglobin should be optimised during the antenatal period. Women who refuse blood or blood product transfusion, e.g. Jehovah's Witnesses, require special considerations.

Timing of Delivery

The optimal timing of delivery remains uncertain, but delivery between 34 and 36 weeks of gestation has been proposed as the timeframe balancing prematurity and the risk of emergency delivery which is associated with more complications than an elective delivery. Antenatal corticosteroids should be considered for lung maturation of the fetus. Administration of magnesium sulphate for neuroprotection of fetus is recommended if delivery is planned before 32 weeks of gestation.

Preoperative Preparation

Women diagnosed with PAS disorder should be counselled about the possibility of haemorrhage and the need for blood transfusion, midline skin incision, hysterectomy or tubal ligation and admission to the intensive care unit, and informed written consent must be obtained. Preoperative or intraoperative placental mapping using ultrasonography is instrumental in planning the skin and uterine incisions. The placement of endovascular catheters or balloon catheters in the anterior division of the internal iliac arteries should be contemplated so that these vessels can be occluded in the event of massive intraoperative haemorrhage. However, these methods are associated with vessel rupture and thromboembolic complications and may even exacerbate bleeding from the collateral circulation. The alternative is to ligate these vessels at surgery as a prophylactic or therapeutic measure. Internal iliac artery ligation has the advantage of being available in resource-poor settings. Some advocate placing a 3-way urinary catheter in preparation for testing of bladder integrity by intraoperative methylene blue dye injection, as well as ureteric stents to identify the ureters in cases of suspected lateral extension of the placenta. During ureteric stent placement, cystoscopy can identify bladder invasion by the placenta. A bed in the intensive care unit should be reserved for cases of PAS disorder.

Caesarean Delivery

Blood warmers, rapid infusion sets and crossmatched blood (4–6 units) should be available in the operating theatre, in preparation for massive transfusion. Instruments needed for caesarean hysterectomy and internal iliac artery ligation should be ready (discussed in Chapters 18 and 19). Although regional anaesthesia is safer and associated with a reduced risk of haemorrhage as compared to general anaesthesia, the majority of surgeries are performed under general anaesthesia. Placing the woman in Lloyd Davis position allows intraoperative assessment of blood loss through the vagina, but this is done at the discretion of the operator. At laparotomy, skin and uterine incisions that would avoid transecting the placenta should be used. A generous low transverse skin incision may be used if the anterior part of the placenta does not reach the upper segment of the uterus. An incision at the rectus sheath curving upwards enables access to the myometrium above the upper border of the placenta in the majority of cases (Figure 13.11).

If the placenta is anterior and extends further upwards, then a midline skin incision may be necessary. Dissection of the bladder first before the delivery of the fetus allows the creation of the vesicouterine plane before bleeding ensues. Bladder dissection is performed by sharp incision inwards from the round ligaments and by using traction and counter traction. It is important to mobilise the bladder as much as possible in anticipation of caesarean hysterectomy which might be necessary in the event of massive bleeding following delivery of the fetus (Figure 13.12). Newly formed vessels may be found between the posterior bladder wall and the invaded placenta, and it is prudent to ligate these vessels rather than to use electrocoagulation (Figure 13.13). The assistance of a urological surgeon may be required in cases of placenta percreta in which the placenta has invaded into the bladder.

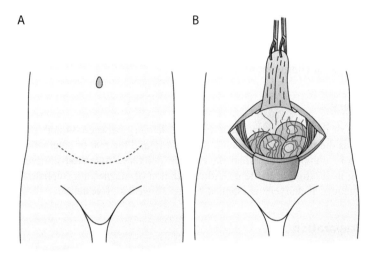

FIGURE 13.11 Transverse incisions on the skin and the rectus sheath.

The uterus may be opened by a transverse incision while avoiding the placenta. In the case of an anteriorly located placenta, the uterine incision may possibly be made in the fundal region. The fetus is then delivered, and the umbilical cord is subsequently clamped. Once the fetus is delivered, separating the abnormally adhered or invaded placenta, which can provoke catastrophic bleeding, should be averted. Uterotonic agents can cause partial separation of the placenta and increase the risk of bleeding, and therefore, should be avoided unless the placenta separates completely from the uterine wall.

Following the delivery of the fetus, three options are available. Caesarean hysterectomy is the most widely accepted and may possibly be the only option available in case of torrential bleeding in these

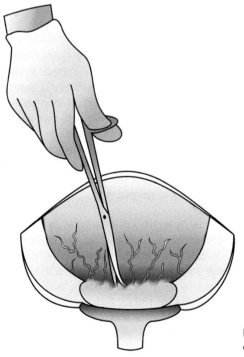

FIGURE 13.12 Bladder dissection in placenta accreta spectrum disorders.

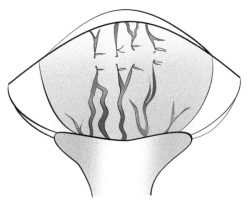

FIGURE 13.13 Ligation of blood vessels between the posterior bladder wall and the invaded placenta.

cases. In recent years, there has been a growing interest in the second option of conservative management, where the affected area is excised, and the uterus conserved after repair of the deficit in order to minimise caesarean hysterectomy-related maternal complications and also to preserve the uterus when future fertility is desired. The third option is expectant management, in which case the placenta is left in situ. The decision when to use each of these management strategies is based, in large part, on the experience of the operator.

Caesarean Hysterectomy

Caesarean hysterectomy, the most widely accepted method of treatment for PAS disorders, may probably be the only option available in case of torrential bleeding in these instances, as discussed earlier. Ironically, hysterectomy itself may lead to uncontrollable bleeding. Caesarean hysterectomy in the setting of PAS disorders is one of the most challenging surgeries due to the presence of intra-abdominal adhesions, a thin, hypervascular and fragile lower segment, pelvic neovascularization, bulky in situ placenta (Figure 13.14) and the invasion of the placenta into bladder, bowel and parametrium. The surgical risks heighten with the depth of placental invasion. In most cases, total hysterectomy is required as the lower segment is usually involved, and subtotal hysterectomy is not sufficient to control bleeding from this site.

Continuous dialogue between the operator/s, the anaesthesiologist and the nursing staff, as well as attention to blood loss, haemoglobin, electrolytes and coagulation parameters are pivotal in ensuring the safety of the woman. Transfusion of blood and blood products can be guided by rotational thromboelastometry, if this is available. The use of an autologous cell saver is also an option, and this reduces the need for allogenic blood transfusion without any adverse sequelae. The antifibrinolytic agent, tranexamic acid 1 g IV should be administered early, but its function as a prophylactic agent against haemorrhage in PAS disorders has not been proven. It is imperative to keep the patient warm, because many clotting factors work poorly in the presence of hypothermia. Manual aortic compression (just above the bifurcation of the aorta, with compression released every 30 minutes) can be utilised to control haemorrhage until hysterectomy is completed (discussed in Chapter 14).

Bladder Injury

The bladder is quite prone to injury in PAS disorders. In case of bladder injury, the edges should be freshened and the bladder must be repaired in two layers using an absorbable suture. If the injury is close to the ureteric orifices, then infant feeding tubes or JJ stents can be placed within the ureters to avoid incorporating the ureters into the repair. Following the reconstruction, the integrity of the bladder can be confirmed by infusing methylene blue into the bladder. Placing an omental flap over the bladder will help to reduce the risk of vesicovaginal fistula. The urinary catheter should be kept for 14 days in

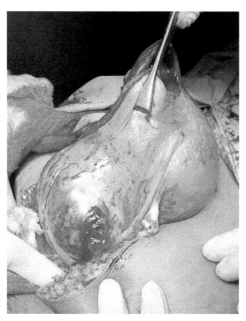

FIGURE 13.14 Bulging of the lower segment due to the placenta. Note the rupture on the right side of the uterus.

the postoperative period. In cases of dense bladder adhesions and in whom bladder dissection is extremely difficult, an intentional cystostomy and subsequent repair may have to be performed.

Postoperative Management

Women with PAS disorders are at an increased risk of secondary haemorrhage, fluid overload, multiorgan damage and VTE in the postpartum period, and therefore, should be managed in an intensive care unit in a multidisciplinary setting. Having experienced the antenatal period with a condition that carries a considerable risk of morbidity and mortality and only to end up with hysterectomy is an exceptionally traumatic experience, and these women should be provided with extensive debriefing. Debriefing of all of the involved staff and accurate documentation are important.

Conservative Management

Conservative management refers to resection of the invasive accreta area (partial myometrial resection) followed by immediate uterine reconstruction (Figure 13.15). This may be appropriate in cases in which the entire placental implantation site is easily accessible (anterior or posterior), and the area of placental invasion is limited in depth and surface area. Once the fetus is delivered following an incision on the uterus while steering clear of the placenta, the uterus is exteriorised. Next, the posterior side of the bladder is dissected. Then, the placenta with the invaded myometrium is removed in one piece. Local haemostatic agents and uterine compression sutures can be applied in order to achieve haemostasis. Once haemostasis has been achieved, the myometrial defect is repaired in two layers of continuous sutures. Additional mattress sutures may be required if the defect is large and an approximation of the cut edges of the uterus is difficult, or if the defect extends considerably to the upper segment. If mattress sutures are deemed necessary, then 3–4 mattress sutures are applied, and their free ends merely held together, instead of tied together, using artery forceps. Afterward, the myometrial defect is repaired using two layers of continuous sutures. Finally, the free ends of the mattress sutures are tied together. Lastly, the bladder should be repaired if necessary.

Another conservative technique described is the 'Triple P procedure', which comprises of *p*erioperative placental localisation and the delivery of the fetus via a transverse uterine incision above the

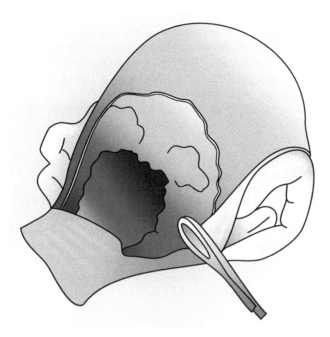

FIGURE 13.15   The defect on the uterus after performing myometrial excision.

upper border of the placenta; *p*elvic devascularization with temporary occlusive balloon catheters in the anterior division of the internal iliac arteries; and *p*lacental nonseparation with myometrial excision and reconstruction of the uterine wall. Modifications of the 'Triple P procedure', such as temporary clamping or ligation of the anterior division of internal iliac arteries, have been tried in centres with no access to interventional radiology. Uterine balloon tamponade has also been used successfully to control bleeding in these cases.

There are substantial complications associated with conservative management. As the uterus is highly vascularised, there may be massive haemorrhage, particularly in cases of lateral implantation of the placenta. When the excision is wide, the approximation of the cut edges will be difficult, leaving room for the formation of a uterine window. In addition, extensive damage to the myometrium increases the risk of scar dehiscence or uterine rupture in subsequent pregnancies.

Expectant Management

In expectant management, the uterine incision is made circumventing the placenta; the cord is ligated and cut near the placental insertion; the whole placenta is left in situ; and the uterine and skin incisions are closed. On the other hand, an attempt may be made to gently remove the placenta in cases of false-positive prenatal diagnosis and lack of clinical evidence of PAS disorder at caesarean delivery. Expectant management is particularly important in cases of lateral parametrial invasion with possible involvement of the ureters or internal iliac vessels with the potential to bleed heavily at hysterectomy.

The success rate and outcome following expectant management depend on the degree of placental invasiveness, both in-depth and laterally. A significant proportion of these women may require an emergency hysterectomy in order to control haemorrhage. These women should be followed up in a centre of excellence with immediate access to the operating theatre, blood bank and expertise in managing these cases. Prophylactic antibiotics (e.g. oral co-amoxiclav) should be administered. Furthermore, they should be counselled about the risk of bleeding and sepsis and advised on immediate admission in case they develop abdominal pain, fever, vaginal bleeding or vaginal discharge. It is important to note that the period of resolution is variable, and this may last several months. Follow-up visits should be arranged weekly during the first two months, and once every two weeks, thereafter. Resorption of the placenta left in situ is assessed by β-hCG levels, size of the placental mass and uteroplacental arterial circulation. Complete placental resorption may not have occurred even when β-hCG has decreased to negligible levels. The follow-up should also include an assessment of the haematological profile for coagulopathy and for infection (e.g. full blood count, C reactive protein, prothrombin time/INR, activated partial thromboplastin time).

Although expectant management appears to have a minimal effect on subsequent fertility, with nearly a quarter of women subsequently becoming pregnant, it does carry a high recurrence risk of PAS disorder.

Adjuvant Therapy in Expectant Management

Although methotrexate has been used as an adjuvant therapy to expectant management, it is not re-commended because it has unproven benefits. In addition, methotrexate acts on dividing cells, and the placental cells no longer divide following delivery. Furthermore, it is associated with neutropaenia which increases the risk of sepsis in these cases, and it is contraindicated in breastfeeding. Routine hysteroscopic resection of placental remnants is also not advised. Also, the benefit of delayed interval hysterectomy is uncertain, although the blood loss in this case is considerably less than that at hys-terectomy performed at the time of caesarean delivery.

Unexpected Diagnosis of Placenta Accreta Spectrum Disorder

Placenta accreta spectrum disorders remain undiagnosed before delivery in half to two-thirds of cases. If the possibility of PAS disorder has been unanticipated and is discovered at laparotomy, caesarean delivery should be deferred until expertise to deal with massive haemorrhage is available and pre-parations have been made to deal with such an eventuality. In case expertise is inaccessible on-site, stabilisation, closing the abdomen and transfer to a facility equipped with the resources to deal with PAS disorders should be considered, provided both maternal and fetal conditions are satisfactory. The possibility of PAS disorder should be suspected in cases of a retained placenta following vaginal delivery, and preparations should be made to deal with haemorrhage before manual removal is attempted.

Vasa Praevia

Similar to placenta praevia, the term 'vasa praevia' is used when vessels lie before the fetus in the birth canal. These vessels traversing the free placental membranes are unprotected by placental tissue or Wharton's jelly of the umbilical cord and are prone to rupture during labour or at amniotomy, parti-cularly when located over or near the cervix. Vasa praevia is classified as type I when the vessels are connected to a velamentous umbilical cord, and type II when the vessels connect the placenta to a succenturiate (accessory) lobe (Figure 13.16). Risk factors for vasa praevia include a low-lying placenta, multiple pregnancy and in vitro fertilisation. Although rare, with an incidence between 1 in 1,200 to 1 in 5,000 pregnancies, it bears a 60% fetal mortality rate, as rapid fetal exsanguination can occur following rupture of these vessels.

Clinical Features

Vasa praevia usually presents with painless vaginal bleeding at the rupture of membranes, either spontaneous or artificial (Figure 13.17). As the blood lost is that of the fetus', fetal distress can be severe. As the blood volume in the fetus is 80–100 ml/kg, loss of even a seemingly small amount of blood may have major implications for the fetus. The presence of painless vaginal bleeding and acute fetal compromise immediately following spontaneous or artificial rupture of membranes should give

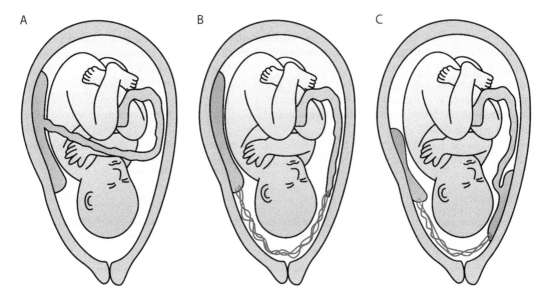

FIGURE 13.16   Vasa praevia; A – normal placenta, B – type I vasa praevia, C – Type II vasa praevia.

heed of the possibility of vasa praevia. Sometimes, the fetal derived blood vessels may be felt pulsating on the membranes prior to amniotomy, in which case amniotomy should be immediately abandoned.

Diagnosis

A diagnosis of vasa praevia is seldom made during the antenatal period. A combination of transabdominal and transvaginal colour Doppler imaging ultrasonography is the most accurate method of detecting vasa praevia in the antenatal period. However, there is insufficient evidence to support routine screening for vasa praevia at the mid-trimester anomaly scan.

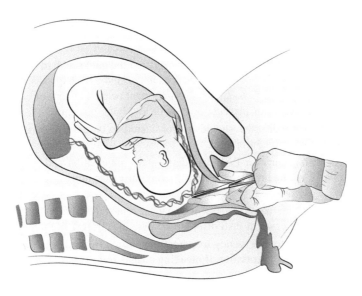

FIGURE 13.17   Vaginal bleeding at amniotomy.

The differential diagnosis includes placental abruption and cord presentation. The fetal blood is usually a darker red colour, and this helps in differentiating between vasa praevia and placental abruption. In cases of doubt, the rapid bedside 'Apt test' which detects fetal haemoglobin can be used to aid the diagnosis of vasa praevia. The process starts with adding a few drops of blood to 10 ml of 0.1% sodium hydroxide. Adult haemoglobin will turn brown within 30 seconds, while fetal haemoglobin, which is resistant to denaturation by alkali, will remain pink. However, in case of bleeding which can be detrimental to the fetus, the diagnosis of vasa praevia is made clinically and treatment should be instituted without delay.

The diagnosis should be confirmed by pathological examination of the placenta, particularly when stillbirth has occurred or there has been sudden fetal compromise during delivery.

Management

In the event of rupture of vasa praevia, immediate caesarean delivery should be performed to prevent fetal death. Following delivery, the neonate should be resuscitated, which includes transfusion of blood to treat hypovolaemic shock.

When vasa praevia has been diagnosed during the antenatal period, elective caesarean delivery should be carried out prior to the onset of labour, while minimising the impact of iatrogenic prematurity. In these cases, delivery is usually performed between 34 and 36 weeks of gestation, after a course of antenatal steroids has been considered. Early delivery is indicated if these women present in labour or with rupture of membranes. Women with a history of vaginal bleeding or with risk factors for preterm delivery may need to receive in-ward care from 30–32 weeks of gestation. Fetoscopic laser ablation of vasa praevia vessels is also an option in antenatally diagnosed cases.

Key Points

- Immediate resuscitation and stabilisation should be the priority in haemodynamically unstable women presenting with APH, irrespective of the diagnosis.
- Vaginal delivery may be feasible in cases of placental abruption or an anterior low lying placenta, provided that both the maternal and fetal conditions are suitable.
- Caesarean delivery is necessary in cases of haemodynamic instability, fetal compromise, placenta praevia, low lying placenta (with the leading edge less than 10 mm from the internal os) and PAS disorders.
- Postpartum haemorrhage should be anticipated in all cases of APH.
- Although ultrasound with colour Doppler is considered the gold standard in the diagnosis of PAS disorders, the absence of ultrasound features does not exclude the diagnosis. The diagnosis should be suspected on clinical risk factors, the most important being a history of one or more caesarean deliveries and the presence of placenta praevia or low lying placenta.
- The possibility of PAS disorder should be considered in cases of retained placenta in which manual removal is not straightforward.
- The essence of management of PAS disorders entails anticipation and preparation for massive haemorrhage, and taking necessary steps to minimise haemorrhage or haemorrhage-related complications.
- Placental transection, uterotonic agents and manual removal of placenta should be avoided in diagnosed or suspected cases of PAS disorder, as these may trigger life-threatening haemorrhage.
- There is no alternative to emergency hysterectomy which by itself carries a considerable risk of maternal morbidity and mortality, if bleeding ensues following delivery of the fetus in PAS disorders.
- Conservative and expectant management options are emerging as an alternative to caesarean

hysterectomy, mainly to alleviate the hysterectomy-related complications and also to preserve fertility, but these strategies are also associated with serious complications.

- The diagnosis of vasa praevia is clinically made when there are painless vaginal bleeding and acute fetal compromise following the rupture of membranes.

BIBLIOGRAPHY

1. Society of Gynecologic Oncology, American College of Obstetricians and Gynecologists and the Society for Maternal–fetal Medicine. Cahill AG, Beigi R, Heine RP, Silver RM, Wax JR. Placenta Accreta Spectrum. *Am J Obstet Gynecol* 2018;219(6):B2–16.
2. FIGO Placenta Accreta Diagnosis and Management Expert Consensus Panel. FIGO consensus guidelines on placenta accreta spectrum disorders. *Int J Gynecol Obstet* 2018;140(3):261–98.
3. Jauniaux E, Alfirevic Z, Bhide AG, Belfort MA, Burton GJ, Collins SL, Dornan S, Jurkovic D, Kayem G, Kingdom J, Silver R, Sentilhes L, Royal College of Obstetricians and Gynaecologists. Placenta praevia and placenta accreta: diagnosis and management: Green top Guideline No. 27a. *BJOG* 2019; 126(1):e1–48.
4. Oppenheimer L. Society of Obstetricians and Gynecologists of Canada Clinical. Practice Guideline: Diagnosis and Management of Placenta Previa. *J Obstet Gynecol Can* 2007;29:261–66.

14

Primary Postpartum Haemorrhage

Sanjeewa Padumadasa and Malik Goonewardene

Postpartum haemorrhage (PPH) is the leading cause of maternal deaths in countries with limited resources, and it is a notable reason for maternal deaths in well-resourced countries as well. It is responsible for a quarter of maternal deaths occurring worldwide and is associated with considerable maternal morbidity, such as multiple blood transfusions, peripartum hysterectomy and multiorgan failure. Almost all deaths due to PPH are considered avertible by the adoption of appropriate interventions for women with risk factors for PPH, as well as anticipation, early detection and appropriate management of bleeding following childbirth.

As a normal delivery can result in a blood loss of up to about 300 mL, primary PPH has traditionally been defined as bleeding from the genital tract in excess of 500 mL within 24 hours of vaginal delivery. However, in clinical practice, there are many variations for this cut-off point and what is considered as 'heavy' blood loss. Some define it as a blood loss of 600 mL for a normal delivery and 750 mL for a caesarean delivery. Others recommend a cut-off of 1,000 mL loss for a caesarean delivery, which is probably rather high except for overweight or obese women. Small women who have a corresponding smaller blood volume as compared to average-sized women, as well as women who are already anaemic, may not endure a blood loss of as little as 500 mL. Therefore, primary PPH could be defined as a blood loss exceeding 500 mL, or any smaller blood loss which causes haemodynamic changes in the woman, within 24 hours of delivery. It has been suggested that blood losses should be estimated at three time periods, i.e. 'at the time of birth', 'after the delivery of the placenta until up to 24 hours', and 'at the time of birth until up to 24 hours'. 'Severe primary PPH' is defined as clinically estimated or measured blood loss that is equal to or greater than 1,000 mL at the time of birth. It would also be prudent to consider any blood loss in excess of 2,000 mL as being 'very severe'. Because of the practical difficulties in measuring blood loss accurately, along with frequent underestimation of it after delivery, a fall in the haematocrit by 10% and the requirement for a blood transfusion have also been suggested as retrospective definitions.

The uterine blood flow may comprise up to 10% of cardiac output at term, and this places the woman at risk of life-threatening haemorrhage unless blood loss is rapidly curtailed. Although maternal physiological adaptations such as an increased blood volume, increased efficiency of clotting and impaired fibrinolysis allow some degree of compensation following blood loss in pregnancy or after delivery, hypovolaemic shock can occur in instances of excessive bleeding.

Causes of Primary Postpartum Haemorrhage

The four Ts mnemonic can be used to recognise the causes of primary PPH (Table 14.1).

The main mechanism of arresting blood loss following delivery is the 'living ligatures' mechanism, where contraction and retraction (permanent shortening) of the uterine muscle fibres, which are arranged in a criss-cross pattern, cause compression of the uteroplacental blood vessels that lie between them. This is vital as the normal uteroplacental vessels are refractory to vasoactive substances, and these also have a poor ability to undergo intrinsic vasoconstriction, as they lack an effective musculo-elastic media

TABLE 14.1

Causes of primary postpartum haemorrhage

Tone – uterine atony

Trauma – of any part of the genital tract which includes genital tract lacerations, haematomas, rupture of uterus and an inverted uterus

Tissue – retained placenta, placenta accreta spectrum disorders

Thrombin – coagulopathy

---

due to the normal extra-embryonic trophoblastic invasion of the spiral arterioles. The 'living ligatures' are supplemented by other haemostatic mechanisms, such as platelet aggregation and clot formation.

Uterine Atony

Anything that interferes with the ability of the uterus to contract and retract, causes uterine atony, the most common cause of primary PPH, and accounts for 80%–85% of cases. Risk factors for uterine atony are listed in Table 14.2. However, the majority of cases of uterine atony occur in women with no risk factors. Therefore, primary PPH is largely unpredictable, and every birth attendant should be able to adopt appropriate preventive measures, anticipate and detect excessive bleeding early on and quickly commence appropriate initial management, if it indeed occurs.

TABLE 14.2

Risk factors for uterine atony

Multiparity

Overdistension of uterus

    Multiple pregnancy

    Polyhydramnios

    Fetal macrosomia

Abnormal labour

    Induced labour

    Prolonged labour

    Precipitate labour

Intraamniotic infection

Antepartum haemorrhage

    Placenta praevia (the lower segment does not contract as well as the upper segment following delivery)

    Placental abruption resulting in a *Couvelaire uterus* (blood which has seeped into myometrial tissue interferes with contraction of the uterus)

Anatomic distortion of uterus

    Uterine fibroids

    Congenital anomalies of the uterus

Material inside the uterine cavity

    Retained placental fragments

    Blood clots

Medication

    Tocolytics

    General anaesthetic agents such as fluorinated hydrocarbons

History of uterine atony in previous pregnancies

Genital Tract Trauma

This is the second most common cause of PPH, and multiple sites of bleeding may coexist. Causes of genital tract trauma include.

- Lacerations in the perineum, vagina and cervix
- Episiotomy
- Paravaginal and broad ligament haematomas
- Extension of uterine incision, especially at second stage caesarean delivery (discussed in Chapter 11)
- Uterine rupture (discussed in Chapter 16)
- Acute uterine inversion (discussed in Chapter 21)

Abnormalities in Tissue

These include retained placenta and placenta accreta spectrum (PAS) disorders and are extensively discussed in Chapters 20 and 13 respectively.

Abnormalities in Thrombin

These include inherited coagulation disorders, secondary coagulopathies including disseminated intravascular coagulation (DIC) and the use of anticoagulants. Inherited coagulation disorders do not contribute significantly to primary PPH, because the main mechanism of arresting bleeding following delivery is the contraction of the uterus. In addition, the changes in the coagulation system which occur during pregnancy favour blood clotting. However, women with inherited coagulation disorders may present with secondary PPH (discussed in Chapter 15).

Disseminated intravascular coagulation which can rapidly lead to massive bleeding is characterised by the following.

- Widespread intravascular coagulation, which results in depletion of the clotting factors in the circulation
- Formation of vascular occlusive thrombi within the body, which in turn leads to multiorgan dysfunction
- Fibrinolysis which destabilises the clots that are formed

Severe pre-eclampsia, amniotic fluid embolism, sepsis and intrauterine fetal demise are associated with DIC. Furthermore, prolonged blood loss and hypovolaemia leading to tissue hypoxia can also result in DIC.

Excessive administration of crystalloids and colloids and failure to replace the coagulation factors which would have been lost as a result of a heavy blood loss can lead to a dilution of coagulation factors and platelets. This results in a 'dilutional coagulopathy' and continued bleeding. Administration of solely packed red cells which lack coagulation factors and platelets may also give rise to a coagulopathy. In placental abruption, a 'consumptive coagulopathy', with an aggregation of clotting factors at the placental site, probably in an attempt by the body to stop the bleeding and save the fetus, leads to a generalised depletion of coagulation factors, which in turn may result in profuse bleeding elsewhere.

Prevention of Primary Postpartum Haemorrhage

Antepartum and intrapartum risk factors which could lead to a PPH should be given due consideration, and appropriate interventions must be adopted. It is important to screen for and treat anaemia during the antenatal period, because this can reduce the morbidity associated with PPH. Every woman's blood group and Rhesus status should be recorded in her case notes before the onset of labour. Adequate amounts of blood should be crossmatched and prepared prior to the delivery of a woman with a high risk of PPH. Ultrasonography to detect placenta praevia and PAS disorders and planning for delivery when there is abnormal placentation are important (discussed in Chapter 13). Women who decline transfusion of blood or blood products are particularly at risk of mortality or serious morbidity in case PPH occurs. Therefore, arrangements must be made for uterine artery embolisation and cell salvage for such women.

Active management of the third stage of labour (AMTSL), which currently includes the administration of a uterotonic agent immediately after the delivery of the baby, delayed cord clamping (unless there is active bleeding that requires attention, the need for neonatal intubation and ventilation or Rhesus iso-immunisation) and delivery of the placenta by controlled cord traction once the uterus contracts reduce the risk of PPH compared to expectant management. Oxytocin, ergometrine or a combination of 5 units of oxytocin and 0.5 mg of ergometrine, can be used for this purpose. Oxytocin is the drug of choice and is given as a dose of 5–10 units intravenously (IV) or by intramuscular (IM) injection. It is associated with a lower risk of an entrapped placenta than with ergometrine, which is administered as a dose of 0.5 mg IV or IM. Ergometrine or the combination of oxytocin and ergometrine, should not be used in AMTSL for women with hypertension. Although carboprost and sulprostone should not be used, 400–600 µg of oral misoprostol could be used for AMTSL. Uterotonic agents should not be administered if there is any suspicion of PAS disorder, because partial separation of the placenta may lead to catastrophic bleeding (discussed in Chapter 13). Early cord clamping, which was formerly included in AMTSL, is no longer recommended, because this is a precursor to increased anaemia and iron deficiency in the infant compared to delayed cord clamping, especially in preterm deliveries. Routine uterine massage after the delivery of the baby, which was originally included in AMTSL, is also no longer advised, as it is of little value if the uterus has contracted significantly. However, it is a very effective, initial measure that complements uterotonics in controlling haemorrhage from an atonic uterus.

Intravenous tranexamic acid (0.5–1 g) should be given to women who have a high risk of developing PPH and are undergoing caesarean delivery. An IV infusion of 20 units of oxytocin in 500 mL of normal saline, at 125 mL/hour, should be administered following delivery in women with a high risk of PPH.

As primary PPH is largely unpredictable, all women should ideally give birth in a hospital. Although this may not reduce the incidence of PPH, early measures can be taken to manage the condition. Early breastfeeding, which stimulates the release of oxytocin, is a simple measure that aids uterine contractions and reduces the risk of uterine atony.

Early Recognition of Postpartum Haemorrhage

Assessment of ongoing blood loss is an important aspect of management in every woman after delivery. Early identification of bleeding allows timely intervention which is pivotal in improving the outcome. However, there is no ideal method used to clinically measure the blood loss accurately. Visual estimation, which is the most convenient method done to assess blood loss, is unreliable and usually leads to underestimations. In a vaginal delivery, the weighing of drapes, pads and swabs before and after use (gravimetric method) or the collection of blood into a plastic drape placed under the woman's buttocks (volumetric method) are more accurate, but an amount of amniotic fluid will invariably be included in the estimation. Estimating blood loss after a caesarean delivery is also challenging due to contamination with liquor, and significant overestimations may occur. Therefore, direct measurements of spilled blood and sucker bottle volumes, and weighing the towels and drapes before and after use (combined method), can be used after a caesarean delivery.

Assessing the uterine size and its tone is essential. A well-contracted uterus is firm and should be below the level of the umbilicus. Massive bleeding is easily recognised. However, the trickling of blood may easily be mistaken for lochia and remain unrecognised. A change in vital signs should prompt a thorough assessment of blood loss, including possibly concealed haemorrhage, e.g. uterine rupture and broad ligament haematoma. Rarely, the bleeding may be of non-genital tract origin, e.g. ruptured spleen, ruptured splenic artery, ruptured hepatic artery.

The Modified Early Obstetric Warning Score (MEOWS) chart facilitates postpartum monitoring and allows the early recognition of any deterioration of the woman's condition, so that appropriate intervention can be instituted. It is important to note that, due to the physiological changes of pregnancy, vital parameters may remain in the normal range for a pregnancy until a significant amount of blood has been lost from the body. Although a rule of 100 (pulse > 100/minute and a systolic blood pressure < 100 mmHg) and a shock index (pulse/systolic blood pressure) of ≥1 are often considered as indicators of severe blood loss, isolated maternal tachycardia could be the first sign of a severe blood loss, and this must not be overlooked.

Identification and Treatment of the Cause

While resuscitation is taking place, two practical points to be initially considered are, 'Is the placenta delivered and if so, is it complete?' and 'Did the bleeding start immediately after the delivery of the baby?'. If the bleeding started during or immediately after the delivery of the baby, then the likelihood of genital tract tears is high.

If the placenta is not delivered, then manual removal of the placenta should be carried out promptly while under cover of a narcotic analgesic or anaesthesia, depending on the feasibility (described in Chapter 20). If the placenta is not complete, then the uterine cavity should be explored for any remaining placental parts. If there is suspicion of PAS disorder, then no attempt should be made to remove the placenta or placental parts, as this may lead to catastrophic bleeding.

Management of Uterine Atony

Uterine atony is the most common cause of PPH and is suggested by a soft, relaxed uterus. Therefore, initial management of PPH should involve measures to stimulate myometrial contractions.

Fundal Massage

Fundal massage, which is the first step in managing uterine atony, should be applied with circular movements of the left hand on the fundus of the uterus. Only gentle rubbing is needed to initiate uterine contractions. Vigorous rubbing is unnecessary and could possibly even be counterproductive. Blood clots within the lower uterine segment, the cervical canal and in the vagina should be simultaneously removed with the index and middle fingers of the right hand in the vagina (Figure 14.1). If these blood clots are not removed, then the uterus would not be able to contract adequately, in spite of high and repeated doses of uterotonics. It is important to identify the uterine fundus carefully in obese women because a roll of abdominal fat may be mistaken for the uterus. A two-handed technique of applying fundal massage is also described.

Emptying of the Bladder

A urinary catheter should be inserted in order to drain the bladder, as a full bladder may inhibit uterine contractions. This also allows the urine output to be measured accurately.

Uterotonic Agents, in a Stepwise Manner

Unless the woman is hypertensive, a bolus dose of IV ergometrine 0.5 mg or a combination of 5 units of oxytocin and 0.5 mg of ergometrine should be the first-line therapeutic uterotonic used in a woman who has a PPH following AMTSL. This should be immediately followed by an IV infusion of 40 units of oxytocin in 500 mL of normal saline over four hours. In the majority of cases of mild atonic PPH, these two interventions combined with continued uterine massage would suffice. If the bleeding is not completely controlled by these methods within five minutes, then rectal or sublingual misoprostol 800 μg, or carboprost 0.25 mg IM or intramyometrially should be added. As uterotonic agents act on the myometrium via

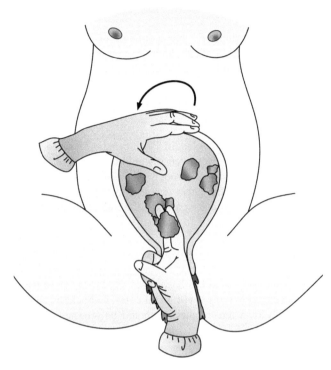

FIGURE 14.1 Fundal massage and removal of blood clots from the lower uterine segment, cervical canal and the vagina.

different receptors, it is vital to quickly move to the next choice if one agent is ineffective. In the presence of hypotension, uterotonic agents may not reach the uterus in adequate doses. Therefore, it is important to administer these early and before the woman goes into a state of haemodynamic instability.

Ergometrine

Ergometrine causes sustained contractions of the uterus, and it can be repeated up to a total dose of 1.5 mg, if necessary. Ergometrine produces peripheral vasoconstriction and can cause hypertension, and although it is usually avoided for women with hypertensive disorders of pregnancy, it may be used even in these very women in case the bleeding is severe and the blood pressure drops.

Oxytocin

Oxytocin causes contractions of the uterus with relaxation in between. Oxytocin receptors may have been downregulated especially after induction and/or augmentation of labour, which in turn reduces the effectiveness of oxytocin in controlling haemorrhage. A bolus dose of oxytocin produces a transient vasodilatory effect, which makes the blood pressure fall by approximately 20 mmHg immediately following administration. Carbetocin, which is an expensive, long-acting synthetic analogue of oxytocin, could be given as a single dose of 100 μg IM or IV, and this would obviate the need for an IV infusion of oxytocin.

Syntometrine

Syntometrine, the combination of oxytocin and ergometrine, provides the benefit of short-acting oxytocin and the more sustained uterotonic effect of ergometrine. The vasodilatory effect of oxytocin balances out the vasoconstrictory effect of ergometrine.

Misoprostol

Misoprostol, an analogue of prostaglandin E1, has a duration of action of about two hours. It has the advantage of not requiring intravenous administration. Women may develop a raised temperature and start shivering at around 1–2 hours following administration, which is usually transient and self-limiting.

Carboprost

Carboprost (15-methyl analogue of prostaglandin F2α) can be repeated at intervals not less than 15 minutes and up to a total dose of 2 g. However, it would be advisable to intervene surgically if the bleeding is not controlled after three doses of carboprost. The duration of action of carboprost is up to six hours, and therefore, it is a useful agent when a prolonged uterotonic effect is required. Nonetheless, it can also cause severe bronchospasm, and therefore, should be avoided in women with bronchial asthma.

Tranexamic Acid

The antifibrinolytic agent, tranexamic acid has been discovered to be effective in the management of primary PPH, irrespective of the underlying cause. In all cases, it should be administered early at a dose of 1 g in 10 mL intravenously over ten minutes. It should be repeated after 30 minutes if bleeding persists.

Refractory Uterine Atony

The majority of cases respond to resuscitation, fundal massage and medical management. However, if these measures fail to control haemorrhage within a maximum of one hour (the concept of the golden hour), and the bleeding continues despite the exclusion of genital tract trauma and placental abnormalities, then refractory atony must be suspected and managed with second-line measures, such as uterine balloon tamponade or surgical measures such as uterine compression sutures (discussed in Chapter 17), uterine devascularization (discussed in Chapter 18) or hysterectomy (discussed in Chapter 19).

Uterine Balloon Tamponade

Formerly, uterine tamponade was achieved by packing the uterus with wide, rolled gauze. This has been superseded by the use of balloon tamponade. Balloon tamponade was first attempted with the Sengstaken-Blakemore oesophageal catheter or the Rusch urological balloon. Subsequently, the Bakri balloon was specifically designed for the purpose of uterine tamponade. Balloon tamponade is a simple and relatively noninvasive procedure that can be performed in the labour room, and it does not require anaesthesia. It will often immediately reduce or stop the bleeding and avert the need for laparotomy. The principle of balloon tamponade is to apply direct pressure on the uteroplacental vessels that are exposed after placental separation so that, once the bleeding stops, blood can clot and form a permanent seal. Therefore, the pressure applied should be greater than the pressure of blood flow in the uteroplacental vessels. The uterine cavity should be empty of blood clots or placental tissue in order for balloon tamponade to be effective.

The balloon is placed inside the uterine cavity and then filled with 250–350 mL of fluid to create a tamponade effect from within the uterus. In some cases, up to 500 mL of fluid may be necessary. Success is judged by a declining loss of blood through the cervix and the drainage channel of the balloon (tamponade test). If bleeding continues, then surgical treatment is necessary, provided that genital tract trauma and retained tissue are excluded. To prevent the displacement of the balloon, the vagina should be packed with iodine or antibiotic-soaked gauze which should not extend into the uterus (Figure 14.2).

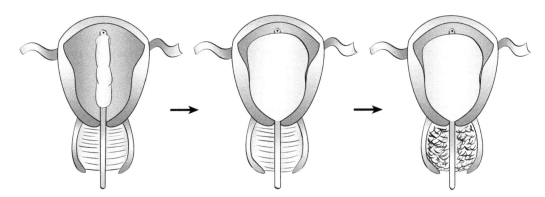

FIGURE 14.2 Bakri balloon.

PROCEDURE – UTERINE TAMPONADE USING A BAKRI BALLOON

Obtain verbal consent from the woman and place her in lithotomy position. Clean and drape the perineal region.

Administer prophylactic antibiotics (e.g. cefuroxime and metronidazole).

Insert a Sim's speculum.

Hold the anterior lip of the cervix with sponge forceps.

Insert the Bakri catheter into the uterus using another set of sponge forceps.

Fill the Bakri catheter with 250–350 mL of normal saline.

Observe for the cessation of bleeding.

Pack the vagina tightly with moistened gauze.

Balloon tamponade has been shown to be effective in controlling haemorrhage which is evident after closing the uterine and abdominal incisions after caesarean delivery. It has also been found to be successful in controlling haemorrhage from the lower segment following caesarean delivery for placenta praevia, after caesarean delivery at full dilatation or subsequent to conservative management of PAS disorder (discussed in Chapter 13), but surgical measures may be a more reasonable option in these situations. It has also been used following manual replacement or O'Sullivan hydrostatic method for acute uterine inversion (discussed in Chapter 21).

Improvised devices which act on the same principle, such as a condom (Figure 14.3) or a surgical glove tied to a urinary catheter, have been successfully used in managing PPH in resource-poor settings.

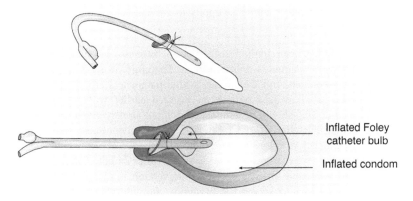

Inflated Foley catheter bulb

Inflated condom

FIGURE 14.3 Condom catheter.

As the usual condom catheter tamponade system does not have a channel for drainage of blood, improvisation with a drainage channel has been described. A vacuum-induced uterine tamponade system has also recently been demonstrated as an alternative to uterine balloon tamponade in the process of managing refractory uterine atony.

PROCEDURE – UTERINE TAMPONADE USING A CONDOM CATHETER

Obtain informed verbal consent from the woman.

Commence intravenous antibiotics (e.g. cefuroxime and metronidazole) and continue administering for at least 48 hours before converting to oral therapy.

Adhere to sterile procedures.

Roll a condom over a No. 22 (preferable) or No. 20 Foley catheter, so that two-thirds of the condom covers the tip of the catheter and one-third is free. Two condoms, one placed over the other, may be used for greater security.

Using a sterile suture, tie the condom to the catheter without obliterating the lumen of the catheter, so that it will be watertight.

Connect an infusion set to a pack of warmed normal saline and attach the other end to the catheter, and fill the condom with warm normal saline.

Make sure the system is watertight and not leaking from the condom attachment by holding the balloon with the catheter tip upwards.

Disconnect the infusion set, empty the condom, place it on a sterile tray and wash it with povidone iodine, because condoms are not sterile.

Place the woman in lithotomy position, clean and drape the perineal region, insert two Sim's specula and hold the anterior lip of the cervix with sponge forceps.

Keeping the condom catheter system between the index and middle fingers, insert the entire system into the uterus, similar to carrying out a pelvic examination, and explore the uterus until the fundus is felt.

Reconnect the infusion set, keep the saline pack about 150 cm above the woman and allow gravity to fill the condom. Usually, around 350 mL is needed.

Stop filling the condom when the catheter balloon is bulging out of the cervical os.

Observe for the cessation of bleeding from the uterine cavity.

Pack the vagina tightly with moistened roller gauze, around the catheter in a circumferential manner, to prevent the condom catheter from being expelled from the uterine cavity.

Continue filling the catheter until the gravity-aided filling stops at approximately 500 mL.

Apply gentle pressure on the fundus and observe the fluid column moving up in the saline pack, confirming an intact pressure system.

Fold the distal end of the catheter and tie it tightly to prevent backflow.

Once balloon tamponade has been applied to the uterus, there is a possibility of bleeding from the uterus going undetected, as the vagina is tightly packed. Therefore, it is essential that the level of the fundus is marked on the abdomen, and the woman's vital parameters are closely monitored. The indwelling urinary catheter which would have been inserted earlier will prevent urinary retention. A second dose of tranexamic acid should be administered, if not already given; the oxytocin infusion of 40 units in 500 mL of normal saline at 125 mL/hour should be continued; and the woman must be monitored in a high dependency or intensive care unit.

When a decision is made to remove the tamponade system after 24 hours, the operating room should be informed and remain accessible in case surgical intervention is required. First, half of the fluid volume is drained, and the woman observed for 30 minutes for any rebleeding. If there is no bleeding through the vaginal pack, then the vaginal pack is removed. The tamponade system is kept in situ for another 30 minutes, and if there is no further bleeding, then the remaining fluid is also drained. The entire tamponade system is kept in situ for a further 30 minutes, and in the absence of any rebleeding, the system is gently removed from the body. Leaving the tamponade system in situ for 30 minutes after draining all the fluid allows the system to be restored with fluid in case bleeding recurs. After the removal of the entire tamponade system, ergometrine 0.5 mg IV and the commencement of an IV infusion of 20 units of oxytocin in 500 mL of normal saline at 125 mL/hour is recommended.

Management of Trauma to the Genital Tract

Vaginal Wall Lacerations

In these cases, it is important to identify the apex of the injury. If the apex is not visible, then a stitch should be placed as high as possible; traction must be applied on that stitch; and a continuous suture needs to be progressively applied until the apex is reached (Figure 14.4). The laceration is then sutured with a layer of a continuous suture. If there are multiple lacerations and oozing, then the need for multiple needle punctures may lead to increased bleeding. In these cases, vaginal tamponade may be applied using a vaginal pack, a Bakri, a similar balloon or an inflated blood pressure cuff inside a surgical glove or sterile plastic bag. It is extremely important to rule out uterine bleeding before applying vaginal tamponade, because blood can collect inside the uterus and cause atony which would aggravate bleeding from the uterus.

Vestibular Tears

Vestibular tears should be sutured after inserting a urinary catheter in order to enable the easy identification of the urethra and to avoid involving it in the sutures (Figure 14.5).

Cervical Lacerations

Vaginal bleeding, which occurs despite a well-contracted uterus and which does not appear to be arising from the vagina or perineum, is an indication that calls for examining the cervix. Furthermore, uterine atony could be secondary to bleeding from a cervical tear (especially an endocervical tear), with blood tracking to the endometrial cavity as the woman is lying supine. Endocervical tears are very difficult to be visualised unless the woman is placed in the lithotomy position with her head placed low. This position is also needed to visualise high vaginal tears. The cervix and vagina should be thoroughly examined with a Sim's speculum and vaginal wall retractors under proper light and under cover of a narcotic analgesic or anaesthesia for an accurate diagnosis. Two ring forceps or Green Armytage forceps should be applied, and their positions must be changed in sequence to 'walk around' the entire cervix in order to identify cervical tears (Figure 14.6). Cervical tears are most common at the lateral angles between the anterior and posterior lips of the cervix, especially at three o'clock and nine o'clock positions (Figure 14.7), but it is possible that multiple lacerations exist at varying sites, especially after instrumental vaginal deliveries, other obstetric interventions or the delivery of a macrosomic baby.

Paravaginal Haematomas

Paravaginal haematomas usually appear a few hours after delivery and are classified into infralevator and supralevator haematomas according to their location relative to the levator ani. A high degree of suspicion is necessary to diagnose these cases, because bleeding may be concealed, and the symptoms may be non-specific.

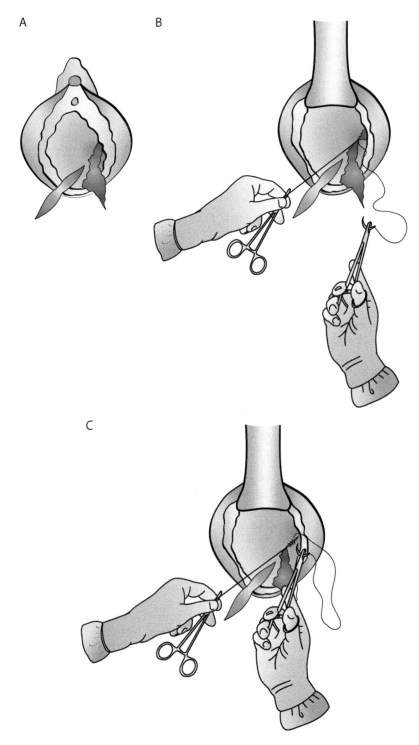

FIGURE 14.4 Suturing of vaginal wall lacerations.

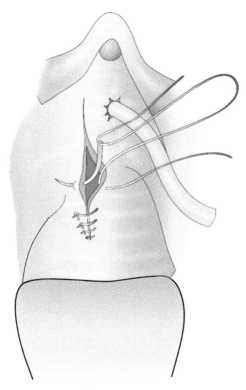

FIGURE 14.5 Suturing of vestibular tears.

Infralevator Haematoma

Vaginal lacerations which continue to ooze despite suturing may lead to the accumulation of blood in the loose areolar tissue below the levator ani muscles, and this dead space can rapidly fill with continued bleeding, even if no frank haemorrhage is visible through the vagina. An episiotomy or perineal injury which has been repaired without achieving proper haemostasis could also result in a paravaginal infralevator haematoma. An infralevator haematoma may be visible, as it would usually cause a bulge into the lower vaginal canal and cause a bluish discolouration of the overlying vaginal epithelium, and it may even be palpable externally as a tender lump (Figure 14.8A). If the haematoma is <5 cm in diameter, then it could be managed expectantly with analgesia, antibiotics and strict monitoring of vital signs. Very often, there is a disparity in visible blood loss and the clinical state of the postpartum woman, and therefore, intervention is necessary. If the haematoma is ≥5 cm in diameter or is rapidly increasing in size, then it should be evacuated via a vaginal incision, made as medially as possible in order to minimise visible scarring. Identification and ligation of an active bleeding point are often difficult, in which case, 'figure of eight' sutures should be applied to the bed, and the dead space must be obliterated. A tight pack into the cavity of the haematoma and another one into the vagina should be applied, and a urinary catheter must be inserted. Perioperative broad-spectrum IV antibiotics, e.g. cefuroxime and metronidazole, should be given. Both packs should be gently removed after 24–48 hours. The insertion of a Foley catheter into the cavity of the haematoma and inflating its bulb with sterile fluid to achieve tamponade has also been sometimes used. In instances where complete haemostasis has been achieved following the evacuation of the haematoma and obliteration of the dead space, suturing of the vaginal incision and applying tight vaginal tamponade has also been documented.

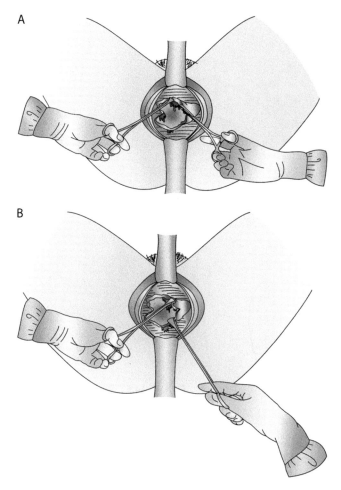

FIGURE 14.6   Examination of the cervix.

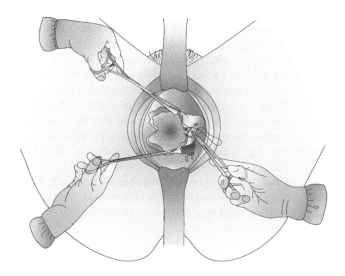

FIGURE 14.7   Repair of cervical tears.

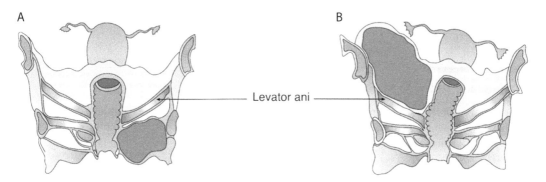

FIGURE 14.8 Paravaginal haematomas; A – Infralevator haematoma, B – supralevator haematoma.

Supralevator Haematoma

A high paravaginal haematoma, which is above the levator ani muscles, is rarer in comparison to an infralevator haematoma, but it could be significantly more dangerous to the woman. Moreover, there could be different presentations. A clue to the diagnosis would be a disparity in the visible blood loss associated with trauma to the upper vagina or the cervix and the clinical state of the postpartum woman. In some cases, it may be possible to feel a nontender, boggy mass protruding into the upper portion of the vaginal canal and causing vaginal or rectal pain and exhibiting pressure symptoms (Figure 14.8B). Sometimes, the haematoma may not be detectable externally. Combined abdominal and vaginal ultrasonography helps in its diagnosis. If it is detected immediately or a few hours after delivery, then it requires emergency laparotomy. It is a very dangerous condition that is often burdensome to manage. The principles of management are the same as for an infralevator haematoma. However, identification of an active bleeding point is even more troublesome, and the application of haemostatic sutures to the bed of the haematoma is also more demanding on account of engorged venous plexuses and the need to prevent injury to the ureters. Ligation of the internal iliac arteries (described in Chapter 18) or pelvic arterial embolisation may be required. Insertion of a tight vaginal pack prior to the laparotomy, tight packing of the pelvis after evacuating the blood clots and achieving haemostasis as much as possible, and reinforcing the vaginal pack after the laparotomy, are measures that could be adopted in these difficult cases. If the woman presents late with no deterioration of her clinical condition, then conservative management is possible.

Treatment with the second dose of tranexamic acid is particularly important in the management of a PPH due to genital tract trauma. Furthermore, broad-spectrum IV antibiotics (e.g. cefuroxime and metronidazole) are indicated, especially in the management of paravaginal haematomas.

Management of Tissue Abnormalities

If the placenta has been delivered, then it should be carefully examined for any obvious missing parts. Even when the placenta appears complete, there is still the possibility of unrecognised retention of a cotyledon or segment of a bipartite placenta. Therefore, exploration of the uterus must be performed in every case of PPH that is unresponsive to standard medical treatment. If the PPH is associated with a retained placenta or PAS disorder, then it should be managed as discussed in Chapters 20 and 13 respectively.

Management of Thrombin Abnormalities

In the presence of thrombin abnormalities, a careful vaginal delivery avoiding lower genital tract trauma is preferred over caesarean delivery, which is associated with causing greater trauma to tissues. A coagulopathy can be a reason as well as a consequence of haemorrhage. This is discussed in the following section.

Management of a Very Severe Primary Postpartum Haemorrhage

The main principles of management are: anticipation and early recognition, multidisciplinary management, resuscitation, early identification and appropriate treatment of the cause, all of which need to be carried out simultaneously.

Multidisciplinary Management

The successful management of a very severe PPH hinges upon teamwork. The early involvement of experienced personnel is key to a successful outcome. The most accomplished obstetrician, obstetric anaesthesiologist and transfusion specialist should be involved at the start. Additional specialties may possibly be involved later, e.g. an intensivist, an interventional radiologist. Effective communication among the specialties as well as with the woman and her partner is essential. Nursing and midwifery staff and other supporting personnel form an important part of the team.

Resuscitation

Assessment of airway, breathing and circulation should be performed, and oxygen must be administered via a face mask at 10–15 l/minute. The woman should be positioned flat. Two large-bore (14 or 16 G) IV cannulae should be inserted and blood must be obtained for crossmatching of at least five units of packed red cells, full blood count and clotting profile which includes prothrombin time (PT) and INR, activated partial thromboplastin time (APTT) and fibrinogen levels, blood urea, serum electrolytes, renal and liver function tests and serum glucose level. Moreover, arterial blood gases must also be done. Two litres of crystalloids should be infused rapidly: the first within 20 minutes and the second within 30 minutes, because it is important to avoid hypotension which can lead to multiorgan damage. Intravenous fluids should be limited to a maximum of 3 L during initial resuscitation in order to prevent a dilutional coagulopathy. Hydroxyethyl starch may be used in resuscitation, while dextran, which has antiplatelet and antithrombotic effects, should not be used. Lost blood is best replaced by blood. Therefore, blood should be transfused as soon as possible. However, if the situation demands immediate transfusion and crossmatched blood is not available, then group-specific (preferable) or O negative blood should be transfused until crossmatched blood is accessible. The administration of more than two packed red cell packs should be supplemented with fresh frozen plasma, ideally in a 1:1 ratio.

The haemoglobin level (obtained by a bedside hemoCue) can be misleadingly normal in cases of acute haemorrhage. Therefore, the infusion of fluids, including blood, is best guided by a combination of the clinical picture and laboratory results. Fibrin degradation products (FDP) and D-dimers, which are end products of fibrinolysis, need to be assayed if DIC is suspected. There is no single laboratory test for the diagnosis of DIC. The PT - INR and APTT are reduced to the lower end of the normal range, and fibrinogen levels are increased in pregnancy. Therefore, a significant amount of blood could be lost before changes are evident in these tests.

Treating the cause of bleeding is one of the most important aspects of resuscitation, as it reduces further blood loss.

Massive Transfusion Protocol

The massive transfusion protocol (MTP) should be adopted if facilities are available. The transfusion of blood and blood components should ideally be guided by rotational thromboelastometry (ROTEM), which provides the opportunity for 'point of care' testing and real-time laboratory data in a setting of dramatically changing haemostasis. Once the MTP is activated, blood products will be dispensed as 'rounds' with each round bearing a specific number of blood products.

- Round 1:4 units packed red cells, 4 units FFP
- Round 2:8 units packed red cells, 8 units FFP, 1 unit platelet, 1 unit cryoprecipitate
- Round 3:8 units packed red cells, 8 units FFP

The aim of MTP is to rapidly replace the volume of lost blood and to prevent the lethal trial of coagulopathy, hypothermia and acidosis (Figure 14.9). Transfused agents have to be warmed, wet and bloody clothes removed promptly and a forced-air warming device used in order to prevent hypothermia. If facilities for ROTEM are not available, then FFP should be administered in a 1:1 ratio. A higher dose of FFP is necessary if the PT and APTT are greater than 1.5 times the normal. In women with suspected coagulopathy, as in cases of amniotic fluid embolism, placental abruption and in cases of delayed detection of PPH, early transfusion of FFP should be considered. Cryoprecipitate or fibrinogen concentrate should be used if the fibrinogen level is less than 2 g/L. Platelet transfusion is indicated if the platelet count is less than 50×10^9/L. Cryoprecipitate, platelets and FFP should ideally be group compatible. In addition, platelets have to be of Rhesus negative type if given to a Rhesus negative woman.

If a Rhesus negative woman has received Rhesus positive blood, then anti D immunoglobulin has to be given. Larger preparations that contain 2,500–5,000 IU of anti D immunoglobulin are more advisable over the usual preparations which contain 500 IU. Exchange transfusion may be considered in reducing the load of Rhesus positive red blood cells in the circulation and the required dose of anti D immunoglobulin in cases of massive transfusion.

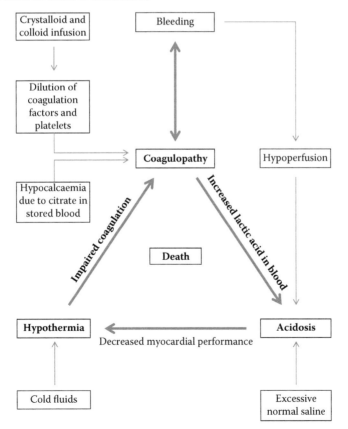

FIGURE 14.9   The triad of death.

Procedures Used in the Management of Very Severe Postpartum Haemorrhage

- Bimanual compression of the uterus
- Aortic compression
- Intraoperative cell salvage
- Pelvic packing
- Radiological procedures
- Uterine compression sutures (discussed in Chapter 17)
- Uterine devascularization (discussed in Chapter 18)
- Hysterectomy (discussed in Chapter 19)

Bimanual Compression of the Uterus

Bimanual compression of the uterus involves placing the operator's fist in the anterior fornix and pushing it upwards while simultaneously pushing down on the posterofundal part of the uterus with the other hand (Figure 14.10). This leads to compression of the bleeding uteroplacental vessels, as well as the stretching of the uterine arteries and the reduction of blood flow within them. This is usually employed as a temporary measure in order to control bleeding while transferring the woman to the operating room. If it is effective in significantly reducing blood loss, then it might be an indication that compression of the uterus by means of compression sutures might be adequate in controlling bleeding.

Aortic Compression

Aortic compression is also a temporary measure used to control massive haemorrhage prior to definitive surgical options (Figure 14.11). It is feasible prior to laparotomy in the postpartum woman whose abdominal wall has been distended, which leads to reduced muscular resistance. The woman may be semi-conscious or drowsy, making it technically easy to perform aortic compression. The arterial pressure within the aorta is low and only little compression on the aorta

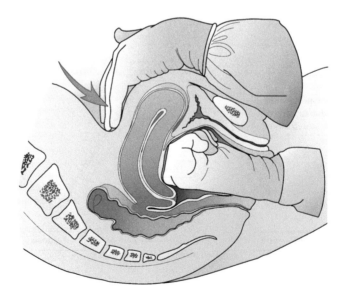

FIGURE 14.10   Bimanual compression of the uterus.

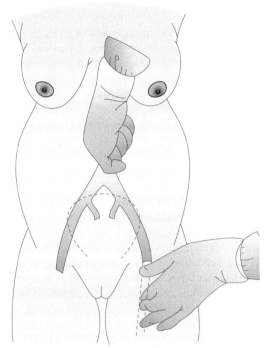

FIGURE 14.11   Aortic compression.

is needed to reduce blood loss. Firstly, the femoral pulse should be palpated in the inguinal area. The fist of the operator's dominant hand should then be closed, with the thumb outside the fingers. Next, the fist should be placed on the umbilicus with the forearm perpendicular to the skin, following which the fist is slowly forced downwards until the aortic pulsations are felt. The fist should be lowered until it reaches the bony surfaces of the vertebral column. The aorta is compressed between two bony surfaces, i.e. the digital bones of the operator's hand and the vertebral column of the woman. Successful compression of the aorta is confirmed by the absence of femoral pulsations. It could also be carried out by an assistant at laparotomy, while definitive surgical measures are in progress.

PROCEDURE – AORTIC COMPRESSION

Feel for the femoral pulse in the inguinal area.

Form a closed fist with the thumb outside the fingers.

Place the fist on the umbilicus with the forearm perpendicular to the skin.

Slowly lower the fist downwards in order to feel the aortic pulsations.

Lower the fist until it reaches the bony surfaces of the vertebral column.

Compress the aorta between the digital bones of the operator's hand and the vertebral column of the woman.

Confirm effective compression of the aorta by the absence of femoral pulsations.

Intraoperative Cell Salvage

If facilities are available, intraoperative cell salvage may be used in the management of PPH. In cell salvage, blood shed within the surgical field is retrieved by an anticoagulated suction apparatus, centrifuged and washed to remove fibrin, debris, plasma, platelets and procoagulant, and subsequently returned to the circulation via a leucocyte depletion filter. It reduces the need for allogenic transfusion and is useful especially in women who refuse blood product transfusion. Although there is a theoretical risk of amniotic fluid embolism and maternal infection from contaminants, in practice, these complications are rare. Sensitisation of a Rhesus negative woman to Rhesus positive fetal blood cells can be prevented by the administration of Anti D immunoglobulin.

Pelvic Packing

This creates a tamponade effect and is useful in the management of broad ligament, high paravaginal (supralevator) or retroperitoneal haematomas, extensive lacerations and oozing from diffuse areas in the pelvis. Historically, pelvic packing has been achieved by placing a plastic bag with wet gauze against the pelvic bleeders, pulling the drawstrings through the vagina and attaching these to a weight. A large, damp, gauze pack could be tightly and directly applied to the oozing areas in the pelvis with the vagina closed. Abdominal drains should not be inserted below the pack, as this will reduce the tamponade effect of the blood clots that may form. The abdominal cavity is then closed in the usual manner. Broad-spectrum IV antibiotics should be administered. The pack should be removed after 48 hours under general anaesthesia, and the pelvic cavity must be examined gently for bleeding. Aggressive exploration of the pelvic cavity, which can dislodge blood clots and provoke rebleeding, should be avoided. Moreover, leaving the pack for longer periods increases the risk of infection.

Radiological Procedures

Pelvic arterial embolisation can be performed for PPH in institutions with access to radiological expertise and equipment. Success rates of around 90% have been reported. Even in these institutions, delay in accessing embolisation should not deny alternate surgical treatment. Complications include those related to the procedure itself, such as anaphylaxis, post-procedure fever and renal toxicity, and those related to dislodgement of emboli, such as necrosis of uterus, bladder and rectum, ischaemic nerve injury, vascular perforation and infection. However, these complications are infrequent and may largely be operator-dependent. Temporary balloon occlusion techniques are being employed to control bleeding from PAS disorders (discussed in Chapter 13).

A major advantage of radiological procedures is the potential to preserve future fertility. However, the limiting factors in employing radiological measures are that it requires round the clock availability of a skilled interventional radiologist and radiological facilities in close proximity to the obstetric department. Invariably, there are delays in setting up the equipment if bleeding has been unanticipated. Therefore, the main use of radiological measures in controlling PPH is when bleeding has been anticipated and expertise is available on site. However, PPH occurs without warning in a considerable number of cases. Therefore, it is crucial that every obstetrician is familiar with the surgical techniques, i.e. uterine compression sutures and devascularization, which can be performed quickly and do not require sophisticated equipment.

Recombinant Factor VIIa

Life-threatening arterial and venous thromboembolic complications have been reported following the administration of recombinant factor VIIa. Therefore, routine use of recombinant factor VIIa is currently not recommended in the management of PPH, unless this is part of a trial.

Monitoring of Vital Signs

The woman should be connected to a multimonitor, and her vital parameters, pulse rate, blood pressure, respiratory rate and oxygen saturation are monitored. An indwelling urinary catheter should be inserted, and an input-output chart maintained. A full bladder may inhibit uterine contractions; therefore, keeping the bladder empty is also useful in the management of uterine atony, as discussed earlier. Treatment should be guided by a combination of estimated blood loss, vital parameters and laboratory investigations. Repeat assessments at specific time intervals that are proportionate to the severity of bleeding are important to evaluate response to ongoing therapy.

Invasive monitoring of arterial blood pressure or central venous pressure in an intensive care setting may be necessary in cases of massive PPH.

Post-Procedure Management

These women are at risk of secondary haemorrhage, multiorgan failure, sepsis, venous thromboembolism (VTE) and death. Appropriate measures such as anti-embolic stockings should be employed and administration of low molecular weight heparin (once bleeding is controlled) considered, in accordance with the local protocols in order to reduce the risk of VTE.

Accurate documentation of the events surrounding the PPH and management, with particular emphasis on timelines, is crucial for future reference. Moreover, debriefing of the woman, her partner and the staff is also a key aspect in the management. Risk management is important in order to highlight the strong aspects as well as shortcomings in the management, and to improve the quality of care. The importance of regular, systematic audits and simulation-based training cannot be undermined in a serious, life-threatening emergency such as a primary PPH.

A practical guide to managing primary PPH is illustrated in Figure 14.12.

The type and timing of the interventions utilised in primary PPH depend mainly on the experience of the lead obstetrician who is in charge the case. Other factors that influence management are the haemodynamic stability of the woman, the extent of blood loss, parity, desire for future fertility and the site of confinement. A combination of mechanical, pharmacological, radiological and surgical measures may be necessary for the management of PPH and should be directed towards the cause of the haemorrhage. The above methods, in no particular order, should be utilised depending on available expertise and the individual clinical circumstances.

Key Points

- Deaths due to PPH are largely preventable.
- All pregnancies are at risk of PPH, even in the absence of predisposing factors.
- Due consideration and adoption of appropriate interventions for risk factors, anticipation, early detection and appropriate management of bleeding after childbirth are essential.
- Early and aggressive treatment by experienced practitioners working closely together as a team, are crucial in the management of a severe PPH.
- In cases of refractory PPH, there could be more than one cause for the aforementioned PPH.

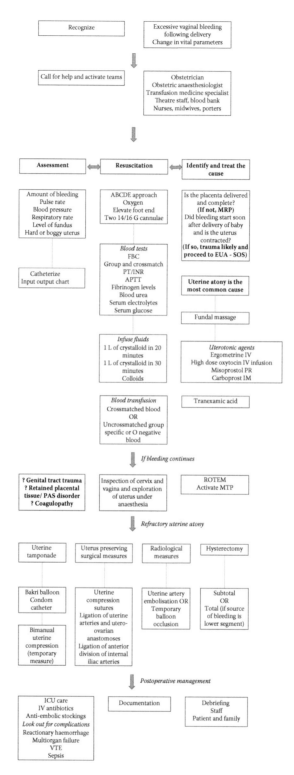

FIGURE 14.12 A practical guide to managing primary PPH; MRP – manual removal of placenta, EUA – examination under anaesthesia, PT/INR – prothrombin time/international normalised ratio, APTT – activated partial thromboplastin time, PAS – placenta accreta spectrum, ROTEM – rotational thromboelastometry, MTP – massive transfusion protocol, VTE – venous thromboembolism.

BIBLIOGRAPHY

1. Begley CM, Gyte GML, Devane D, McGuire W, Weeks A, Biesty LM. Active versus expectant management for women in the third stage of labour. *Cochrane Database Syst Rev* 2019;2(2). Art. No.: CD007412. DOI: 10.1002/14651858.CD007412.pub5.
2. Women's Health Committee (RANZCOG). Management of Postpartum Haemorrhage C-Obs 43. Sydney, Australia: Royal Australian and New Zealand College of Obstetricians and Gynaecologists, 2017.
3. American College of Obstetricians and Gynecologists. Practice Bulletin No. 183: postpartum hemorrhage. *Obstet Gynecol* 2017;130(4):e168–86. doi:10.1097/AOG.0000000000002351.
4. Mavrides EAS, Chandraharan E, Collins P, Green L, Hunt BJ, Riris S, Thomson AJ on behalf of the Royal College of Obstetricians and Gynaecologists. Prevention and management of postpartum haemorrhage Green-top Guideline No 52. *BJOG* 2016;6(124):e106–49.
5. WHO Recommendations: Uterotonics for the Prevention of Postpartum Haemorrhage. Geneva: World Health Organization, 2018. Licence: CC BY-NC-SA 3.0 IGO
6. WHO Recommendations for the Prevention and Treatment of Postpartum Haemorrhage Geneva, Switzerland: World Health Organization, 2012.
7. Withanathantrige M, Goonewardene M, Dandeniya R, Gunatilake P, Gamage S. Comparison of four methods of blood loss estimation after caesarean delivery. *Int J Gynaecol Obstet* 2016;135:51–55. http://dx.doi.org/10.1016/j.ijgo.2016.03.036.
8. Mavis N., Schorn CNM. Measurement of blood loss: review of the Literature. J *Midwifery Women's Health* 2010;55(1):20–27.
9. Rishard MRM, Galgomuwa VMP, Gunawardane K. Improvised condom catheter with a draining channel for management of atonic postpartum haemorrhage. *Ceylon Med J* 2013;58:124–25.
10. Purwosunu Y, Sarkoen W, Arulkumaran S, Segnitz J. Control of postpartum hemorrhage using vacuum-induced uterine tamponade. *Obstet Gynecol* 2016;128(1):33–36. doi:10.1097/AOG.0000000000001473.
11. Arulkumaran S, Karoshi M, Keith LG, Lalonde AB, B-Lynch C, eds. A Comprehensive Textbook of Postpartum Hemorrhage. Duncow: Sapiens Publishing, 2012.

15

Secondary Postpartum Haemorrhage

Sanjeewa Padumadasa

Secondary postpartum haemorrhage (PPH) is defined as excessive vaginal bleeding from 24 hours after delivery up to 12 weeks postpartum. Less emphasis is made regarding the amount of blood loss, in contrast to primary PPH. It occurs in just under 1% of women and commonly presents in primary care as prolonged or extreme bleeding once the woman has returned home after delivery. Therefore, every practitioner caring for women in the postpartum period should be aware of this condition. Although mortality is rare, morbidity associated with this condition is considerable, and it is the leading cause of readmission in postpartum patients.

Causes of Secondary Postpartum Haemorrhage

The main causes of secondary PPH are retained placental tissue and endometritis and, often, a combination of the two. There are other causes, which are rare and diverse, as listed below (Table 15.1).

Diagnosis

Prolonged rupture of membranes, prolonged labour, multiple vaginal examinations, internal monitoring, emergency delivery, manual removal of placenta, maternal anaemia and poor socioeconomic status are risk factors for endometritis, while a history of retained placenta and placenta accreta spectrum (PAS) disorder are risk factors for retained placental tissue. Retained placental tissue, endometritis or a combination of the two, leads to subinvolution of the uterus and failure of obliteration of blood vessels underlying the placental site. Sloughing of an infected area may expose a bleeding vessel and can subsequently lead to a sudden gush of bleeding. Missed genital tract lacerations and haematomas and infected episiotomy sites may also present as secondary PPH. A uterine polyp or fibroid may get infected or prevent the uterus from involuting and lead to bleeding in the postpartum period.

Rarely, delayed presentations of broad ligament haematomas and bleeding from the dehiscence of caesarean scar have been reported. Abnormalities of uterine vasculature, such as arteriovenous malformations or pseudoaneurysms, are rare causes of secondary PPH. Massive haemorrhage can take place in cases of expectantly managed PAS disorder (discussed in Chapter 13). Although the inversion of uterus is usually an acute condition presenting immediately following delivery, subacute inversion may present with secondary PPH. Although the majority of choriocarcinomas occur following molar pregnancy, a minority of choriocarcinomas may develop after nonmolar pregnancy as well. These cases can present with secondary PPH or irregular vaginal bleeding.

Women with congenital haemorrhagic disorders such as von Willebrand's disease, carriers of haemophilia A (factor VIII deficiency), haemophilia B (factor IX deficiency) and factor XI deficiency are at an increased risk of secondary PPH. These women are usually not at heightened risk of antepartum haemorrhage or primary PPH, as there is a surge of clotting factors and a decrease of anticoagulation factors during pregnancy. These women may present with secondary PPH, as the pregnancy-induced changes in clotting and anticoagulant factors normalise following delivery.

TABLE 15.1

Causes of secondary postpartum haemorrhage

Retained placental tissue

Endometritis

Lower genital tract lacerations/haematoma

Uterine polyp/fibroid

Dehiscence of caesarean scar

Arteriovenous malformations in the uterus/pseudoaneurysms

Expectantly managed placenta accreta spectrum (PAS) disorder

Subacute inversion of uterus

Choriocarcinoma

Coagulation disorders

Use of anticoagulants

Management of Secondary Postpartum Haemorrhage

The main aims of management are resuscitation (if indicated), investigating whether the woman is septic or not and identifying and treating the cause of secondary PPH.

Resuscitation

Although the amount of blood loss at presentation varies in secondary PPH, it is usually not as severe as observed in a primary PPH. However, some will have massive haemorrhage which can rapidly lead to hypovolaemic shock, and immediate resuscitative measures should be instituted in these women (discussed in Chapter 14).

Investigation for Sepsis

The possibility of sepsis should be borne in mind, and rapid assessment along with aggressive treatment are important if sepsis is suspected (discussed in Chapter 6).

Identification of the Cause of Secondary Postpartum Haemorrhage

A thorough history should be obtained to ascertain parity, circumstances around labour, mode of delivery, details of the third stage and puerperal complications. The symptoms of offensive lochia, lower abdominal pain or maternal pyrexia should alert the clinician with the possibility of endometritis. Uterine tenderness, which is usually a sign of endometritis, or subinvolution of the uterus with an open cervical os, which is usually a sign of retained placental tissue may be detected by an abdominal and vaginal examination. A sterile speculum examination should be carried out to assess the bleeding, to visualise the cervix and vagina to exclude lacerations and to obtain high vaginal and endocervical swabs for culture and antibiotic sensitivity studies. A bimanual pelvic examination should be performed thereafter, which should help in the diagnosis of subinvolution, uterine fibroids and subacute uterine inversion.

Blood should be taken for full blood count, C reactive protein, coagulation studies, blood urea, serum electrolytes, culture and group and crossmatching. Blood should also be taken for serum beta hCG levels if choriocarcinoma is suspected and for clotting factor assays if a clotting disorder is possible. A midstream urine sample must be obtained for culture and antibiotic sensitivity.

A pelvic ultrasound scan should be performed in order to identify retained placental tissue. An echogenic mass within the uterine cavity or a thickened endometrium is associated with the afore-mentioned retained placental tissue. Retained placental tissue is unlikely if a normal endometrial stripe is observed. However, pelvic ultrasound is not an entirely reliable method of identifying retained placental tissue as it has a high false-positive rate, and overdiagnosis may lead to unnecessary surgical interventions with a significant risk of serious consequences. However, ultrasound does have a good negative predictive value and is, therefore, particularly helpful in excluding retained placental tissue. Ultrasound is also useful in detecting uterine polyps or fibroids. Colour Doppler will help distinguish retained placental tissue from blood clots and debris, as retained placental tissue will usually maintain a blood supply unlike necrotic decidua and blood clots. Nonetheless, the absence of vascularity of these tissues does not exclude retained placental tissue. Colour Doppler also offers the advantage of detecting arteriovenous malformations or pseudoaneurysms which are rare but otherwise recognised causes of secondary PPH. Additional imaging such as chest x-ray and a computerised tomography (CT) scan of abdomen and pelvis for suspected choriocarcinoma, magnetic resonance imaging for PAS disorders and CT angiography for suspected arteriovenous malformations should be considered in appropriate cases.

Treatment for the Cause

Retained Placental Tissue

Management in cases of retained placental tissue includes the administration of tranexamic acid and antibiotics followed by an exploration of the uterine cavity. Unlike in the case of a primary PPH, uterotonic agents are not effective in controlling haemorrhage in this case. Examination under anaesthesia and surgical evacuation of the uterus should be performed if there is retained placental tissue. It may be prudent to defer surgery for 24 hours after the commencement of broad-spectrum intravenous antibiotics in haemodynamically stable patients. However, an immediate surgical evacuation of the uterus is indicated in haemodynamically unstable patients and in cases of continuous bleeding. Digital removal of retained placental tissue (Figure 15.1), suction evacuation, ovum forceps (Figure 15.2) or blunt curettage (Figure 15.3) can be used to evacuate the uterus of retained placental tissue. If the uterus is enlarged well above the pubic symphysis, then the operator could stabilise the fundus of the uterus with their non-dominant hand, while the assistant holds on to the sponge forceps that are attached to the anterior lip of the cervix. Uterotonic agents may be used at the time of evacuation and afterward, to aid uterine contractions. Care should be taken as the risk of uterine perforation is increased, because the uterus is thinner and softer postpartum, and the risk is even greater in the presence of endometritis. Also, a history of caesarean delivery increases the risk of uterine perforation at surgical evacuation. Surgical

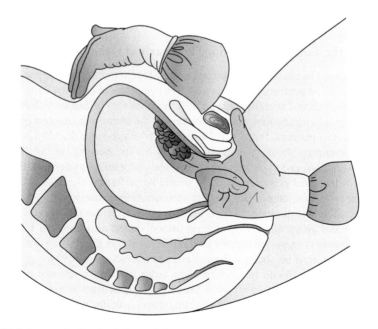

FIGURE 15.1   Digital removal of retained placental tissue.

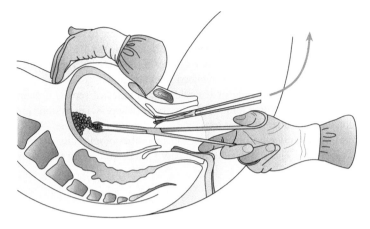

FIGURE 15.2 Removal of retained placental tissue using ovum forceps.

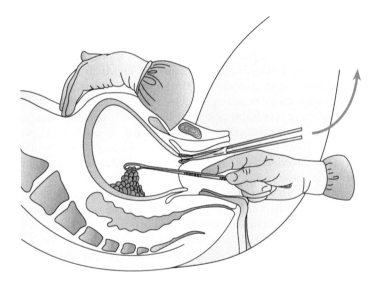

FIGURE 15.3 Blunt curettage.

evacuation of the uterus should be carried out only by a competent obstetrician. If the curettage is too vigourous, then it could be associated with secondary amenorrhoea (Asherman syndrome). Surgical evacuation of the uterus could be performed under ultrasound guidance if facilities are available.

The tissue removed should be sent for culture and antibiotic sensitivity testing, as well as for histopathological examination to rule out trophoblastic disease. Also, balloon tamponade of the uterus can be used to control bleeding following the evacuation of retained placental tissue (discussed in Chapter 14). Uterine artery embolization is also an option if expertise is available. Very rarely, the woman may need laparotomy and other surgical procedures in the form of uterine devascularization, internal iliac artery ligation or hysterectomy in order to control bleeding (discussed in Chapters 18 and 19).

Endometritis

As endometritis is a significant cause or an important contributor to secondary PPH, intravenous broad-spectrum antibiotics play a major role in the management of these distinct women. The organisms that are commonly identified are Group B Streptococcus, *Bacteroides sp.*, *Escherichia coli*, *Clostridium perfringens* and Group D Streptococcus. Cephalosporins, a combination of carbapenem and clindamycin, or a combination of gentamicin and clindamycin are effective in the treatment of endometritis. However, local guidelines should be followed. The antibiotic can be changed according to the results of the sensitivity tests. Parenteral antibiotics are continued until the woman has been afebrile for at least 24 hours, following which oral antibiotics are prescribed to complete a 7-day course of antibiotic therapy. Routine curettage of the uterine cavity is not advised in the absence of retained placental tissue.

Endometritis can be complicated by sepsis if neglected. In cases of sepsis, if there is no response to antibiotics, then treatment may involve removal of the focus of sepsis, i.e. hysterectomy. In these cases, hysterectomy is challenging due to adhesions and friable necrotic tissue. An experienced multi-disciplinary team, which includes an obstetrician, an anaesthesiologist and an intensivist, should be involved in the management. The woman should receive intensive care in the postoperative period.

Treatment of Rare Causes

If the cause is a genital tract laceration or haematoma, then repair of the laceration or evacuation of haematoma is necessary. If dehiscence of the caesarean scar is suspected, then laparotomy followed by repair of the defect should be performed.

Pelvic angiography to assess the internal iliac, uterine and vaginal arteries and subsequent selective arterial embolization are proven to be successful in some cases of ongoing haemorrhage, especially those that are associated with arteriovenous malformations or pseudoaneurysms. In these cases, the involvement of interventional radiologists or vascular surgeons is crucial.

Emergency secondary hysterectomy may have to be performed if a woman with PAS disorder managed expectantly, presents with secondary PPH (discussed in Chapter 13). If a subacute uterine inversion is diagnosed, then it should be managed accordingly. Unlike in acute uterine inversion, where an immediate manual replacement or hydrostatic methods are effective in the management (discussed in Chapter 21), surgical measures are necessary if subacute uterine inversion is diagnosed. Women with choriocarcinoma are treated with methotrexate with folinic acid rescue. Other chemotherapeutic agents, such as etopside, actinomycin, vincristine, cyclophosphamide and 6-mercaptopurine are administered along with methotrexate to medium and high-risk patients.

The opinion of a haematologist should be sought if a coagulation disorder is suspected. Women with von Willebrand's disease and carriers of haemophilia A and B are treated with desmopressin (DDAVP), recombinant clotting factor concentrates, tranexamic acid and combined oral contraceptives. Women with acquired haemophilia in the postpartum period that is caused by antibodies to factor VIII are treated with immunosuppressive drugs such as corticosteroids, cyclophosphamide and azathioprine in order to expedite the disappearance of factor VIII inhibitors. Bleeding due to warfarin should be treated with vitamin K, while that due to heparin is treated with protamine sulphate.

Management of secondary PPH is summarised in Figure 15.4.

Prevention of Secondary Postpartum Haemorrhage

Strict aseptic conditions should be maintained when performing vaginal examinations and uterine manipulations, and unnecessary and repeated vaginal examinations must not be carried out. Prophylactic antibiotics should be considered following instrumental vaginal delivery, manual removal of placenta and intrauterine manipulations. If necessary, the cervix should be dilated with a finger at antepartum caesarean delivery, especially in a nullipara, in order to prevent the accumulation of blood clots inside the uterine cavity. As women with secondary PPH usually present to healthcare practitioners in the community, it is important that every practitioner caring for women in the postpartum period is aware of this condition.

Key Points

- Women with secondary PPH commonly present to healthcare practitioners in the community.
- Secondary PPH is associated with significant morbidity, and it can sometimes result in haemodynamic instability.

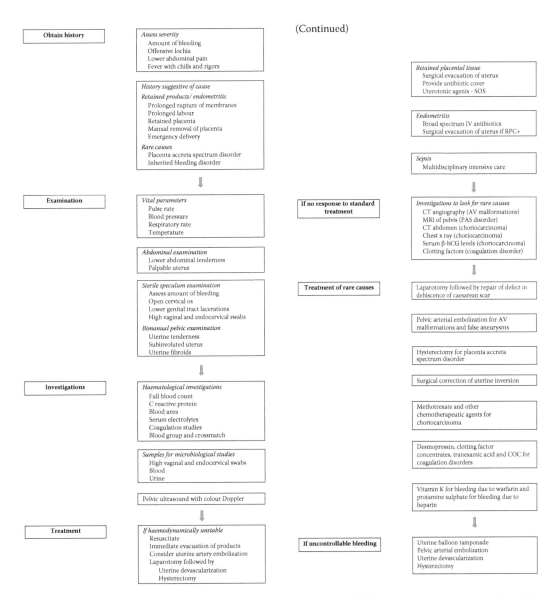

FIGURE 15.4 Summary of secondary postpartum haemorrhage management: RPC – retained products of conception, AV - arteriovenous, COC – combined oral contraceptives.

- The leading causative factors, i.e. retained placental tissue and endometritis, usually coexist in the same patient. Therefore, treatment is essentially done with intravenous broad-spectrum antibiotics and removal of retained placental tissue after resuscitation, if needed. Uterotonic agents are of insignificant value.
- Rare causes should be investigated in cases of secondary PPH with no evidence of retained placental tissue or endometritis or if there is no response to standard therapy.

BIBLIOGRAPHY

1. Groom KM, Jacobson TZ. The management of secondary postpartum haemorrhage. In: Arulkumaran S, Karoshi M, Keith LG, Lalonde AB, B-Lynch C, eds. A comprehensive textbook of postpartum hemorrhage. Duncow: Sapiens Publishing, 2012, pp. 466–73.

16

Uterine Rupture

Malik Goonewardene

Uterine rupture is a rare obstetric emergency but is associated with significant maternal and perinatal morbidity and mortality. Its incidence varies widely due to inconsistencies in reporting but happens in approximately 1 in 2,000 pregnancies. Rupture at the site of a previous uterine surgery is the most common cause in well-resourced centres, while obstructed labour resulting from mismanagement may continue to occur in centres with limited resources.

Uterine rupture may be complete when the tear extends up to and includes the serosal surface or considered incomplete when the serosa remains intact (Figure 16.1). Complete uterine rupture may present as a dramatic emergency jeopardising the lives of both the woman and the fetus, whereas incomplete rupture, which could occur due to dehiscence of a lower segment caesarean scar, could be asymptomatic and may even be incidentally diagnosed at a subsequent caesarean delivery.

Causes of Uterine Rupture

- Scarred uterus
- Inappropriate use of uterotonic agents to induce or augment labour
- Grand multiparity
- Trauma resulting from intrauterine manipulation, instrumental vaginal delivery, fundal pressure or external forces
- Placenta accreta spectrum (PAS) disorders
- Compression sutures on the uterus
- Obstructed labour
- Congenital uterine anomalies

Rupture of a previous caesarean delivery scar is the most frequently encountered uterine scar rupture. A classical midline upper segment scar, which is rarely seen today, is about eight times more likely to have a complete rupture than a lower segment transverse scar, and it may rupture even during the antenatal period. The risk of rupture is heightened in a hysterotomy scar and in a low vertical incision, which is used at extreme preterm gestations, as these scars are likely to involve the upper segment. In contrast, partial or complete dehiscence is more prevalent in a lower segment transverse scar. The risk of uterine rupture increases with the number of previous caesarean deliveries, induction or augmentation of labour and a short time interval since the previous caesarean delivery. Any extensions of the lower segment incision to the upper segment increase the risk of uterine rupture, especially if it is in an inverted T shape compared to a J-shaped extension. It is uncertain whether the risk is still raised when the extension to the incision is confined to the lower segment of the uterus. There is conflicting evidence as to whether single-layer closure of the uterine incision as compared to double-layer closure heightens the risk of rupture in a subsequent pregnancy. However, the double-layer closure is preferred by most obstetricians. Uterine rupture has been reported following myomectomy, metroplasty and cornual resection for ectopic pregnancy. There is no evidence that either supports or refutes the suggestion that the risk of

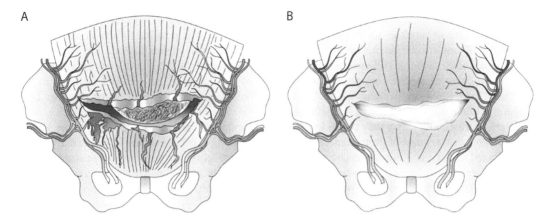

FIGURE 16.1 Types of uterine rupture; A – complete, B – incomplete.

uterine rupture is only increased if the previous uterine surgery had involved the full thickness of the uterine wall. Laparoscopic myomectomy, when performed by a skilled surgeon, does not raise the risk of uterine rupture in subsequent pregnancies over that of open myomectomy.

Induction or augmentation of labour carries a higher risk of uterine rupture as compared to spontaneous labour, especially with increasing parity. A combination of pharmacological methods used to induce labour have been found to be associated with the highest risk, followed by prostaglandins, oxytocin and rarely, mechanical methods. It is rather unusual to encounter uterine rupture in a primigravida even with the frequent use of oxytocic agents used to induce or augment labour. Uterine rupture in a primigravida, or a woman with no previous history of any form of uterine surgery, raises the suspicion of an undisclosed uterine perforation, which could possibly be following an illegal surgical abortion.

Uterine manipulations and instrumental vaginal deliveries may cause uterine rupture, especially when strict protocols are not adhered to and when performed by inexperienced personnel. The application of fundal pressure in case of difficult delivery has been shown to be associated with uterine rupture and therefore, this practice is not recommended. Rarely, PAS disorders may cause uterine rupture in the antepartum period and, when conservative management has been adopted, even in the postpartum period. Rarely, uterine rupture may occur as a result of ischaemia following the application of uterine compression sutures to control obstetric haemorrhage. With recent advancements in the monitoring of labour, patient education and improvement of maternity care, obstructed labour is gradually dwindling as a cause of uterine rupture, but this may still occur in unsupervised labours in low-resource settings.

Clinical Presentation of Uterine Rupture

The majority of uterine ruptures occur during labour, but these may also occur during the antenatal and postpartum periods. Complete uterine rupture at the site of a previous lower segment caesarean scar may happen with minimal warning signs as the scar is relatively avascular. If the rupture is incomplete, which is usually the case, then the woman may be asymptomatic or the symptoms may appear as mild and gradual. Incomplete uterine rupture is often diagnosed incidentally at a subsequent caesarean delivery as a window in the uterine wall. One of the first indications of uterine dehiscence or impending rupture is an abnormality of the fetal heart rate. Prolonged fetal bradycardia occurs in two-thirds of cases. The initial symptoms of impending rupture are abdominal pain and vaginal bleeding. If there is an atypical pattern of pain, especially persisting between contractions, or if the pain which was controlled with analgesia earlier becomes more severe, then impending uterine rupture should be suspected, particularly in the presence of a scarred uterus. However, there is no basis for withholding intrapartum analgesia on the premise that it may mask the symptom of pain in impending uterine rupture. Bleeding may be intra-abdominal rather than vaginal, and uterine rupture should be anticipated in any situation in which the degree of shock is not proportionate to the blood loss. It is possible for the woman to have tachycardia. Complete uterine rupture may present with sudden, severe abdominal pain and collapse, but this is rare. The clinical signs of a recession of the presenting part of the fetus, easily palpable fetal parts and the cessation of uterine contractions are also seldom encountered. The presence of blood in the peritoneal cavity and the irritation of the diaphragm could cause referred pain in the shoulder tips. Rupture into the bladder may cause haematuria.

Rarely, uterine rupture may only be evident following the delivery of the fetus. Uterine rupture should be considered in every case of postpartum collapse. A Bandl's ring may be observed before uterine rupture in obstructed labour, but it is rarely encountered today. Tenderness over the previous uterine scar has poor sensitivity and specificity as a diagnostic sign of a 'weak' scar or impending uterine rupture. Similarly, intrauterine catheter monitoring of uterine activity is not a reliable method of preventing or detecting uterine rupture.

Management of Uterine Rupture

General Principles

The early diagnosis and treatment of uterine rupture are pivotal to a successful outcome. The early involvement of a senior obstetrician, an anaesthesiologist, a neonatologist and a transfusion medicine specialist forms an essential part of management. The aims of management are resuscitation (discussed in Chapter 14) and laparotomy followed by repair of the uterine tear (with or without tubal ligation) or hysterectomy. Verbal consent for either of the surgical interventions should be obtained from the woman. The urgency of the situation necessitates general anaesthesia to be administered.

Surgical Technique

In the majority of cases, the abdominal cavity may be entered via a low transverse incision along a skin crease and a similar curved incision on the rectus sheath. A midline incision may be necessary in cases of traumatic uterine rupture and suspected injury to abdominal viscera. Following laparotomy, the fetus and placenta should be delivered, if this has not already been done previously. The most common site of rupture is the anterior lower part of the uterus consistent with the previous lower segment caesarean incision. Ruptures due to previously unrecognised uterine perforations typically occur in the fundal and postero-fundal part of the uterus. These can be difficult to manage, because there may be extensive lacerations extending in various directions.

Control of Bleeding until Definitive Treatment is Instituted

The uterus should be exteriorised. This leads to the stretching of uterine vessels and reduction of blood loss, and enables the identification of the extent of injury, including extension into the broad ligament. Correct orientation of the uterus is crucial, and the remnants of the uterus should be positioned in what would be the normal anatomical position (Figure 16.2). Temporary haemostasis can be achieved swiftly by applying Green Armytage forceps on the bleeding edges until definitive treatment is instituted (Figure 16.3). Furthermore, two long, straight clamps can be applied over the round ligament, Fallopian tube and ovarian ligament on each side in order to reduce bleeding from the ovarian blood supply, and a tourniquet can be applied over the lower segment of the uterus to occlude the uterine vessels.

Repair of the Uterine Tear

Repair of the uterine tear should be attempted provided that haemostasis can be achieved, especially when there is a need to preserve future fertility. If the rupture is confined to the lower segment, then repair of the tear is appropriate as the risk of rupture in a subsequent pregnancy is similar to that

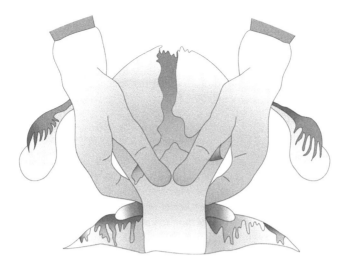

FIGURE 16.2 Orientation of the uterine remnants in the normal anatomical position.

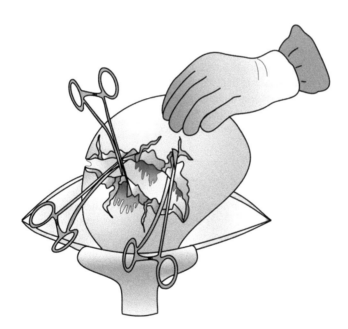

FIGURE 16.3 Application of green armytage forceps to the torn edges.

following another lower segment caesarean delivery. The tear can be sutured in two layers of continuous sutures using No. 1 polyglycolic acid suture material. Additional mattress sutures may be needed, especially in cases of ruptures extending to the upper segment. When future fertility is not an issue, repair of the uterine tear is usually followed by sterilisation.

Hysterectomy

Hysterectomy may be necessary if successful haemostasis cannot be achieved by repairing the uterine tear and in the presence of haemodynamic instability (discussed in Chapter 19). Extensive lacerations in the upper segment are challenging to be repaired and are a contraindication to subsequent pregnancy, and therefore, hysterectomy may be appropriate in these cases. Subtotal hysterectomy may be performed if the rupture is confined to the body of the uterus and offers the advantages of a shorter operating time, as well as a lower morbidity and mortality rate over total hysterectomy. If the cervix or paracolpos is part of the rupture, then a total hysterectomy is necessary. Internal iliac artery ligation may be performed as an adjunct to hysterectomy (discussed in Chapter 18). The insertion of an abdominal drain is at the discretion of the obstetrician.

Involvement of the Urinary Tract

The bladder may possibly be damaged due to the rupture itself or as a result of the intervention (i.e. repair or hysterectomy). Bladder damage can be identified as well as avoided by careful dissection of the bladder from the site of injury. In case of doubt, sterile methylene blue dye can be injected via the Foley catheter. Bladder injury is repaired in two layers of continuous sutures using 3.0 polyglycolic acid suture material. Determining the ureters by opening the pelvic peritoneum at the pelvic brim in front of the sacroiliac joint and tracing downwards is crucial in cases of broad ligament haematomas.

Postoperative Management

Following the treatment of uterine rupture, the woman should receive intensive care due to the risk of secondary haemorrhage, infection and multiorgan failure. Peri-operative broad-spectrum antibiotics should be prescribed. Preventive measures against venous thromboembolic disease should be instituted, and this involves thromboembolic deterrent stockings and the administration of low molecular weight heparin when haemostasis has been achieved. Future fertility is not possible if hysterectomy or sterilisation had been performed, and it is likely that the uterine rupture has resulted in a perinatal death of the fetus. Thus, extensive debriefing should be provided in the postpartum period. Accurate documentation of the events that led to the uterine rupture, the degree of the rupture as well as the interventions performed, is essential for future reference.

Pregnancy Following Uterine Rupture

It is important to provide contraception for at least two years to women who have had their fertility preserved following uterine rupture. There is a paucity of studies on the management of a subsequent pregnancy following uterine rupture. These women should be counselled about the risk of recurrent uterine rupture and managed in a tertiary centre. Generally, the maternal and neonatal outcome are satisfactory. These women will usually undergo an elective caesarean delivery between 34 and 37 weeks of gestation or even earlier in the presence of symptoms suggestive of impending uterine rupture, after a course of antenatal steroids has been considered.

Prevention of Uterine Rupture

Careful selection of cases for a trial of labour after caesarean or any other uterine surgery is important, and an accomplished obstetrician should be involved in the decision-making. These women should deliver in a hospital with the expertise and facilities used to manage uterine rupture. It must be kept in mind that ultrasound measurement of uterine scar thickness has not been found to be sufficiently predictive of uterine rupture for it to be useful in clinical practice. In labour, intravenous access should be obtained and blood must be crossmatched. Oxytocin may be used to induce or augment labour in these cases, after careful consideration by an experienced obstetrician, but prostaglandins should not be used. Progress of labour should be assessed at least every four hours, with close observation for any signs of vaginal bleeding. Maternal symptoms and signs should be monitored regularly. The fetus should be monitored using continuous electronic fetal monitoring.

The early identification of fetopelvic disproportion, judicious use of prostaglandins or oxytocin for induction, and oxytocin for augmentation of labour especially in multigravida and in the second stage of labour are essential in reducing the risk of uterine rupture in women with no previous uterine surgery. An early resort to caesarean delivery should be considered before labour becomes obstructed, because obstructed labour could lead to uterine rupture. Women with PAS disorders should be counselled about the risk of uterine rupture antenatally as well as postpartum (if managed conservatively) and advised on immediate admission to a hospital, if they developed vaginal bleeding or abdominal pain. Manual removal of placenta (discussed in Chapter 20), exploration of the uterus (discussed in Chapter 15), instrumental vaginal delivery (discussed in Chapter 9) and uterine manipulations such as external cephalic version (discussed in Chapter 27) and internal podalic version followed by breech extraction (discussed in Chapter 28) should be performed or directly supervised by a competent obstetrician. If an extension to the uterine incision is necessary to deliver the fetus, such as when the head is impacted within the pelvis in the second stage, then a J-shaped incision, which is likely to heal better, should be made instead of an inverted T-shaped incision. It is important to avoid excessive tension on the sutures, which could lead to ischaemia of the uterine walls, when applying compression sutures on the uterus.

Key Points

- An experienced obstetrician should be involved in the selection of cases for a trial of labour after a previous uterine surgery.
- A competent obstetrician should also be involved in the decision-making process for induction or augmentation of labour in all women.
- Oxytocin is highly advantageous, and is frequently used in labour, but it may also cause devastating effects if it is not used cautiously.
- Uterine manipulations should either be performed or overseen by an experienced obstetrician.
- Silent (asymptomatic), partial dehiscence of a previous lower segment uterine scar may occur prior to the onset of labour.
- In many cases of complete uterine rupture, the classical triad of continuous abdominal pain, vaginal bleeding and fetal heart rate abnormalities may not be observed.
- Uterine rupture should be considered in all cases of obstetric haemorrhage where the degree of haemodynamic instability is out of proportion to the amount of blood loss.

BIBLIOGRAPHY

1. American College of Obstetricians and Gynecologists' Committee on Practice Bulletins—Obstetrics. ACOG Practice Bulletin No. 205: vaginal birth after cesarean delivery. *Obstet Gynecol* 2019;133(2):e110–27.
2. Berhe Y, Wall LL. Uterine rupture in resource-poor countries. *Obstet Gynecol Surv* 2014;69(11):695–707.
3. Landon MB. Uterine rupture in primigravid women. *Obstet Gynecol* 2006;108:709–10.
4. Royal College of Obstetricians and Gynaecologists. Birth After Previous Caesarean Birth. Guideline No. 45. London: RCOG, 2015.
5. Turner MJ. Uterine rupture. *Best Pract Res Clin Obstet Gynaecol* 2002;16:69–79.

17

Uterine Compression Sutures

Sanjeewa Padumadasa

Applying compression sutures to the uterus in order to reduce blood loss was first described by Christopher B-Lynch and colleagues in 1997. Since then, modifications to the original technique have been recommended by several other experts. Although the main use of uterine compression sutures is in refractory uterine atony, these have also been utilised in placenta praevia and placenta accreta spectrum (PAS) disorders, and also applied as a prophylactic measure in acute uterine inversion in order to prevent a reinversion.

General Principles

Similar to any other method used in the management of postpartum haemorrhage (PPH), it is important to note that, if uterine compression sutures are to be applied, this should be done as soon as possible before disseminated intravascular coagulation sets in. Before insertion of these compression sutures, the uterus is exteriorised and the compression test performed by applying pressure on the anterior and posterior surfaces of the uterus using both hands to gain information whether compression sutures would be effective in controlling haemorrhage. Placing the woman in the Lloyd-Davis position allows an assessment of bleeding. An absorbable suture material is used to minimise the risk of bowel herniation through the remaining loops of the suture during the involution of the uterus in the postpartum period. It is essential to avoid excessive tension on the sutures, as this can lead to ischaemia of the uterine walls and increase the risk of uterine rupture. When multiple sutures are used, it is crucial to leave some room between the sutures and to also not occlude the lower segment completely in order to allow the passage of blood and lochia within and out of the uterus.

B-Lynch Suture

The B-Lynch suture was originally described for the management of uterine atony refractory to medical treatment at caesarean delivery, and therefore, the uterine cavity should already be open for it to be applied. After its application, it resembles the braces which are used to hold up the trousers of a man, hence it is also referred to as 'Brace Sutures'. A No.1 absorbable suture of sufficient length (at least 90 cm) is passed back and forth over the anterior and posterior surfaces of the uterus using a large (>70 mm) round-bodied needle while the assistant maintains compression of the uterus (Figure 17.1). If a large round-bodied needle is unavailable, then an 8–10 cm long straight needle can be used as an alternative. While the assistant manually compresses the uterus incrementally, the suture is progressively tightened. Once adequate compression and tightening are achieved, the two ends of the suture are tied together. The uterine incision is then closed in the routine fashion.

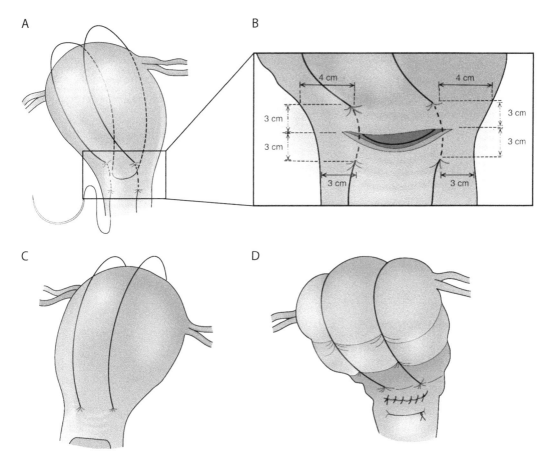

FIGURE 17.1 B-Lynch Suture. A. Anterior surface of the uterus, B. Entry and exit points of the suture on the anterior surface of the uterus, C. Posterior surface of the uterus, D. The appearance of the uterus after applying the B-Lynch suture.

PROCEDURE – B-LYNCH SUTURE

1. Exteriorise the uterus.
2. Apply compression on the anterior and posterior surfaces of the uterus.
3. Check whether bleeding is controlled.
4. If bleeding is controlled with the compression of the uterus, proceed to the application of the B-Lynch suture.
5. Pass a No.1 absorbable suture into the uterine cavity using a large (>70 mm) round-bodied needle 3 cm below the caesarean incision and 4 cm from the lateral wall of the uterus.
6. Let the suture exit at a similar point above the uterine incision.
7. Loop the suture over the uterine fundus to the back of the uterus.
8. Pass the suture again into the uterine cavity from the posterior surface of the uterus at the same level as in step 6 above, apply moderate traction and ensure that the suture is tight while the assistant manually compresses the uterus.

9. Take the suture horizontally within the uterine cavity to the other side of the uterus and make it exit the uterus at a similar point on the posterior surface on the other side.

10. Loop the suture back over the uterine fundus and over the anterior surface of the uterus.

11. Pass the suture into the uterine cavity 3 cm above the uterine incision and 4 cm from the lateral wall of the uterus, at the same level as in step 6 above.

12. Exit the uterine cavity through a similar point 3 cm below the uterine incision, at the same level as in step 5 above.

13. At this point, both free ends of the suture should be recognized on the anterior side of the uterus below the uterine incision.

14. Progressively tighten the suture while the assistant manually compresses the uterus.

15. Tie the free ends together below the uterine incision.

16. Finally, close the uterine incision with a separate suture.

Other Types of Compression Sutures

The other methods of achieving uterine compression are listed below.

- Modifications to the B-Lynch suture, such as the use of two separate sutures for the two sides of the uterus
- The application of two or more separate vertical compression sutures to the upper uterine segment that are horizontally tied together across the fundus without opening into the uterine cavity
- The application of multiple square compression sutures
- A combination of vertical and square compression sutures

Vertical Compression Sutures

In the application of vertical compression sutures, 2–4 sutures depending on the width of the uterus, are passed from the front to the back of the uterus at a level just above the reflection of the bladder using a straight 10 cm needle, and a knot is tied over the fundus of the uterus after progressive tightening of the suture while an assistant manually compresses the uterus. The sutures should be tied together at the fundus in order to prevent these from sliding down off the sides of the uterus. A couple of horizontal compression sutures are also often inserted just above the reflection of the bladder (Figure 17.2).

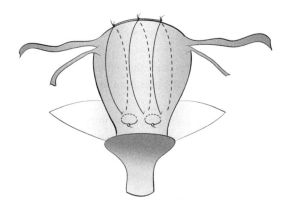

FIGURE 17.2   Vertical compression sutures on the uterus, as described by Hayman and colleagues.

The advantages of this method over the B-Lynch procedure are that it is faster and does not require a hysterotomy.

PROCEDURE – VERTICAL COMPRESSION SUTURES ON THE UTERUS

- Pass a No.1 absorbable suture through the uterus from front to back just above the reflection of the bladder using a straight 10 cm needle.
- Loop the suture on each side of the uterus to the fundus and tie the free ends of the suture at the fundus while an assistant maintains compression on the uterus.
- Insert 2–4 sutures depending on the width of the uterus.
- Horizontally tie the sutures together at the fundus to prevent these from sliding down laterally.
- Insert two horizontal compression sutures on either side of the uterus just above the reflection of the bladder.

Square Compression Sutures

Square compression sutures involve passing a threaded straight needle through the anterior and posterior walls of the uterus in the configuration of a square with roughly 3 cm spacing and tying down the suture in order to approximate the anterior and posterior walls of the uterus (Figure 17.3). Usually, around 4–5 sutures are applied. These sutures can also be utilised to control troublesome bleeding from the lower segment of the uterus in cases of placenta praevia and conservatively managed PAS disorders (discussed in Chapter 13). Targeted compression to specific areas of bleeding is possible. As mentioned previously, it is important to leave some room between the sutures and to not completely occlude the lower segment in order for collected blood and lochia to drain out of the uterus. Multiple needle punctures, around 16–20 in total, may give rise to increased bleeding which may be difficult to control.

PROCEDURE – SQUARE COMPRESSION SUTURES ON THE UTERUS

- Pass a No.1 absorbable suture on a 10 cm straight needle back and forth through the anterior and posterior surfaces of the uterus in a square configuration with approximately 3 cm spacing.
- Tie the free ends of the suture while an assistant maintains compression on the uterus.
- Repeat the procedure at several sites to be able to cover the whole uterus.
- Leave some room between sutures for collected blood and lochia to drain out of the uterus.

Combined Techniques

The 'Uterine sandwich' technique is a method in which the uterine walls are sandwiched between the B-Lynch procedure and an intrauterine balloon. However, vertical compression sutures or square compression sutures cannot be combined with an intrauterine balloon, because the sutures traverse the uterine cavity. The combination of uterine compression sutures, ligation of uterine arteries and utero-ovarian anastomoses or internal iliac arteries has also been described. It is important to note that the combination of uterine compression sutures and devascularization may be associated with a higher risk of uterine ischaemia as compared to the combination of uterine compression sutures and balloon tamponade.

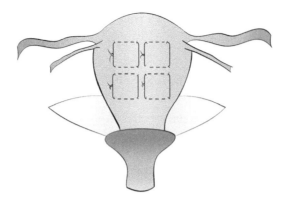

FIGURE 17.3   Square compression sutures on the uterus, as described by Cho and colleagues.

Complications of Uterine Compression Sutures

Complications are rare after compression sutures are applied on the uterus. Isolated cases of haematometra, pyometra, intrauterine synechiae and myometrial necrosis have been reported. Data on menstruation or fertility is limited, but cases of uterine rupture in subsequent pregnancies have been reported.

Key Points

- Uterine compression sutures are effective in cases of refractory uterine atony, placenta praevia and conservatively managed PAS disorders.
- The B-Lynch procedure is appropriate in the management of uterine atony at caesarean delivery, while vertical or square compression sutures are advisable for refractory uterine atony following vaginal delivery, after mechanical and medical management and the application of intrauterine balloon tamponade have failed to control the haemorrhage.
- It is important to leave some room between the sutures for collected blood and lochia to drain out of the uterus and also to avoid excessive tension on the sutures in order to minimise complications associated with uterine compression sutures.
- Although the application of uterine compression sutures is an attractive uterus-preserving management option in refractory PPH, more evidence is necessary for long-term outcomes.

BIBLIOGRAPHY

1. B-Lynch C, Shah H. Conservative surgical management. In: Arulkumaran S, Karoshi M, Keith LG, Lalonde AB, B-Lynch C, editors. A Comprehensive Textbook of Postpartum Hemorrhage. Duncow: Sapiens Publishing, 2012. Pp. 433–40.
2. Cho JH, Jun HS, Lee CN. Hemostatic suturing technique for uterine bleeding during cesarean delivery. *Obstet Gynecol* 2000;96(1):129–31. doi:10.1016/s0029-7844(00)00852-8.
3. Condous GS, Arulkumaran S, Symonds I, Chapman R, Sinha A, Razvi K. The "tamponade test" in the management of massive postpartum hemorrhage. *Obstet Gynecol* 2003;101(4):767–72. doi:10.1016/s0029-7844(03)00046.
4. Hayman RG, Arulkumaran S, Steer PJ. Uterine compression sutures: surgical management of postpartum hemorrhage. *Obstet Gynecol* 2002;99(3):502–06. doi:10.1016/s0029-7844(01)01643.

18

Uterine Devascularization

Sanjeewa Padumadasa and Prasantha Wijesinghe

Uterine devascularization is utilised to control bleeding of uterine origin, such as refractory uterine atony, placenta praevia, placenta accreta spectrum (PAS) disorder, uterine rupture and that due to trauma, such as vaginal lacerations and haematomas. Uterine devascularization is used if mechanical methods and medical treatment fail to control haemorrhage following vaginal delivery. However, in haemorrhage following caesarean delivery, it is logical to resort to uterine devascularization much earlier, because the abdominal cavity is already open. If uterine devascularization alone fails to manage haemorrhage from the uterus, then it may be combined with uterine compression sutures or hysterectomy depending on the urgency of the clinical situation.

Blood Supply to the Uterus

The uterus has two distinguishable blood supplies (Figure 18.1).

- The body of the uterus (referred to as the S1 segment), supplied by the ascending branch of the uterine arteries and the descending branch of the ovarian arteries.
- The lower uterine segment, cervix, upper vagina and respective parametria (referred to as the S2 segment), supplied by branches of the uterine, cervical, upper vesical, vaginal and pudendal arteries.

Uterine devascularization and radiological measures (embolisation or balloon occlusion) used to treat postpartum haemorrhage (PPH), are aimed at controlling blood flow in one or both of these circulations. Bilateral ligation of uterine arteries and the utero-ovarian anastomoses (quadruple ligation) and bilateral internal iliac artery ligation (IIAL) are two commonly used uterine devascularization techniques.

Ligation of Uterine Arteries and Utero-Ovarian Anastomoses

As there is a rich anastomosis between branches of the uterine arteries and branches of the ovarian arteries, ligation of uterine arteries and utero-ovarian anastomoses should be performed on both sides in order for this procedure to be effective in controlling haemorrhage from the uterus. This procedure is likely to be effective only for haemorrhage from the S1 segment of the uterus and will not reduce bleeding from the S2 segment of the uterus.

Procedure

The uterus should be exteriorised, and the urinary bladder should be pushed down in order to avoid injury to the urinary tract. An assistant should retract the uterus away from the side the ligation is performed. An absorbable No.1 suture on a large curved needle is passed through the

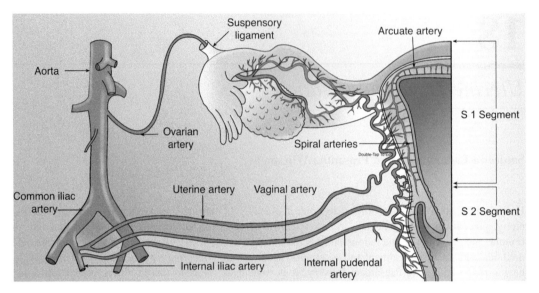

FIGURE 18.1 Blood supply to the uterus.

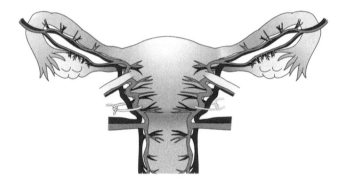

FIGURE 18.2 Uterine artery ligation.

myometrium from front to back at around 2 cm medial to the lateral edge of the uterus and at a level which would be approximately 2 cm below a lower segment caesarean incision, or if the uterovesical fold of peritoneum is intact, as low down as possible and above the bladder (Figure 18.2). The myometrium is included in the stitch in order to provide a firm base for the ligature. The needle is brought back through an avascular portion of the broad ligament to encircle the uterine vessels, and the free ends of the suture are tied together. The procedure is then repeated on the other side.

When ligating the utero-ovarian anastomoses, a common practice is to place sutures on either side, just below the ovarian ligament, in the same manner as described for uterine artery ligation (Figure 18.3A). However, this ligature will not include the arcuate vessel that branches off just under the tubal implantation site. If the suture is placed in between the tubal implantation site and the blood vessel running underneath it, then blood flow not only to the body of the uterus, but also to its fundus, will be impeded (Figure 18.3B). It is important to take the needle medially and include part of the myometrium in the suture, similar to what was done for the uterine artery ligation.

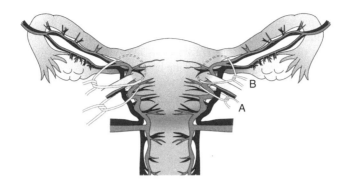

FIGURE 18.3   Ligation of anastomosing branches of uterine and ovarian arteries.

PROCEDURE – LIGATION OF UTERINE ARTERIES AND UTERO-OVARIAN ANASTOMOSES

- Push the bladder down.
- Pass an absorbable No.1 suture on a large round-bodied needle through the myometrium, from front to back about 2 cm medial to the lateral edge of the uterus and at a level which would be approximately 2 cm below a lower segment caesarean incision, or if the uterovesical fold of peritoneum is intact, as low down as possible and above the bladder.
- Bring the needle back through an avascular portion of the broad ligament to encircle the uterine vessels, and tie the suture firmly to compress the uterine vessels.
- Repeat the procedure on the other side.
- Pass a suture between the tubal implantation site and the arcuate vessel running underneath it, take the needle medially to include part of the myometrium, and tie the suture.
- Alternatively, tie the utero-ovarian anastomoses on both sides just below the ovarian ligament.

Internal Iliac Artery Ligation

The procedure of bilateral IIAL came into the limelight in the field of obstetrics and gynaecology, when Sir Howard Kelly performed it to control intraoperative bleeding from cervical cancer in 1893. However, it was not until the late 1960s, when RC Burchell demonstrated that the procedure did not entirely shut the blood supply from the pelvis, that this procedure began to emerge as a useful tool in the management of PPH.

Indications for Internal Iliac Artery Ligation

Internal iliac artery ligation is useful either as a therapeutic or prophylactic measure when there is a desire to preserve fertility, or when hysterectomy alone fails to control the haemorrhage. It is used to manage haemorrhage due to placenta praevia, PAS disorders, uterine atony refractory to medical treatment and genital tract trauma. It is effective in arresting blood loss in cases of deep tears of the vaginal fornices and haematomas, because the vaginal artery is a direct branch of the anterior division of the internal iliac artery. It is also used to control haemorrhage from areas of diffuse bleeding within the pelvis without a clearly identifiable vascular bed.

In complete placenta praevia, as the lower segment of the uterus receives a considerable proportion of its blood supply from the descending cervical and vaginal arteries, IIAL is more effective than uterine artery ligation in terms of controlling haemorrhage, as the blood supply from both the uterine and vaginal arteries is reduced following IIAL. Following hysterectomy, IIAL lessens the risk of reactionary haemorrhage, thereby reducing the chances of the woman having to return to the operating theatre.

Current Role of Internal Iliac Artery Ligation

The introduction of numerous uterotonic agents for the management of uterine atony, and relatively non-invasive techniques such as uterine artery embolisation and balloon tamponade of uterus have almost sidelined this invaluable technique. It is not as difficult to perform as it is commonly perceived. It can be conducted quickly without a need for the involvement of other healthcare professionals and their corresponding additional expertise and facilities as in the case of uterine artery embolisation, which is equally successful in some instances (discussed in Chapter 14).

Although it seems that the skill of performing IIAL is deserting the present-day obstetrician, it will remain a major life-saving tool in the armamentarium of an obstetrician, especially in under-resourced settings with no access to or expertise in techniques such as uterine artery embolisation and in the event of torrential bleeding from the genital tract. The necessity to perform IIAL can be expected to increase in the future due to the escalating rates of caesarean delivery and the concomitant increase in the incidence of placenta praevia and PAS disorders, which are potentially lethal conditions associated with caesarean delivery.

Anatomy of the Internal Iliac Artery

The common iliac artery bifurcates in front of the sacroiliac joint at the level of the intervertebral disc between the L5 and S1 vertebrae and into two main branches: the external iliac artery and the internal iliac artery. The bifurcation of the common iliac artery stands out as an inverted Y. The internal iliac artery branches off from the common iliac artery at a right angle and courses medially and inferiorly to supply the pelvic viscera. The continuation of the common iliac artery is the external iliac artery, which courses laterally and superiorly over the psoas muscle to continue into the lower limb at the inguinal ligament, as the femoral artery (Figure 18.4).

The internal iliac artery divides into anterior and posterior divisions. The posterior division branches off just beyond its origin, is not easily visible and gives off the branches, iliolumbar, lateral sacral and superior gluteal, which supply the gluteal region. The anterior division gives off the umbilical, which in turn provides for the superior vesical, obturator, vaginal (i.e. the equivalent of inferior vesical in males), middle rectal, internal pudendal, inferior gluteal and uterine arteries. Although there are a lot of anatomical variations in the branches of the anterior division, the anatomy is relatively constant at the distal end of the common iliac artery, its bifurcation and the first few centimetres of the internal iliac artery,

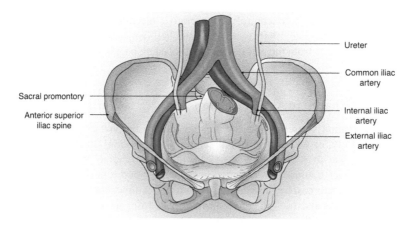

FIGURE 18.4 Anatomical relationships of the internal iliac artery.

the site of relevance for IIAL. The ureter crosses the common iliac artery from its lateral to the medial side just proximal to its bifurcation into the external and internal iliac arteries.

Physiology of Internal Iliac Artery Ligation

The internal iliac arteries supply all of the pelvic organs – uterus, vagina, urinary bladder, rectum and anal canal – with extensive collateral circulations among these viscera. As a result, even bilateral IIAL does not shut the blood supply to the pelvis completely. Therefore, the internal iliac arteries can be ligated without fear of ischaemic necrosis of these pelvic viscera. However, at the same time, IIAL fails to arrest bleeding from the pelvis completely, especially in the case of PAS disorder, in which marked collateral circulations develop in the pelvis. Bilateral IIAL is necessary in almost all the cases where IIAL is performed. Unilateral IIAL may be successful in controlling bleeding only in limited situations, such as bleeding from one side of the pelvic wall.

The effect of IIAL is the near abolition of arterial pulse pressure, leading to a circulation similar to that of a venous system, with slow and sluggish flow, which provides the normal clotting mechanisms of the body an opportunity to achieve haemostasis.

Procedure of Internal Iliac Artery Ligation

The following are needed to perform IIAL (Figure 18.5).

a. Two Kelly retractors
b. Two Mixter right-angled forceps
c. Long toothed forceps
d. Fine dissecting scissors
e. Dental cotton pellets mounted on Allis forceps
f. No. 0 or 1.0 polyglycolic acid suture

There are three approaches to the internal iliac artery: direct approach, the broad ligament approach and extraperitoneal approach.

The obstetrician mainly uses the direct or the broad ligament approach. The direct approach involves the identification of the bifurcation of the common iliac artery, making an incision in the peritoneum and tracing the internal iliac artery in a longitudinal direction. The broad ligament approach involves tracing the external iliac artery to the bifurcation of the common iliac artery, and subsequently, to the internal iliac artery caudally via an opening between the two leaves of the broad ligament. In both of these approaches, the ureter should be taken on the medial fold of peritoneum and retracted medially with the blades of a long retractor. An obstetrician should master both the direct and the broad ligament approaches as the two may be needed depending on the clinical situation. If the uterus is already removed, then the broad

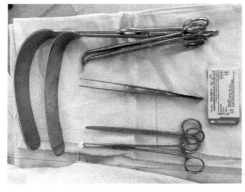

FIGURE 18.5 Instruments needed to perform internal iliac artery ligation.

ligament will already be open, in which case the broad ligament approach could be adopted. If the uterus is intact, then either approach could be used. If pelvic pathology prevents the internal iliac artery from being approached via the broad ligament, then the direct approach has to be adopted.

The extraperitoneal approach, which is via a skin incision on the inguinal area and a muscle-splitting incision in the external oblique muscle (Rutherford-Morrison technique), is mainly adopted by general surgeons in cases of traumatic bleeding from the pelvis.

Surgical Technique

Although IIAL can easily be performed with a suprapubic transverse incision, the presence of PAS disorder may necessitate a midline incision (discussed in Chapter 13). Some recommend changing sides during the operation, because visualisation of the pelvic vessels is better from the opposite side of the pelvis. Some also recommend performing ligation of the internal iliac artery on the right side first and later move to the left side, as the sigmoid mesocolon may hinder the approach to the artery on the left side. These recommendations could be adopted, at the discretion of the operator. The safety and effectiveness of the procedure depend on meticulous surgery, a technique of which is described below.

Exteriorisation of the Uterus and Packing Off the Abdominal Viscera

If the uterus is still intact, then the uterus must be exteriorised. This not only provides access to the posterior pelvic wall, but also reduces further blood loss due to the stretching of uterine vessels. The abdominal viscera are subsequently packed away from the pelvis. This can be achieved by moving the abdominal viscera above the pelvic brim, supporting them with one hand in order to prevent them from falling into the sacral hollow, and then with the other hand, inserting a soaked abdominal pack from one side to the other above the pelvic brim (Figure 18.6). A head-down tilt also helps in clearing the surgical site of abdominal viscera. It also has the advantage of reducing the blood supply to the pelvis, thereby reducing blood loss. However, placing the woman in a head-down tilt may not be feasible in case spinal anaesthesia has been administered.

Opening into the Retroperitoneal Space

The retroperitoneal space on the pelvic side wall is opened using long-toothed forceps (or artery forceps) and fine dissecting scissors at about 2 cm below the bifurcation of the common iliac artery, just lateral to the ureter (Figure 18.7). The bifurcation of the common iliac artery can be identified using two landmarks; the sacral promontory and an imaginary line through the anterosuperior iliac spines. However, the woman may be placed in a head-down tilt position, and this should be considered when using these landmarks to identify the bifurcation of the common iliac artery. Although pulsations of blood vessels can be used in identifying the bifurcation of the common iliac artery, these may be very weak in the case of haemodynamic shock.

Alternatively, the internal iliac artery can be accessed at the base of the broad ligament between the two leaves of the broad ligament (broad ligament approach). The broad ligament may already be open, if a hysterectomy has been previously performed.

Extending the Incision on the Posterior Pelvic Peritoneum

Next, the incision on the pelvic side wall should be extended by about 3–4 cm longitudinally (Figure 18.8). This can easily be done using fingers lateral to the ureter.

Identifying the Internal Iliac Artery

The loose areolar tissue around the blood vessels is cleared in the direction of the vessels, and not across them, in order to avoid trauma to these blood vessels. This is best done by blunt dissection using fingers.

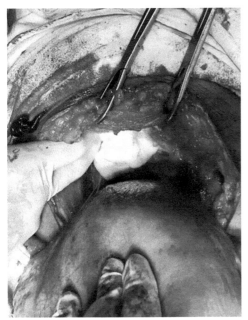

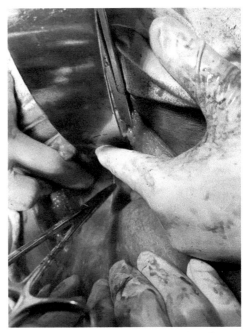

FIGURE 18.6 Exteriorisation of the uterus and packing off abdominal viscera.

FIGURE 18.7 Opening into the retroperitoneal space.

Clearing of loose areolar tissue should be continued until the bifurcation of the common iliac artery comes into view as an inverted Y (Figure 18.9).

Determining the internal iliac artery, its relationship to the common and external iliac arteries and visualisation of the inverted Y throughout the surgery are of utmost importance to avoid accidental ligation of the common iliac and external iliac arteries, as well as the ureter.

Ensuring that the Ureter is on the Medial Flap of the Peritoneum

It must be ensured that the ureter is on the medial flap of the peritoneum. Gravity makes the ureter deviate away from the surgical site, but it should also be manually retracted medially and away from the surgical site with the help of long retractors (e.g. Kelly retractors). Kelly retractors are used to not only retract the peritoneal flaps, but also to apply slight pressure on the blood vessels directed cranially on top and caudally at the bottom (but not downwards), because a blood vessel that is not lax makes it more convenient to clear the loose areolar tissue around the vessel (Figure 18.10). Excessive pressure, which can cause damage to these blood vessels, must be avoided.

Clearing the Areolar Tissue around the Internal Iliac Artery

Using small cotton pellets (similar to dental pellets) mounted on Allis tissue forceps, the loose fibroareolar tissue, which contains lymphatics, lying around the internal iliac artery should be cleared in the direction of the vessels rather than across them. Next, the internal iliac artery could be carefully separated from the internal iliac vein which lies beneath it (Figure 18.11). Clearing the areolar tissue around the internal iliac artery is important, not only to create a safe pathway between the internal iliac artery and the vein, but also to prevent the incorporation of the lymphatics contained within it in the ligature.

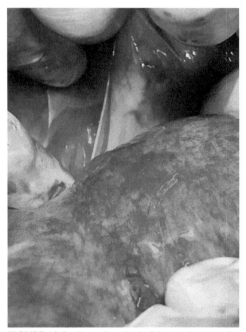

FIGURE 18.8 Extending the incision on the posterior pelvic peritoneum.

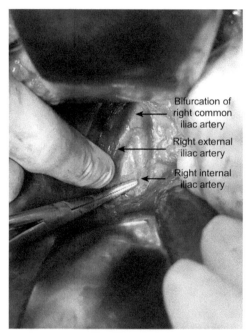

FIGURE 18.9 Identification of the internal iliac artery.

Passing a Fine Right-Angled Forceps beneath the Internal Iliac Artery

Once a clear plane is identified between the internal iliac artery and the vein, a Mixter or any other fine right-angled forcep is passed beneath the internal iliac artery from the lateral to the medial side (Figure 18.12). This should be done approximately 2 cm below its origin in order to leave the posterior

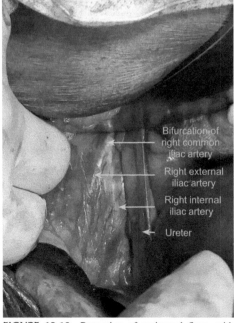

FIGURE 18.10 Retraction of peritoneal flaps, with the ureter placed medially.

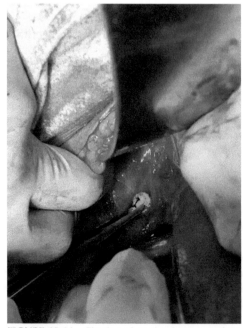

FIGURE 18.11 Clearing of areolar tissue around the internal iliac artery.

division of the internal iliac artery intact. It is not necessary to locate the posterior division, because it is time-consuming and can also potentially damage the internal iliac vein. The right-angled forcep is passed from the lateral to the medial side in order to avoid damaging the external iliac vein. If tissue is still present beneath the internal iliac artery, then careful, sharp dissection could be used to separate them.

If the fine right-angled forcep is used to clear the tissue around the internal iliac artery and the vein, then this should be done conscientiously by placing the forcep at the lateral border of the internal iliac artery and gently opening its tips without forcing it between the two vessels. Extreme caution must be exercised in order to avoid damage to either the internal iliac artery or the internal iliac vein by the tip of the instrument. Some experts advocate the use of Babcock forceps in order to elevate the internal iliac artery to facilitate the passage of the right-angled forcep under the internal iliac artery. However, the Babcock forceps itself could obstruct the operative field.

Preparation of the Suture for Ligation

An assistant should grasp a doubled No. 1.0 or 0 polyglycolic acid or polyglactin suture on another Mixter right-angled forcep. The free ends of the suture should be caught between the tips of the right-angled forcep, and the loop of the suture should be held up without twisting (Figure 18.13).

The assistant should then direct the tips of the second right-angled forcep (with the ends of the suture held between its tips) towards the tips of the first right-angled forcep, and then gently underneath it afterwards (Figure 18.14).

By gently opening the tips, the ends of the suture should then be caught between the tips of the first right-angled forcep which is directly underneath the internal iliac artery (Figure 18.15).

The assistant should then release the ends of the suture from the second right-angled forcep by lightly opening its tips. The doubled polyglycolic acid suture should now be between the tips of the first right-angled forcep situated underneath the anterior division of the internal iliac artery (Figure 18.16).

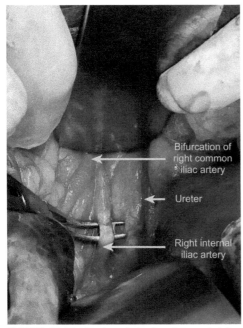

FIGURE 18.12 Passing of the fine right-angled forceps beneath the internal iliac artery.

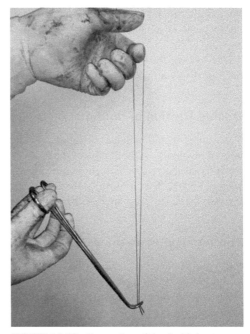

FIGURE 18.13 Preparation of the doubled suture.

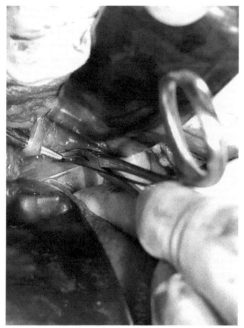

FIGURE 18.14   Positioning the suture underneath the
internal iliac artery.

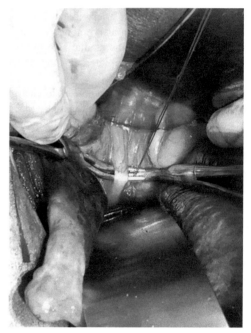

FIGURE 18.15   Feeding the suture.

Swaying of the instruments during the feeding of the suture should be avoided, as this can cause injury to the blood vessels.

The doubled suture, which is situated underneath the internal iliac artery, should then be delicately pulled laterally. Although feeding the loop of the doubled suture is easier for the assistant and catching the loop is easier for the operator as compared to with the ends of the suture, the technique described above helps to maintain a gap of 5 mm between the two arms of the suture and prevents possible twisting of the suture.

The loop of the suture should be cut into two in order to obtain two separate sutures beneath the anterior division of the internal iliac artery (Figure 18.17).

Double Ligation of the Anterior Division of the Internal Iliac Artery

The sutures should be tenderly pulled upwards and in the lateral direction (Figure 18.18). This further helps to avoid the incorporation of the ureter or tissues around it in the ligature. The anterior division of the internal iliac artery is then doubly ligated with sutures that are 5 mm apart, but it is not divided (Figure 18.19). The division of the internal iliac artery is unnecessary and could even be dangerous, because the underlying internal iliac vein could get damaged.

Confirmation of an Intact External Iliac Artery

It is paramount to ensure that the external iliac artery has not been accidentally ligated by using a saturation probe on toes, because ligation of this vessel leads to ischaemia, resulting in loss of the lower limb. Although checking for femoral pulsations is possible, these pulsations could be weak in case of shock.

The procedure must be repeated on the other side. At the end of the procedure, the site of surgery must be examined to exclude bleeding and also to confirm that the ureters are intact.

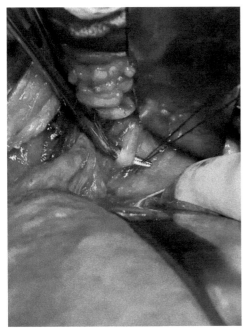

FIGURE 18.16 The doubled suture between the tips of the right-angled forceps situated underneath the anterior division of the internal iliac artery.

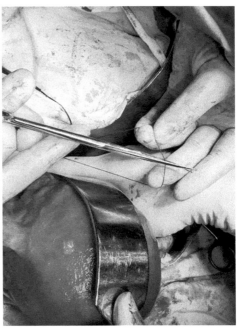

FIGURE 18.17 Cutting the loop of the suture and obtaining two sutures.

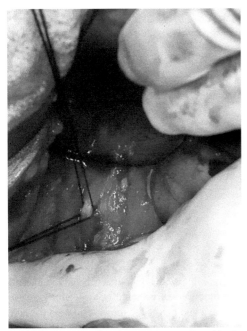

FIGURE 18.18 Pulling the sutures upwards and in the lateral direction.

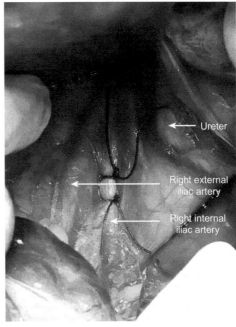

FIGURE 18.19 Double ligation of the internal iliac artery.

PROCEDURE – INTERNAL ILIAC ARTERY LIGATION

- Exteriorise the uterus and pack the abdominal viscera away from the pelvis. A head-down tilt may help.
- Identify the bifurcation of the common iliac artery directly or via an opening between the two leaves of the broad ligament.
- If the direct method is employed, make an incision on the peritoneum of the pelvic side wall at about 2 cm below the bifurcation of the common iliac artery and just lateral to the ureter so that the ureter will lie on the medial fold of peritoneum and extend the incision by approximately 3–4 cm longitudinally.
- Clear the loose areolar tissue from the internal iliac artery by blunt dissection using fingers in the direction of the major vessels rather than across them so as not to cause damage to them.
- Use Kelly retractors not only to retract the peritoneal flaps, but also to apply slight pressure on the blood vessels.
- Clear the loose fibroareolar tissue around the internal iliac artery and separate the internal iliac artery from the internal iliac vein which lies beneath it.
- Once a clear plane is identified between the internal iliac artery and the vein, pass a Mixter or another fine right-angled forcep beneath the internal iliac artery from the lateral to medial side roughly 2 cm below the origin of the internal iliac artery. This avoids including the posterior division of the internal iliac artery in the ligature.
- The assistant should then pass the ends of a doubled No. 1 or 0 polyglycolic acid or polyglactin suture on another Mixter right-angled forcep towards the tips of the first right-angled forcep, and then gently underneath it.
- Catch the ends of the doubled suture with the tip of the right-angled forcep which is beneath the internal iliac artery.
- Pull the doubled suture, which is situated medial to the internal iliac artery under it, in the lateral direction.
- Cut the loop of the suture into two, and tie the anterior division of the internal iliac artery with two ligatures that are 5 mm apart.
- Repeat the procedure on the other side.
- Ensure that the external iliac artery has not been accidentally ligated by using a saturation probe on the foot. Confirm that the ureters are intact.

Complications of Internal Iliac Artery Ligation

The most common adverse complication is damage to the internal iliac vein which lies beneath the internal iliac artery. If there is damage to the internal iliac vein, then direct pressure should be applied in order to prevent haemorrhage. Vascular clamps can then be applied above and below the injury, and with the help of a vascular surgeon, the tear should be repaired with a figure of eight suture using a non-absorbable vascular suture material, such as 4.0 polypropylene on a round-bodied needle. Incorporating the adventitia of the internal iliac artery into the suture adds support to the vein at the site of injury. Meticulous separation of the internal iliac artery from the internal iliac vein should prevent this complication.

Rarely, damage to the internal iliac artery itself may occur before the ligation is completed. This is easily dealt with by applying direct pressure on the site of the injury, then applying vascular clamps on either side of the injury and finally, ligating the vessel.

Inadvertent ligation of the common iliac and external iliac arteries, involvement of the posterior division of the internal iliac artery in the ligature and damage to the ureters are unlikely complications. These can easily be avoided by giving careful consideration to the anatomical relationships of the iliac vessels.

Accidental ligation of the external iliac artery leads to ischaemia of the lower limb, thus risking the loss of that limb. Therefore, it must be ensured that the external iliac artery is intact before ligating the internal iliac artery. If the external iliac artery has accidentally been tied, then the ligature should be immediately removed. However, even if the ligature is removed, the inner layer of the artery wall may have been damaged, and if adequate blood flow in the external iliac artery is not restored, then the help of a vascular surgeon should be sought in order to perform an end-to-end anastomosis or a short vascular graft.

Involvement of the posterior division of the internal iliac artery in the ligature may lead to ischaemia of the gluteal region resulting in corresponding gluteal pain, although in practice, cases like this are few and far in between. This can be avoided by ligating the anterior division of the internal iliac artery about 2 cm from its origin, as the posterior division branches off just distal to the origin of the internal iliac artery. Identification of the ureter and retracting the ureter medially using long retractors prevents accidental injury to the ureter and also makes surgery easier to perform.

It is important not to spend too much time when performing IIAL, as every second is precious in the event of profuse bleeding. Mastering this technique and rehearsing the feeding of the suture by the assistant will help in carrying out this procedure swiftly and safely.

Key Points

- As a result of the extensive anastomotic network in the uterus, ligation of both uterine arteries and utero-ovarian anastomoses is necessary to devascularize the uterus.
- Careful consideration of the anatomical relationships of the internal iliac artery and a meticulous surgical technique prevent complications of IIAL.
- The procedure of IIAL is easy to learn, simple to perform and will continue to be an essential life-saving manoeuvre in the armamentarium of an obstetrician.

BIBLIOGRAPHY

1. Bangal V, Kwatra A, Raghav S. Role of internal iliac artery ligation in control of pelvic haemorrhage. *Pravara Med Rev* 2009;1(2):23–25.
2. Burchell RC, Olson G. Internal iliac artery ligation: aorto-grams. *Am J Obstet Gynecol* 1966;94:117.
3. Burchell RC. Internal iliac artery ligation: haemodynamics. *Obstet Gynecol* 1964;24:737.
4. Burchell RC. Physiology of internal iliac artery ligation. *J Obstet Gynaecol Brit Cwlth* 1968;75:642–51.
5. Clark SL, Phelan JP, Yeh S-Y, et al. Hypogastric artery ligation for obstetric hemorrhage. *Obstet Gynecol* 1985;66:353–56.
6. Padumadasa S. Internal iliac artery ligation – time to revive a dying art. *SLJOG* 2020;42:45–52.

19

Emergency Obstetric Hysterectomy

Sanjeewa Padumadasa and Prasantha Wijesinghe

'The priority in the face of catastrophic bleeding from the uterus should be to preserve the woman's health and life, rather than to preserve her uterus'

Emergency obstetric hysterectomy is usually performed as a last resort for severe postpartum haemorrhage (PPH) that is not responding to other modalities of treatment. Conditions that may require this procedure include placenta praevia, placenta accreta spectrum (PAS) disorder, Couvelaire uterus associated with placental abruption, uterine rupture, uterine atony refractory to uterotonic agents and uterus-conserving measures and extensive uterine sepsis uncontrolled with aggressive treatment. Uterine inversion and rare varieties of abnormal pregnancy, such as cornual, cervical and caesarean scar pregnancies are rare obstetrical causes that might necessitate hysterectomy. Although the incidence of peripartum hysterectomy for refractory uterine atony and uterine rupture has fallen over the years, there has been a dramatic rise in the incidence of peripartum hysterectomy for abnormal placentation, and it can be expected to increase further in the future due to the escalating rates of caesarean delivery and the associated increase in the incidence of placenta praevia and PAS disorders.

Although it is a life-saver, it could result in maternal death, especially in the hands of the inexperienced. Severe maternal morbidity such as haemorrhage, injury to bladder and ureter, disseminated intravascular coagulation (DIC), re-operation and sepsis have been associated with emergency obstetric hysterectomy. Emergency obstetric hysterectomy is a universal indicator of severe acute maternal morbidity. It is one of the surgeries that demands the highest skill and judgement of the obstetrician under the most trying circumstances, and it is imperative that every obstetrician is experienced in this life-saving procedure.

Surgical Principles of Emergency Obstetric Hysterectomy

Management of obstetric haemorrhage entails effective communication, resuscitation, looking for and treating the cause and close monitoring, all of which should occur concurrently. The involvement of an experienced obstetrician, anaesthesiologist, a transfusion medicine specialist, assistants, nursing staff and other supporting staff is important to ensure a favourable outcome.

Timing of Hysterectomy

The timing of hysterectomy is critical to an optimal outcome. It is vital that an experienced obstetric team is involved in both the decision-making process and the surgery itself. There should be a fine balance between resorting to hysterectomy too early and too late, which could result in the death of the woman. Indecisiveness regarding hysterectomy and persisting with non-effective uterus-conserving measures can push the woman to an irreversible stage with tissue hypoxia, acidosis and DIC. Although it would be ideal to proceed with hysterectomy when the woman is resuscitated and is haemodynamically stable, this may not always be feasible as resuscitation could be ineffective until the source of bleeding is removed, which may entail hysterectomy. The woman's desire for future childbearing also plays a dominant role in the decision-making process.

Mode of Anaesthesia

General anaesthesia is preferred. Regional anaesthesia takes more time to be administered and this may exacerbate maternal haemodynamic instability. Furthermore, regional anaesthesia is contraindicated in the presence of coagulopathy, because it increases the risk of spinal or epidural haematoma.

Abdominal Entry

The skin incision is at the discretion of the operator and depends on the circumstances. Although the majority of peripartum hysterectomies can be performed utilising a suprapubic transverse incision, a midline incision may be necessary in case of PAS disorder. When the abdominal cavity is opened, uterine compression sutures (discussed in Chapter 17) and uterine devascularization procedures (discussed in Chapter 18) may be attempted to conserve the uterus, if these measures are considered as appropriate.

Steps to Control Haemorrhage until Hysterectomy is Performed

Once a decision is made to perform hysterectomy, uterotonic agents should not be administered in cases of PAS disorder, because the partial separation of placenta may provoke uncontrollable bleeding.

The uterus should be exteriorised. Exteriorisation of the uterus stretches the uterine arteries and leads to a reduction in blood loss. The assistant could bimanually compress the anterior and posterior walls of the uterus, which would further aid in reducing bleeding. In case of trauma to the uterus, Green Armytage or sponge forceps could be applied to the bleeding edges of the uterine muscle to contain the bleeding. Alternatively, the torn or cut edges may be sutured.

Long straight clamps should be applied on each side of the uterus in order to include the base of adnexal structures, the round ligament and the ovarian ligament to be able to control the collateral blood flow to the uterus from the ovarian vessels. These clamps can also be used to apply traction on the uterus and must be placed slightly away from the lateral border of the uterus to prevent the tips of the clamps from causing injury to the uterine vessels (Figure 19.1). Some prefer to apply a tourniquet (red rubber catheter or plastic intravenous tubing) on the lower part of the uterus in order to reduce blood flow in the ascending branch of the uterine arteries. However, it is vital that no precious time is lost before definitive hysterectomy is performed.

General Principles

The anatomical and physiological changes in the uterus and the pelvis during pregnancy pose technical difficulties when performing hysterectomy in the peripartum period compared to that in a nonpregnant

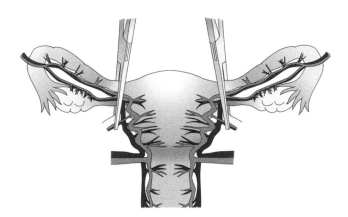

FIGURE 19.1 Application of long straight clamps on either side of the uterus.

woman. In advanced pregnancy, the uterine and ovarian blood vessels are enlarged, distended and tortuous, and the divided pedicles would be thick, oedematous, more vascular and friable. In addition, these pedicles shrink in size as oedema subsides following delivery, which could lead to slippage of the ligatures and subsequent bleeding.

Historically, it was recommended to double clamp the pedicles and apply a third clamp medially to control backflow from the uterus. The pedicles were then cut and doubly ligated. The rationale of the double clamping of the pedicles was to prevent the formation of a haematoma within the pedicle in case a vessel was pierced during transfixation and also to reduce the risk of slippage of the ligature. However, this technique was cumbersome and increased the risk of ureteric injury from the laterally placed clamps. A more feasible approach to achieve the same objectives is to use only two clamps, cut, transfix and ligate each pedicle and then apply a free tie proximal to the transfixing ligature in order to ligate the pedicle for a second time (Figure 19.2). The pedicle should not be held by the transfixing ligature when placing the free tie, as this may loosen the ligature. An atraumatic artery forceps can be used to hold the pedicle when placing the free tie. When applying clamps, the pedicle should be accommodated within the distal two-thirds of the clamp, because the portion of the pedicle within the proximal one-third of the clamp may not be secure. Next, the pedicles should be held in the normal anatomical position without twisting while clamping and tying, as the unraveling that occurs after the clamp has been released and the pedicle has been tied leads to slippage of the suture and corresponding bleeding. An assistant should pull the uterus upwards and towards the opposite side when clamping, cutting and ligating the pedicles.

Surgical Technique

Development of the Round Ligament and Fallopian Tube and Ovarian Ligament Pedicles

The round ligaments should be clamped and cut about 3 cm from its point of attachment to the uterus, followed by a clearing of the areolar tissue within the broad ligament. The anterior leaf of the broad ligament should be incised inferomedially. If a caesarean delivery has been performed, then this incision should join the incision on the uterovesical peritoneum, or if not, this incision should combine with that on the opposite side. The posterior leaf of the broad ligament should now be opened using the middle finger. A curved clamp should be applied medial to the ovary, to the presently exposed pedicle containing the ovarian ligament and Fallopian tube in order to preserve the ovaries, and the pedicle should be incised. With further dissection of the areolar tissue within the broad ligament with finger and gentle sharp dissection when necessary, the uterine vessels should be exposed. Alternatively, a long straight clamp can be applied between the uterus and ovary to include the round ligament, Fallopian tube and ovarian ligament, followed by cutting and ligating the pedicle. This clamp is applied slightly lateral to the clamp that has been applied to control the blood flow from the uterine branches of the ovarian artery. This technique avoids the possibility of troublesome bleeding which may arise from dissection of the broad ligament.

A   B

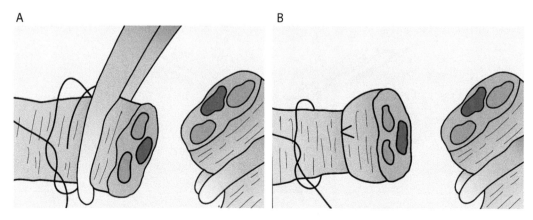

FIGURE 19.2   Double ligation of pedicles; A – transfixing the pedicle, B – free tie.

Bladder Dissection

In most cases necessitating peripartum hysterectomy, the bladder may have adhered to the lower part of uterus as a result of previous surgery and abnormal placentation. The urinary bladder should be dissected down by elevating the uterovesical peritoneum and using sharp dissection. Blunt dissection with gauze is not recommended, because this may result in more bleeding and increase the risk of bladder damage. The bladder dissection should be adequate for the safe placement of clamps which would avoid the urinary tract. Excessive dissection, especially laterally, which can damage the vascular bladder pillars and lead to bleeding that is difficult to be controlled, should be avoided. Excessive dissection is not necessary anyway, if a subtotal hysterectomy is performed. It is important to secure haemostasis while dissecting the bladder from the uterus and upper vagina. This will help in avoiding troublesome bleeding from the bladder base.

Development of the Uterine Vessel Pedicles

On either side of the uterus, at the junction of the cervix and body, large curved clamps should be placed horizontally and perpendicular to the uterine vessels, with the curved end facing upwards. The pedicles should then be cut and ligated (Figure 19.3).

Although each pedicle could be cut and ligated as it is developed (concurrent ligation), it is also possible to apply clamps on both sides of the uterus, cut and proceed until the uterine artery pedicles on both sides are clamped and cut, and then continue to ligating the pedicles (delayed ligation), especially in unstable patients. The delayed ligation technique clamps the main blood supply to the uterus quickly and effectively controls bleeding.

Development of the Utero-Sacral and Cardinal Ligament Pedicles

The utero-sacral and cardinal ligaments should be clamped using straight clamps. Using curved clamps for the utero-sacral and cardinal ligaments may increase the risk of injury to the urinary tract. Ureteric injury should be avoided by placing clamps against the lateral wall of the cervix, medial to those used to secure uterine arteries (Figure 19.4). Lastly, these pedicles should then be cut and ligated. This ligature is applied slightly lateral to and incorporating the uterine artery pedicles. This results in a double ligation of the uterine arteries.

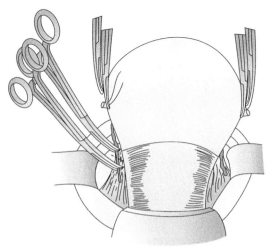

FIGURE 19.3 Clamping of uterine vessels.

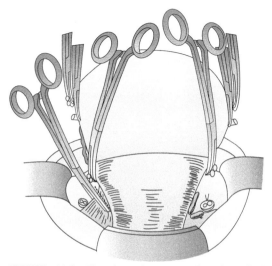

FIGURE 19.4 Clamping of utero-sacral and cardinal ligaments.

Identification of the Cervix

If a total hysterectomy is deemed necessary, then the cervix may be difficult to be identified especially if it has dilated fully. If the uterus is already open, then the rim of the cervix can be identified by inserting a finger through the uterine incision and into the vagina (Figure 19.5). This is not possible if the placenta is still in situ and occupying the lower segment (in case of PAS disorder). The cervix and the anterior fornix can also be identified by inserting a sponge forcep (with a mounted swab) into the vagina and applying pressure on the anterior fornix.

Securing the Angles of the Vagina and Closure of the Vaginal Cuff

The angles of the vagina should be secured by placing curved clamps horizontally, with the curved end facing upwards (Figure 19.6). These pedicles should be cut and ligated with a transfixing suture. Hysterectomy should be completed by cutting the vagina above these pedicles, preferably by using heavy, curved scissors or a scalpel. The vaginal cuff should then be closed with either a continuous suture or interrupted figure-of-eight sutures. All layers of the vagina, some of which may have slipped underneath, must be included in the stitch. Some recommend leaving the vault of the vagina open in order to allow drainage, but this leaves a route for infection in a surgery that already has the potential of being complicated by postoperative infection. Many surgeons insert a drain into the pelvic cavity to aid in postoperative monitoring and also to prevent pelvic haematoma or abscess formation. However, there is no evidence that supports routine insertion of a drain. Although the absence of the drainage of blood can be reassuring, it could also give a false sense of security in case of blockage of the drain.

Total versus Subtotal Hysterectomy

If the source of haemorrhage is not the cervix or paracolpos, then a subtotal hysterectomy would be adequate in order to achieve haemostasis. In this case, the uterus is excised above the ligated uterine vessels (Figure 19.7). The cervical stump is then sutured with figure-of-eight sutures. The advantages of subtotal over total hysterectomy are that it is safer, faster, easier to perform and less likely to injure the bladder and the ureters. However, if the lower uterine segment and paracolpos are involved in hae-morrhage, such as in placenta praevia, PAS disorder or trauma, then total hysterectomy is necessary to achieve haemostasis. Currently, the number of hysterectomies performed for uterine rupture and uterine atony not responding to medical and uterus-conserving surgical measures has decreased. In these cases,

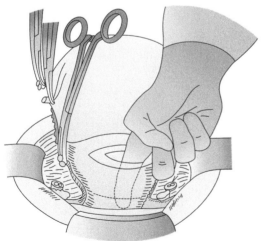

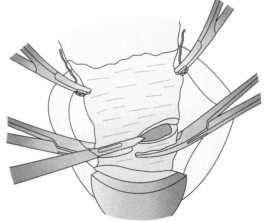

FIGURE 19.6 Securing the vaginal angles with curved clamps.

FIGURE 19.5 Identification of the rim of the cervix through the uterine incision.

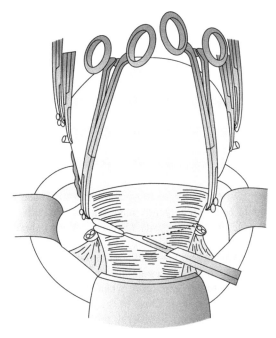

FIGURE 19.7   Subtotal hysterectomy.

subtotal hysterectomy would suffice in controlling the bleeding. In contrast, the number of hyster-ectomies performed for placenta previa and PAS disorders is increasing. Therefore, it is more likely that a total hysterectomy has to be performed if removal of the uterus is considered necessary in current obstetric practice.

Additional Measures to Control Haemorrhage

The pedicles have to be carefully examined for haemostasis before the closure of the abdomen. As some degree of oozing is likely from raw tissue exposed during hysterectomy and which were not included within the clamps, it is advisable that peripartum hysterectomy is accompanied by ligation of the anterior division of both internal iliac arteries. Alternatively, internal iliac artery ligation may be per-formed before embarking on hysterectomy. A good practice point is to extraperitonealize the cut edges of the pedicles, because any oozing from the surgical site may be confined to the extraperitoneal space, creating a tamponade effect which may possibly aid in reducing further bleeding. This can be done by suturing the cut edges of the broad ligament with a continuous suture. A bite has to be taken from the pedicles in order to provide a firm base for the suture as well as to facilitate approximation of the peritoneal edges. Traction on the pedicles which would lead to loosening of the ligatures should be avoided. It is important to be aware of the haemodynamic status of the woman before closing the abdomen, because hypotension will mask bleeding that would manifest later when the blood pressure rises. To reiterate, the role of pelvic drainage is debatable.

Postoperative Management

The woman should receive intensive care in the postoperative period. She should be observed for bleeding and peri-operative antibiotic prophylaxis should be continued for 24–48 hours. As the risk of venous thromboembolism (VTE) is increased in the postpartum period, especially following major surgery such as an emergency obstetric hysterectomy, preventive measures should be taken – such as ensuring adequate hydration and the usage of anti-thrombotic stockings. Thromboprophylaxis with heparin may be initiated once haemostasis is achieved, depending on the woman's risk profile for the development of VTE.

Complete documentation of the events that led to the performing of the emergency obstetric hysterectomy is vital. A post-event analysis session with everyone involved in the management is mandatory. It is imperative that the woman and her partner are extensively debriefed on all the events that led to this situation, which probably would have been completely unanticipated prior to the event.

Complications of Emergency Obstetric Hysterectomy

Bladder and Ureteric Injury

The risk of bladder injury is higher in an emergency obstetric hysterectomy compared to that in a nonpregnant woman. The integrity of the bladder should be tested by gently manipulating the bulb of the Foley catheter through the bladder wall so that an injury can be easily identified. Some experts recommend filling the bladder with methylene blue to be able to identify any bladder injury. If any tear in the bladder is identified, then it should be repaired using two layers of continuous sutures with 3.0 polyglycolic acid or polyglactin suture material. The ureteric orifices should be identified and it must be ensured that these are not incorporated within the repair, especially when dealing with injuries on the posterior wall of the bladder. If the ureteric orifices are close to the site of injury, JJ ureteric stents or infant feeding tubes can be placed within the ureters in order to protect them during bladder repair. Following bladder reconstruction, a Foley catheter should be left in situ for 7–10 days to prevent the formation of a vesicovaginal fistula. The ureters are vulnerable to injury at three sites: when clamping the uterine vessels as the ureters lie just underneath the uterine vessels at this point, at the site of entry into the bladder and when clamping the infundibulo-pelvic ligaments in the rare instance when salpingo-oophorectomy has to be performed. Injuries to the ureters can be avoided by identifying the ureters at the pelvic brim and tracing the course of the ureters downwards, applying clamps medially to those used to secure uterine vessels and careful dissection of the bladder down from the cervix. In case of injury to the ureter, involvement of a urological surgeon is vital. In case of PAS disorder with suspected invasion of the placenta into the parametrium, the preoperative placement of ureteric stents can help in determining the pathway of ureters and preventing accidental ligation or intraoperative injury to ureters.

Disseminated Intravascular Coagulation

The antifibrinolytic agent, tranexamic acid may be administered early, at a dose of 1g intravenously in order to help achieve haemostasis. Oozing may result from DIC which may be a consequence of the condition that necessitated hysterectomy rather than a result of the surgery itself. This should be managed with transfusion of blood products, guided by rotational thromboelastometry, if available (discussed in Chapter 14). Ligation of anterior division of internal iliac arteries (discussed in Chapter 18), extraperitonealization of pedicles and pelvic packing (discussed in Chapter 14) are pertinent measures to control bleeding in this case.

PROCEDURE – EMERGENCY OBSTETRIC HYSTERECTOMY

- Exteriorise the uterus.
- Apply clamps on either side of uterus, commencing from the fundus.
- Mobilise the bladder.
- Cut and proceed until the uterine artery pedicles on both sides are clamped.
- Doubly ligate the pedicles.

- Clamp, cut and doubly ligate the utero-sacral and cardinal ligaments.
- Similarly, clamp, cut and doubly ligate the vaginal angle pedicles.
- Accomplish the hysterectomy.
- Suture the vault of the vagina.
- Exrtraperitonealize the pedicles.
- Observe for bleeding.
- Administer prophylactic intravenous antibiotics.
- Take preventive measures against venous thromboembolic disease.

Key Points

- The decision to proceed to peripartum hysterectomy should be made in a timely manner, not too late and not too early.
- The type of hysterectomy, total or subtotal, is determined by the cause of haemorrhage.
- Doubly ligating the cut pedicles, achieving haemostasis and avoiding damage to the urinary tract are paramount when performing a peripartum hysterectomy.
- Intensive care in the postoperative period is vital.

BIBLIOGRAPHY

1. Baskett TF, Peripartum hysterectomy. In: Arulkumaran S, Karoshi M, Keith LG, Lalonde AB, B-Lynch C, editors. A Comprehensive Textbook of Postpartum Hemorrhage. Duncow: Sapiens Publishing;2012. Pp. 462–65.
2. Baskett TF. Epidemiology of obstetric critical care. *Best Pract Res Clin Obstet Gynaecol* 2008;22: 763–64.
3. Cunningham FG. Peripartum hysterectomy. In: Yeomans ER, Hoffman BL, Gilstrap LC, Cunningham FG, editors. Operative Obstetrics. US: McGraw-Hill publishing;2017. Pp. 979–1015.
4. Knight M, Kuriuczuk JJ, Spark P, Brocklehurst P. Cesarean delivery and peripartum hysterectomy. *Obstet Gynecol* 2008;111:97–105.

20

Retained Placenta

Malik Goonewardene

With expectant management, the placenta is usually delivered within 10–20 minutes of delivery of the baby, and within 5–10 minutes with active management. Active management of the third stage of labour (AMTSL) involves the administration of a uterotonic agent after delivery of the baby, delayed cord clamping and delivery of the placenta by controlled cord traction once the uterus contracts. Although a 60–minute interval after the vaginal delivery of the baby has been suggested, there is no consensus on when a retained placenta should be diagnosed. Most intrapartum caregivers will resort to intervention if the placenta has not been delivered within 30 minutes after vaginal delivery and AMTSL, as the risk of a significant postpartum haemorrhage (PPH) has been shown to increase after 30 minutes into the third stage. The incidence of retained placenta is 2%–4% at 30 minutes and half this value at 60 minutes. Although mortality due to retained placenta is extremely rare, it is associated with considerable maternal morbidity, such as primary PPH, retained placental parts, endometritis and secondary PPH.

Causes of a Retained Placenta

After the delivery of the fetus, inadequate myometrial contractions, especially in the placental bed, have been implicated in the pathogenesis of retained placenta. Inadequate myometrial contractions are also observed in preterm deliveries and atonic PPH. Therefore, the risk factors for a retained placenta parallel those for uterine atony (discussed in Chapter 14). While a history of a retained placenta in a previous pregnancy is a risk factor, current infection of the uterus may also predispose to a retained placenta. It has been shown that a retained placenta is associated with pre-eclampsia, stillbirth and delivery of a small for gestational age infant, raising the suspicion of a common pathophysiologic pathway between defective disorders of placentation, poor obstetric outcome and placental retention.

Frequently, parts of the placenta, rather than the whole, may be adhered to the myometrium (i.e. morbid adherence) (Figure 20.1A). Sometimes, a previously separated placenta may be trapped within the uterus without being expelled. It has been suggested that the use of ergometrine for AMTSL could result in the rapid onset of uterine contractions, placental separation and simultaneous contraction of the cervix, thus predisposing to a 'trapped placenta' within a dilated lower segment of the uterus and an empty upper segment (Figure 20.1B). A deficient decidual reaction leading to invasion of the myometrium by the trophoblast, i.e. placenta accreta spectrum disorder, is a risk factor for a retained placenta (discussed in Chapter 13) (Figure 20.1C).

Management of a Retained Placenta

General Measures

If the retained placenta is associated with uterine atony, or is detached and entrapped, then haemorrhage is highly probable. In such instances, resuscitation should take priority while arrangements are simultaneously being made for immediate manual removal of the placenta (discussed in Chapter 14). Although uterotonic agents may be administered, these are unlikely to be effective until the uterine

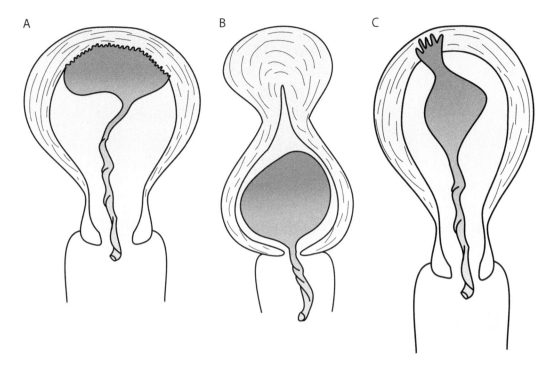

FIGURE 20.1 Types of retained placenta: (A) morbid adherence, (B) trapped placenta, (C) partial accreta.

cavity is completely emptied of any placental parts or blood clots. Uterotonic agents should not be used if placenta accreta spectrum (PAS) disorder is suspected, as these may lead to a partial separation of the placenta and consequently, may aggravate bleeding.

Even if there is no bleeding, if the placenta has not been expelled within a few minutes, then an intravenous infusion should be started and blood crossmatched, because of the risk of haemorrhage while awaiting expulsion or manual removal of the placenta. In the case of PAS disorders, as long as the placenta remains attached to the wall of the uterus, there may be minimal or no bleeding at all, but attempts at manual removal of the placenta may trigger severe bleeding.

Manual Removal of a Retained Placenta

Currently, manual removal is the definitive treatment for a retained placenta. Adequate pain relief is essential, because the procedure is painful and may even cause a vasovagal attack. General, spinal or epidural anaesthesia may be feasible if the woman is haemodynamically stable and can be transferred to an operating room. Manual removal of the placenta may be attempted in the labour room after narcotic analgesia has been administered, if there is massive bleeding and the woman is haemodynamically unstable, or if the operating room is not immediately available.

The woman should be placed in either lithotomy or dorsal position, cleaned and draped and the bladder must be emptied. A well-lubricated gloved (preferably elbow-length) hand should be introduced into the vagina, and the umbilical cord followed through the cervix until the edge of the placenta is identified (Figure 20.2). The fingers and thumb should be extended and approximated in the shape of a cone while entering the cervix. Inside the uterine cavity, the fingers should be separated and flattened in the shape of a spade and inserted into the plane of cleavage between the placenta and its bed, starting from the leading edge of the placenta. The hand should then be gradually moved upwards using side-to-side 'seesaw' movements of the hand, and the placenta must be separated from its bed. The other hand, which should be on the maternal abdomen, should firmly cradle the uterus and push the uterine fundus downwards, towards the woman's feet (Figure 20.3). This will reduce the risk of perforation of the uterine wall. Once the placenta has been completely separated, it should be grasped and removed through the cervix. Any attempts

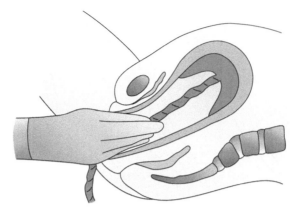

FIGURE 20.2   Use the umbilical cord as a guide to locate the edge of the placenta.

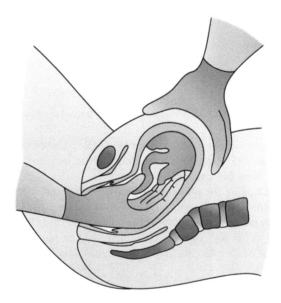

FIGURE 20.3   Manual removal of placenta.

to deliver the placenta while parts of it may still be attached to the uterus may lead to acute uterine inversion (discussed in Chapter 21). In cases where the placenta has pathologically adhered to the uterine wall at certain places, it should be removed piecemeal from these sites.

Ultrasound with or without colour Doppler may be used as an adjunct to clinical examination in order to identify retained placental parts. However, its ability to differentiate between placental parts and blood clots may possibly be low (discussed in Chapter 15). Although manual removal is the fundamental method for removal of the retained placenta, additional suction or sharp curettage may have to be performed in some cases. Excessive or vigorous curettage which can aggravate bleeding or cause uterine perforation and even Asherman's syndrome, should be avoided. Following the procedure, the placenta must be examined carefully to be able to ensure that it has been removed completely. An exploration of the uterus may have to be performed in order to exclude any retained placental parts, especially in the presence of ongoing bleeding. Trauma to the genital tract should be excluded. An oxytocin infusion (e.g. 20 units in 500 mL of normal saline) should be started to maintain uterine contractions, and broad-spectrum antibiotics (e.g. intravenous cefuroxime and metronidazole) administered to prevent infection. If bleeding continues despite completely removing the placenta, then uterine balloon tamponade (discussed in Chapter 14), and laparotomy followed by uterine compression sutures (discussed in Chapter 17), uterine devascularization (discussed in Chapter 18) and even hysterectomy (discussed in Chapter 19), may have to be performed.

PROCEDURE – MANUAL REMOVAL OF PLACENTA

- Anticipate PPH and resuscitate if bleeding is present.
- Consider the possibility of PAS disorder. If in doubt, abandon attempts at the manual removal of the placenta until preparations are made for dealing with a possible massive haemorrhage.
- Provide analgesia/anaesthesia.
- Place the woman in lithotomy or dorsal position, clean and drape her and empty the bladder.
- Use the umbilical cord as a guide to locate the edge of the placenta.
- Use side-to-side movements of the hand to separate the placenta from its bed.
- Use the other hand on the maternal abdomen to firmly cradle the uterus and push down the uterine fundus towards the woman's feet.
- Once the placenta is completely separated, grasp the placenta and remove it through the cervix.
- Observe for genital tract tears.
- Commence an oxytocin infusion.
- Provide broad-spectrum antibiotics.

Intraumbilical Vein Injection of a Uterotonic Agent

It has been postulated that the delivery of a uterotonic agent directly onto the placental bed could induce retroplacental myometrial contractions that are necessary for the separation of the placenta from the uterine wall. An injection of 50 units of synthetic oxytocin dissolved in 30 mL of normal saline into the umbilical vein was recommended by the WHO, and this intervention has been implemented in many centres worldwide, if the placenta has not been delivered within 30 minutes of AMTSL. For this intervention, direct injection is preferred over the use of an infant feeding tube (Figures 20.4–20.6). The main advantage of this intervention is that, although it may not have a 100 percent effectiveness, it is a noninvasive, simple technique with no demonstrable adverse effects, and it reduces the number of manual removal of placentae carried out after 30 minutes of a vaginal delivery. Recent evidence suggests that the intraumbilical vein injection of carbetocin and prostaglandins, such as misoprostol, could have better results than with oxytocin. However, further research is necessary regarding the optimum drug and the corresponding dosage which should be used for this intervention. This intervention is not recommended if there is active bleeding with a retained placenta. If this intervention fails, manual removal of the placenta is indicated. Furthermore, this intervention is contraindicated in the presence of PAS disorder, because the delivery of the uterotonic agent directly into the placental bed may lead to a partial separation of the placenta and could induce catastrophic bleeding.

Trapped Placenta

A trapped placenta should be suspected if there have been signs of placental separation, such as the lengthening of the umbilical cord, a gush of blood and a contracted, globular shaped uterine body rising

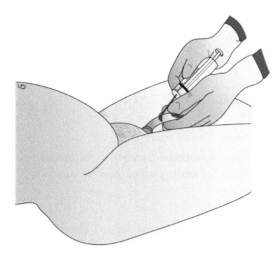

FIGURE 20.4 Direct injection of the uterotonic agent into the umbilical vein.

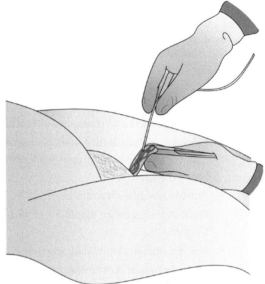

FIGURE 20.5 Injection of the uterotonic agent into the umbilical vein via an infant feeding tube.

up within the abdomen, but the placenta remains undelivered. The trapped placenta may be palpable through the cervical os. Draining the blood trapped in the placenta by releasing the cord clamp, as well as further attempts at controlled cord traction, may achieve placental delivery in this case. Uterine relaxation, especially with nitroglycerin (1 mg sublingually, or 50 micrograms intravenously up to a maximum of 200 micrograms) may be useful as supplementary to manual removal in difficult cases of trapped placenta, although by itself it may not be effective.

Placenta Accreta Spectrum Disorder

Placenta accreta spectrum disorder should be suspected if a clear plane of cleavage between the placenta and the uterine wall cannot be identified (Figure 20.7). In this case, manual removal should be abandoned, and preparations to deal with major haemorrhage, which includes crossmatching of 4–6 units of blood and preparing the woman for an emergency hysterectomy, should be instituted. The involvement

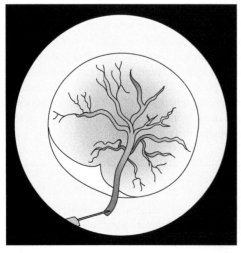

FIGURE 20.6 Distribution of the uterotonic agent in the placental bed.

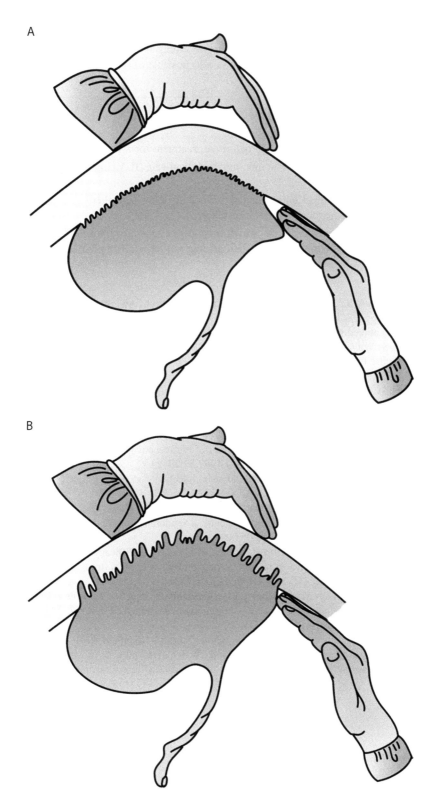

FIGURE 20.7   Plane of cleavage in morbid adherence (A) and its absence in placenta accreta spectrum disorder (B).

of an experienced obstetrician, an anaesthesiologist, a transfusion medicine specialist, nursing and other supporting staff is vital. Although an emergency hysterectomy is the mainstay of treatment for PAS disorders, expectant or conservative management is also possible (discussed in Chapter 13).

Key Points

- At the present, manual removal is the definitive treatment for a retained placenta.
- In the absence of active vaginal bleeding, intraumbilical vein (IUV) injection of a uterotonic agent could be considered.
- In the presence a retained placenta with active bleeding, there is no alternative to resuscitation and immediate manual removal of the retained placenta.
- The possibility of PAS disorder, in which attempts at manual removal of a placenta may be detrimental, should be borne in mind when dealing with a retained placenta.

BIBLIOGRAPHY

1. Endler M, Saltvedt S, Cnattingius S, Stephansson O, Wikstrom AK. Retained placenta is associated with pre-eclampsia, stillbirth, giving birth to a small-for-gesttaional-age infant, and spontaneous pre-term birth: a national register-based study. *BJOG* 2014;121:1462–70.
2. Greenbaum S, Wainstock T, Dukler D, Leron E, Erez O. Underlying mechanisms of retained placenta: evidence from a population based cohort study. *Eur J Obstet Gynecol Reprod Biol* 2017; 216:12–17.
3. Grillo-Ardila CF, Amaya-Guio J, Ruiz-Parra AI, Amaya-Restrepo JC. Systematic review of pros-taglandin analogues for retained placenta. *Int J Gynaecol Obstet* 2018;143(1):19–23.
4. Duffy JM, Mylan S, Showell M, Wilson MJ, Khan KS. Pharmacologic intervention for retained placenta: a systematic review and meta-analysis. *Obstet Gynecol* 2015;125:711–18.
5. Lowenwirt IP, Zauk RM, Handwerker SM. Safety of intravenous glyceryl trinitrate in management of retained placenta. *Aust N Z J Obstet Gynaecol* 1997;37:20–24.
6. Nardin JM, Weeks A, Carroli G. Umbilical vein injection for management of retained placenta. *Cochrane Database Syst Rev* 2011;11(5):CD001337.
7. Salem MAM, Saraya YS, Badr MS, Mohammad AZ. Intra-umbilical vein injection of carbetocin versus oxytocin in the management of retained placenta: a randomized controlled. *J Obstet Gynecol Res* 2019;21:21–25. doi: 10.1016/j.srhc.2019.05.002.
8. Samanta A, Roy SG, Mistri PK, Mitra A, Pal R, Naskar A, et al. Efficacy of intra-umbilical oxytocin in the management of retained placenta: a randomized controlled trial. *J Obstet Gynecol Res* 2013;39(1):75–82. doi: 10.1111/j.1447-0756.2012.01974.x.
9. Harara R, Hanafy S, Zidan MSA, Alberry M. Intraumbilical injection of three different uterotonics in the management of retained placenta: a randomized controlled trial. *J Obstet Gynecol Res* 2011;37(9):1203–07. doi: 10.1111/j.1447-0756.2010.01499.x.
10. World Health Organisation – Reproductive Health Library. *Umbilical Vein Injection for Retained Placenta: Why and How?* Geneva, Switzerland: WHO;2016. https://extranet.who.int/rhl/resources/videos/umbilical-vein-injection-retained-placenta-why-and-how

21

Acute Uterine Inversion

Sanjeewa Padumadasa and Kapila Gunawardana

When the uterine fundus collapses into the endometrial cavity, thus turning the uterus partially or completely inside out, it is referred to as uterine inversion. Acute uterine inversion occurs rarely, in approximately 1 in 15,000 vaginal deliveries, and it reflects suboptimal management of the third stage of labour. Its early recognition and management reduce maternal mortality and morbidity. Acute uterine inversion refers to uterine inversion occurring within 24 hours following vaginal delivery. Uterine inversion occurring after 24 hours and up to four weeks following delivery is referred to as 'subacute', while that occurring after four weeks following delivery or in the non-pregnant state is indicated as 'chronic'. Acute uterine inversion is a life-threatening obstetric emergency and will be described in detail in this chapter.

Degrees of Uterine Inversion

Uterine inversion is classified into various degrees according to the location of the inverted fundus in relation to the rest of the female genital tract (Figure 21.1).

Causes of Uterine Inversion

Mismanagement of the third stage of labour, mainly inappropriate traction on the umbilical cord while the placenta is attached to the uterus is the most common cause of acute uterine inversion (Figure 21.2). Pressure on the uterine fundus before placental separation can also lead to acute uterine inversion.

Localised atony, mainly in the fundal placental site, with active contractions of the rest of the uterus, rapid manual removal of the placenta while a portion of the placenta remains attached to the uterus, and the presence of placenta accreta spectrum disorder (discussed in Chapter 13) can also lead to uterine inversion. A sudden increase in the intra-abdominal pressure, as a result of coughing, sneezing, vomiting or straining, as well as connective tissue disorders such as Marfan syndrome and Ehlers-Danlos syndrome, are also risk factors for uterine inversion. An abnormally short umbilical cord or a cord which was, in effect, shortened by being wrapped around the fetal body, can theoretically cause uterine inversion, and a number of such cases have been reported. Precipitate labour can also give rise to uterine inversion. In half of the women with uterine inversion, there is no identifiable risk factor. Therefore, for all practical purposes, uterine inversion is largely unpredictable. Chronic uterine inversion occurs as a result of unrecognised inversion or as a result of a submucous fibroid or a retained placental cotyledon prolapsing through the cervix.

Prevention of Acute Uterine Inversion

Active management of the third stage of labour, which currently includes administration of a uterotonic agent after the delivery of the baby, delayed cord clamping and the delivery of the placenta by controlled cord traction (CCT), has resulted in a marked reduction in the incidence of acute uterine

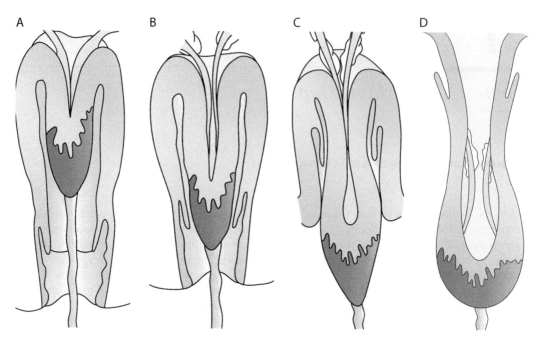

FIGURE 21.1 Degrees of uterine inversion. A - First degree (incomplete) - Dimpling of the uterine fundus with the inverted fundus still above the cervix, B - Second degree (complete) - The inverted fundus extends through the cervix, but remains inside the vagina, C - Third degree (complete) - The inverted fundus extends outside the vagina, D - Fourth degree (complete) - The uterus is completely outside the vagina. In this case, the vagina also inverts. This is also referred to as 'total uterine inversion'.

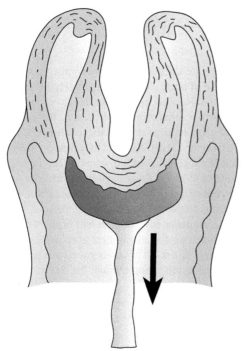

FIGURE 21.2 Inappropriate traction on the umbilical cord is the most common cause of uterine inversion.

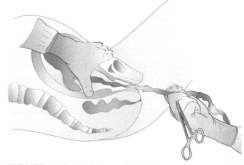

FIGURE 21.3 Delivery of the placenta by controlled cord traction.

inversion. Traction should be applied to the umbilical cord, but only when the woman's uterus has contracted after the birth of her baby, and counter pressure should be applied on her uterus just above the pubic bone until the placenta is delivered (Figure 21.3). It is important to avoid traction on the umbilical cord before the uterus has contracted, as well as to avoid fundal pressure during the third stage of labour. As a result of the uterotonic, the uterus would have contracted, and sometimes, the placenta would have separated by the time CCT is embarked upon after the delayed cord clamping. If the placenta does not detach at the initial attempt at CCT, then it should be repeated after an interval of 2–3 minutes. If the placenta still remains attached to the uterus, placental separation should be awaited. If the placenta is still not delivered after 30 minutes from the time of delivery, then CCT should be repeated, and if this still fails, then it would be considered a case of retained placenta, and should be managed as discussed in Chapter 20. Contraction of the uterus should be confirmed before each attempt at repeat CCT, and excessive traction must not be applied during CCT. Excessively vigorous manual removal of the placenta should also be avoided.

There is a risk of recurrence of uterine inversion in subsequent pregnancies. Therefore, women with a history of acute uterine inversion should be advised to deliver in a hospital, and the third stage of labour must be actively managed.

Diagnosis

Severe and sustained pain in the suprapubic area due to stretching of the infundibulo-pelvic ligaments and other viscera is the most common initial symptom. Vaginal bleeding is usually present, unless the placenta is completely adherent to the uterine wall. Shock is the outstanding sign, which is initially disproportionate to the amount of blood loss, as a result of neurogenic shock due to the initiation of a strong vasovagal reflex from stretching of viscera before hypovolaemic shock sets in. Therefore, there may be bradycardia and hypotension consistent with a neurogenic type of shock during the initial stages. Later, signs of hypovolaemic shock, such as rapid, thready pulse and cold clammy extremities, develop as a result of significant bleeding due to poor retraction and congestion of the inverted uterus and partial separation of the placenta.

In third degree uterine inversion, the uterus is not palpable abdominally and is observed outside the vagina as a polypoidal purplish-red mass with the broader end pointing downwards. Although this is the most dramatic of the clinical presentations of uterine inversion, it is rare. A vaginal examination would reveal the inverted body of the uterus with the ring of the cervix encircling it, in case of second degree uterine inversion. In first degree uterine inversion, a dimple may be palpated on the uterine fundus on abdominal examination.

Management

The foot end of the bed should be elevated in order to reduce the tension on the viscera. This reduces pain as well as the degree of shock. Assistance must be summoned and immediate resuscitation measures for shock should be carried out (discussed in Chapter 14). As hypovolaemic shock would ensue after the initial neurogenic shock, two 14 or 16 G intravenous cannulae should be inserted, and blood must be drawn for crossmatching and other tests for postpartum haemorrhage. Up to 2 litres of crystalloids should be infused rapidly. If the placenta is still attached, then it should not be removed at this stage, as this would increase blood loss. Uterotonic agents are not effective and should not be administered until the uterine inversion is corrected. The procedures which could be done to correct the uterine inversion are described below.

Successful replacement of the inverted uterus in the abdominal cavity should be followed by manual removal of the placenta once the uterus has contracted, if the placenta is still attached. It is important to delicately explore the uterine cavity in order to ensure that there are no placental fragments remaining and also to ascertain that the uterine wall is intact. Bimanual compression of the uterus may be necessary to control haemorrhage until the uterus is well contracted (discussed in Chapter 14). A bolus dose of intravenous (IV) ergometrine 0.5 mg should be administered, and an oxytocin infusion (40 units in 500 mL of normal saline over four hours) must be commenced to be able to maintain uterine contractions in order to control haemorrhage as well as to prevent a re-inversion. The woman should be observed for postpartum haemorrhage. Broad-spectrum IV antibiotics should be administered as prophylaxis against infection.

Manual Replacement of the Uterus

If the inversion is detected soon after the delivery, then the inverted uterus should be manually replaced in the abdominal cavity as soon as possible, as the cervical ring would still be sufficiently relaxed to allow successful reduction (Figure 21.4). Therefore, the birth attendant is the ideal person to manage the case. However, in most instances, a skilled medical officer would not be in attendance. Therefore, immediately calling for help is essential. Any delay will lead to oedema and congestion of the inverted fundus due to the constricting cervical ring, thus making repositioning of the uterus increasingly difficult over time.

The bladder should be catheterised, and adequate analgesia/anaesthesia should be instituted. Because it is important to perform manual replacement as soon as possible, a combination of intravenous narcotics, paracervical and pudendal block and inhalational analgesia is useful to be able to provide effective analgesia. If anaesthesia should be given, it is important to note that general anaesthesia with fluorinated hydrocarbons (sevoflurane and isoflurane) is preferred in order to aid uterine relaxation. Halothane, which is associated with myocardial irritability, arrhythmias and hepatotoxicity is rarely used today. If the woman is on an epidural, it may be continued or spinal anaesthesia may be administered, provided vital signs are normal.

The first-line manoeuvre to reposition the inverted uterus was first described by Johnson in 1949, hence it is termed 'Johnson's manoeuvre'. The portion of the uterus that came down last should be replaced first. Therefore, the lower segment of the uterus should be replaced initially, followed by the fundus of the uterus. The inverted uterine fundus should be cupped in the palm of the hand. Thereafter, pressing on the lower uterine segment at the utero-cervical junction with the thumb and fingers, the uterus should be first pushed into the vagina and then, further upwards towards the umbilicus. Excessive force should not be used, as the thinned out lower segment can tear. Once the uterus has been completely replaced, it should be held in place for a few minutes, while the other hand on the abdomen supports the fundus.

In cases in which initial replacement is unsuccessful, measures to relax the cervical ring by the administration of tocolytics have been tried. Subcutaneous terbutaline at a dose of 0.25 mg is a popular method of providing acute tocolysis. Magnesium sulphate IV and nitroglycerin IV or sublingually, have also been used as agents for acute tocolysis. However, there is controversy surrounding the use of acute tocolysis for treating uterine inversion, as it could further increase the risk of postpartum haemorrhage due to uterine atony. In addition, beta-agonists can cause cardiovascular effects, thereby further compromising the woman who is already at risk of cardiovascular instability.

A   B   C

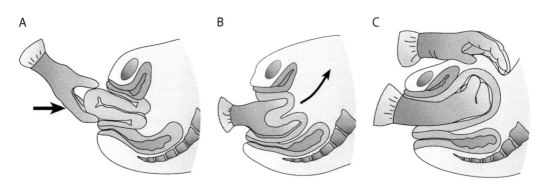

FIGURE 21.4   Manual replacement of the uterus.

PROCEDURE – MANUAL REPLACEMENT OF THE INVERTED UTERUS

- Do not attempt to remove the placenta, if it is still attached to the uterus.
- Catheterise the bladder.
- Provide analgesia/anaesthesia and administer tocolytics, if necessary.
- Cup the inverted uterine fundus in the palm of the hand.
- Press on the lower segment of the uterus with the thumb and the fingers.
- Push the inverted uterus towards the umbilicus and correct the uterine inversion.
- Once the uterus has been replaced inside the abdominal cavity, hold it in place for a few minutes with the other hand abdominally supporting the fundus, and finally remove the placenta manually.
- Gently explore the uterine cavity for any retained products and for integrity of the uterine wall.

Hydrostatic Methods for Correction of Uterine Inversion

Hydrostatic methods have been used successfully in cases in which manual replacement has failed to correct the uterine inversion.

The woman should be placed in lithotomy position. It is vital to exclude uterine or vaginal tears before using a hydrostatic method. If there are tears, these should be sutured. The vaginal fornices are distended with isotonic sodium chloride solution via an infusion set or a rubber tube, and the vulva is sealed (with the wrist, silastic vacuum extractor cup (Figure 21.5) or Green Armytage forceps) in order to prevent the fluid from seeping out. If a vacuum extractor cup is used, then it should be directed towards the posterior fornix. The bag of fluid should be brought to body temperature and must be placed at a height of around 1.5 m above the level of the vagina, in order for sufficient pressure to build up for insufflation. Around 5 L of fluid may be necessary for successful correction of uterine inversion.

The constricting cervical ring is pulled outwards, and the fluid applies pressure on the fundus, which leads to successful replacement of the uterus in the abdominal cavity. Once the uterine inversion has been corrected, the fluid should be allowed to escape slowly from the vagina. Although theoretically, there is a risk of developing TURP syndrome (fluid overload and pulmonary oedema), this has not been reported in the literature. When either manual replacement or O'Sullivan hydrostatic replacement technique fails, laparotomy is required to replace the inverted uterus.

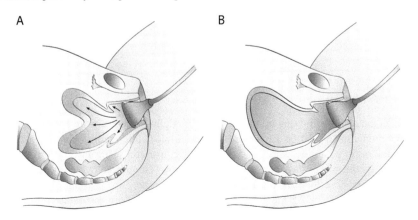

A   B

FIGURE 21.5 Hydrostatic method for correction of uterine inversion.

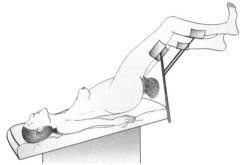

FIGURE 21.6 Patient position during laparotomy for management of acute uterine inversion.

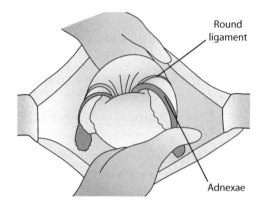

FIGURE 21.7 Atraumatic stepwise reduction of an inverted uterus.

Laparotomy

At laparotomy, the woman should be placed in Lloyd Davis (frog-legged) position with a Trendelenburg (head-down) tilt (Figure 21.6). She should be catheterised, and broad-spectrum IV antibiotics (e.g. cefuroxime) should be administered. The bowels should be packed away from the uterus.

A. Non-instrumental Atraumatic Stepwise Reduction of an Inverted Uterus

In this technique, the hands of the obstetrician should be placed in front and the back of the lower segment, with the fingertips below the level of the inverted fundus. With progressive pressure by the fingertips of both hands, the internal dimple should be sequentially replaced by the rising uterine fundus (Figure 21.7).

B. Huntington's Technique

At laparotomy, upward traction is applied on both round ligaments sequentially using Allis forceps, ring forceps or tenacula. Care must be taken in order to avoid tearing the round ligaments. An assistant may aid the procedure by applying persistent and progressive pressure on the inverted fundus of the uterus from the vagina, using his/her fingertips (Figure 21.8).

C. Use of a Vacuum Cup to Correct Uterine Inversion

An alternative to the use of potentially traumatic forceps is to use a soft silastic vacuum extractor cup (Figure 21.9). The vacuum cup should be placed through the dimple on the inverted uterine fundus, a vacuum must be created and the inverted fundus brought out through the dimple by applying traction on the vacuum cup.

D. Haultain's Technique

In cases in which the constricting ring on the cervix is too tight to proceed with Huntington's operation, Haultain's operation can instead be performed (Figure 21.10). Following laparotomy, a longitudinal incision is made on the posterior aspect of the cervical constricting ring in order to relieve the constriction and increase the size of the ring. Afterward, the uterus is replaced in the abdominal cavity using any of the techniques described as for Huntington's technique. An assistant should exert upward pressure on the inverted parts of the uterus from the vagina below to aid its replacement in the

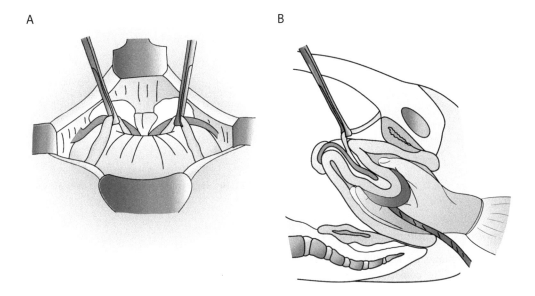

FIGURE 21.8   Huntington's technique; A – abdominal view, B – sagittal view.

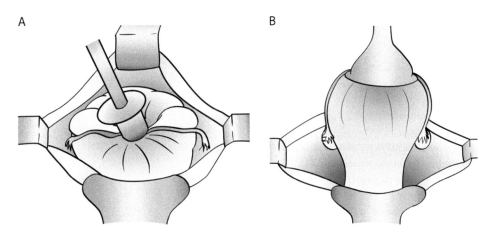

FIGURE 21.9   Use of a vacuum extractor cup at laparotomy to correct uterine inversion.

abdominal cavity. Following correction of the uterine inversion, the incised portion of the lower uterine segment should be repaired with interrupted sutures.

Infrequently, uterine inversion can recur. This can be prevented by uterine balloon tamponade (discussed in Chapter 14) in cases in which manual replacement or hydrostatic replacement technique has been utilised, or otherwise, by application of uterine compression sutures (discussed in Chapter 17) in cases in which laparotomy has been performed.

E. Hysterectomy

Hysterectomy is reported as a last resort, in case of failure of conservative surgical measures to correct uterine inversion, as well as in late presentation with ischaemic changes of the uterus. Hysterectomy may also be indicated in cases of intractable haemorrhage resulting from uterine atony following inversion, which does not respond to medical treatment and conservative surgical measures (discussed in Chapter 19).

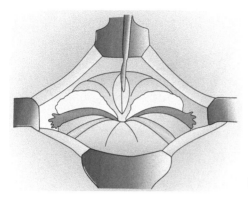

FIGURE 21.10   Haultain' operation to correct uterine inversion.

F. Combined Abdomino-vaginal Procedures

Spinelli's technique, i.e. anterior colpotomy, and Kustner's technique, i.e. posterior colpotomy, along with incision of the constricting cervical ring and the wall of the uterus on the corresponding side vaginally are possible procedures, but these are seldom used today. Historically, these methods have been used in cases of uterine inversion in which the uterus and the adnexae were absent within

TABLE 21.1

Summary of management of uterine inversion

Immediate management

    Resuscitation for shock

    DO NOT remove the placenta (if it is still attached)

    DO NOT administer uterotonic agents before replacement of the inverted uterus

    Elevate the foot end of the bed

    Provide analgesia/anaesthesia

    Insert urinary catheter

Replace the inverted uterus in the abdominal cavity

    Manual replacement of the inverted uterus

    O'Sullivan hydrostatic manoeuvre

    Laparotomy, followed by

    Non-instrumental atraumatic stepwise reduction of the inverted uterus

    Huntington's technique using Allis tissue forceps, ring forceps or tenacula

    Correction of uterine inversion using a vacuum cup

    Haultain's technique

Hysterectomy

    Combined abdomino-vaginal procedures

    Spinelli's technique

    Kustner's technique

Subsequent management

    Manual removal of the placenta through the vagina (if the placenta is still attached)

    Initiate and maintain uterine contractions by uterine massage and uterotonic agents

    Prevent recurrence of uterine inversion by insertion of intrauterine tamponade balloon or application of uterine compression sutures

    Administer broad-spectrum intravenous antibiotics

    Observe for postpartum haemorrhage

---

the pelvis at laparotomy, thus making it impossible to correct the uterine inversion using any of the surgical manoeuvres previously described. In these methods, the uterus is separated into two pieces, and along with adnexae, is pushed into the abdomen from below. Later, the incisions on the uterus and vagina are repaired.

Management of acute uterine inversion is summarised in Table 21.1.

Key points

- Acute uterine inversion is largely preventable with proper active management of the third stage of labour, but it is imperative that every birth attendant is competent with its initial management.
- Acute uterine inversion should be excluded in all cases of postpartum collapse.
- The degree of shock in the initial stages is out of proportion with the amount of blood loss.
- Immediate replacement of the inverted uterus in the abdomen is the key to a successful outcome.

BIBLIOGRAPHY

1. Antonelli E, Irion O, Tolck P, Morales M. Subacute uterine inversion: description of a novel replacement technique using the obstetric ventouse. *BJOG* 2006;113:846–47.
2. Baskett TF. Acute uterine inversion: a review of 40 cases. *J Obstet Gynaecol Can* 2002;24:953–56.
3. Dickson MJ, Anders NK. Acute puerperal uterine inversion: a report of five cases. *J Obstet Gynaecol* 2000;20:426–27.
4. Haultain FWN. The treatment of chronic uterine inversion by abdominal hysterectomy, with a successful case. *BMJ* 1901;2:974.
5. Huntington JL, Boston MD. Acute inversion of uterus. *Med Surg J* 1921;184:376–80.
6. Majd HS, Pilsniak A, Reginald PW. Recurrent uterine inversion: a novel treatment approach using SOS Bakri balloon. *BJOG* 2009;116:999–1001.
7. Matsubara S, Yano H. Uterine compression suture for acute recurrence of puerperal uterine inversion: Hayman suture? *J Obstet Gynaecol Res* 2012;38(10):1272–73.
8. O'Sullivan J. Acute inversion of the uterus. *BMJ* 1945;2:282–83.
9. Ogueh O, Ayida G. Acute uterine inversion: a new technique of hydrostatic replacement. *BJOG* 1997;104:951–52.
10. Wendel MP, Shnaekel KL, Magaan EF. Uterine inversion: a review of a life-threatening obstetrical emergency. *Obstet Gynecol Surv* 2018;73(7):411–17.

22

Amniotic Fluid Embolism

Sanjeewa Padumadasa

Amniotic fluid embolism (AFE) is perhaps the most catastrophic of all of the emergencies in the field of obstetrics. First reported by Meyer in 1926 and later described by Steiner and Lushbaugh in 1941, it is rare, with a reported incidence of 2–3 per 100,000 deliveries. However, the true incidence is unknown because of inaccurate diagnosis and inconsistent reporting of cases. Amniotic fluid embolism can be fatal in up to 80% of cases; the main reasons are cardiac arrest, intractable haemorrhage due to coagulopathy, acute respiratory distress syndrome (ARDS) and multiple organ failure. The case-fatality rate has recently reduced due to early diagnosis and high-level supportive care, but the degree of hypoxia associated with this condition is quite profound that even if the woman survives the initial episode, she is likely to suffer from permanent neurological damage.

Pathophysiology

The underlying pathophysiology of AFE, which has eluded both clinicians and researchers alike, involves an abnormal response to fetal tissue that has gained entry into the maternal circulation. It has been postulated that, in some women rather than all, this leads to the activation of the complement pathway and mast cell degranulation resulting in the release of inflammatory vasoactive mediators such as prostaglandins, leukotrienes, histamine and interleukins among others, which initiates a cascade of events similar as those observed in anaphylactic and septic shock. Therefore, some have proposed the term 'anaphylactoid syndrome of pregnancy' in order to emphasise that the clinical features are secondary to biochemical mediators and not because of a pulmonary embolic phenomenon, as previously believed.

There is a biphasic haemodynamic response in AFE, which leads to right and left ventricular failure, profound hypotension and shock. This is followed by a phase of coagulopathy, triggered by the activation of coagulation factors by procoagulant products contained in the amniotic fluid and fetal cells. It is also speculated that coagulopathy may be compounded by massive hyperfibrinolysis because of the increased concentrations of urokinase-like plasminogen activator and plasminogen activator 1 present in the amniotic fluid. Coagulopathy leads to profound bleeding. It is also hypothesised that the entry of amniotic fluid into the maternal circulation increases the plasma concentration of endothelin, which acts as a bronchoconstrictor as well as a pulmonary and coronary vasoconstrictor, and this may contribute to cardiorespiratory arrest.

Risk Factors

Amniotic fluid embolism commonly occurs immediately after delivery or during labour. However, AFE has been reported as early as the second trimester and as late as a few hours following delivery. Studies have revealed minor associations with increased maternal age (>35 years), multiparity, induction or augmentation of labour with oxytocin, uterine hyperstimulation, polyhydramnios, multiple pregnancy, instrumental vaginal delivery, caesarean delivery, second-trimester miscarriage, uterine rupture, cervical lacerations, placental abruption, amniotomy and other intrauterine procedures such as amnioinfusion and amniocentesis. The connection of AFE in these conditions has been attributed to strong uterine contractions, excessive amniotic fluid or disruption of vessels supplying the uterus. However, these correlations are rather common, and the condition of AFE, in contrast, is quite rare. Therefore, for all practical purposes, AFE is neither predictable nor preventable and can occur at any time in any pregnant woman.

Clinical Features

There is a wide spectrum of clinical presentations in AFE ranging from asymptomatic to dramatic symptoms and signs. Sudden onset cardiorespiratory arrest immediately following delivery or during labour should warn the clinician of a possible diagnosis of AFE.
Other clinical features are listed below.

- Non-specific prodromal symptoms such as restlessness, shivering, lightheadedness, paraesthesia, nausea and vomiting
- Dyspnoea, tachypnoea, frothy sputum, cyanosis, chest discomfort and bronchospasm
- Loss of consciousness, seizures and coma
- Disseminated intravascular coagulation and postpartum haemorrhage, which may be the clinical presentation in atypical cases
- Fetal heart rate abnormalities and fetal death (in cases of AFE occurring during the antepartum and intrapartum periods) – fetal distress may even precede maternal symptoms as blood is shunted from the uterus to the maternal circulation in order to preserve cardiac and neurologic function. Therefore, it is essential to exclude AFE in all cases of unforeseen and unexplained fetal distress.

The relationship between the pathophysiology and clinical features of AFE is summarised in Figure 22.1.

Differential Diagnosis

In a woman who develops sudden onset cardiorespiratory arrest following delivery, the diagnosis of AFE depends more or less on the exclusion of all other possible conditions that could materialize in a similar fashion, because there is no specific test for the diagnosis of AFE (Table 22.1).

Investigations

Blood Tests

Most tests including cardiac enzymes and electrolytes are nonspecific. The white blood cell count may be elevated and, depending on the presence of DIC, the haemoglobin and haematocrit values may be low. Thrombocytopenia is an unusual finding. Arterial blood gas levels will be consistent with hypoxia with reduced pH and PO_2 levels and increased PCO_2 and base excess. Prolonged prothrombin time (PT), international normalised ratio (INR) and activated partial thromboplastin time (APTT), decreased fibrinogen levels together with elevated fibrin degradation products (FDP) and D-dimer levels may be useful in the diagnosis of DIC. However, D-dimer levels may be elevated in normal pregnancies as well.

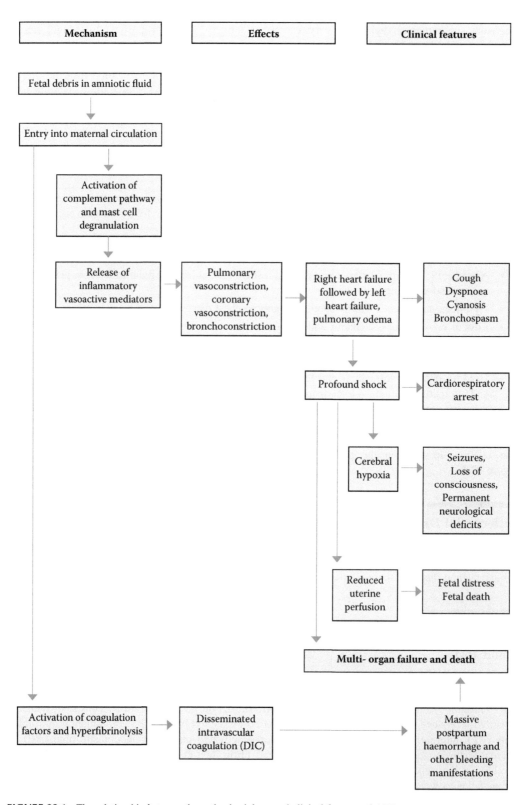

FIGURE 22.1   The relationship between the pathophysiology and clinical features of AFE.

TABLE 22.1

Causes for sudden onset cardiorespiratory arrest following delivery

Obstetric causes
    Postpartum haemorrhage
    Acute uterine inversion
    Amniotic fluid embolism
    Pre-eclampsia/eclampsia
    Peripartum cardiomyopathy

Non-obstetric causes
    Pulmonary/air embolism
    Acute myocardial infarction
    Cardiac arrhythmias
    Heart failure
    Aortic dissection
    Intracerebral haemorrhage
    Septic shock
    Status asthmaticus
    Anaphylactic shock/transfusion reaction

Anaesthetic causes
    Aspiration of gastric contents
    High spinal anaesthesia/epidural block
    Local anaesthetic/magnesium toxicity

Tests to Assess Cardiovascular and Respiratory systems

In the early stages of AFE, the electrocardiogram may reveal a right ventricular strain pattern with ST and T wave abnormalities and tachycardia. Cardiac arrhythmias or asystole can occur in severe cardiovascular collapse. Pulse oximetry may show a sudden drop in oxygen saturation, and this may be the presentation of AFE during caesarean delivery. The chief radiographic abnormalities in AFE are diffuse bilateral heterogeneous and homogeneous areas of increased opacity, which are indistinguishable from acute pulmonary oedema resulting from any other cause. It may also show evidence of effusions and cardiomegaly. Echocardiography is useful in evaluating left ventricular function and compliance. Computerised tomography of lungs and ventilation-perfusion scan will be advantageous in excluding thromboembolism.

Confirmatory Tests

The diagnosis of AFE is confirmed in living subjects by the presence of amniotic fluid debris and fetal squames within the maternal circulation that are tested with blood obtained from the right side of the heart via a central line. The definitive diagnosis is made at postmortem by the existence of fetal squames and amniotic fluid debris in the pulmonary arterioles. In addition to conventional haematoxylin and eosin staining, special fatty staining and immunohistochemical staining for fetal epithelial cells should be performed in order to assess the severity of AFE more precisely. However, morphological findings, which were once considered pathognomonic for AFE, do not correlate with the clinical picture and may still be found in normal pregnancies but not in certain cases of AFE.

In conclusion, a diagnosis of AFE depends on a combination of the clinical picture, postmortem examination and immunohistochemical techniques. At present, there is no test that can reliably confirm nor refute the diagnosis of AFE in suspected cases. Initial studies on serum diagnostic markers such as zinc coproporphyrin, tryptase, sialyl-Tn (a fetal antigen present in meconium and amniotic fluid) and C3 and C4 complement are promising, but larger studies are necessary in order to recommend the aforementioned tests in clinical practice.

Management

Initial Management

Irrespective of the diagnosis, immediate and effective cardiopulmonary resuscitation (CPR), with the aim of preventing hypoxia and maintaining vascular perfusion, should be the priority in any woman who develops cardiorespiratory arrest during pregnancy. The woman must be intubated with 100% oxygen administered along with intermittent positive pressure ventilation.

The patient should be transferred to an intensive care unit and managed by a multidisciplinary team including an obstetrician, an anaesthetist, an intensivist, a transfusion specialist, a neonatologist and other relevant personnel as the clinical situation demands. In the absence of specific therapy, the management of AFE is largely resuscitative and supportive. Two large-bore intravenous cannulae should be inserted and blood must be drawn for the pertinent haematological investigations mentioned above as well as for crossmatching at least six units of blood. Rapid infusion of crystalloids at a rate of 1 litre within 20 minutes and another litre within 30 minutes is crucial in order to counteract hypotension and cardiovascular instability. Vasopressors such as epinephrine, norepinephrine and vasopressin may be used. Vasopressin has the advantage of sparing the pulmonary vasculature from vasoconstriction, particularly at low doses. Maintaining cardiac output, which includes inotropic support with dopamine, constitutes an integral part of management. Dopamine also dilates the renal vasculature, thereby increasing renal blood flow and glomerular filtration rate.

Central venous pressure monitoring is useful in diagnosing right ventricular overload and in guiding fluid and vasopressor therapy. This also provides a means for obtaining blood from the right side of the heart for diagnostic purposes. Pulmonary artery catheterisation and the measurement of pulmonary artery and capillary wedge pressures along with placement of arterial catheters are useful to guide therapy for haemodynamically unstable women. After correction of hypotension, restriction of fluid to maintenance levels is important because there is a risk of ARDS. Steroids have not been proven to be beneficial.

Management of Coagulopathy

Disseminated intravascular coagulation (DIC) will almost always arise if the woman survives the initial incident. The antifibrinolytic agent, tranexamic acid, should be administered early. Management of DIC should be guided by the patient's haemodynamic status as well as the platelet count, prothrombin time and INR, activated partial thromboplastin time and fibrinogen level. If facilities are available, then rotational thromboelastometry (ROTEM) can be used to guide the transfusion of red blood cell concentrates and blood products in the management of DIC. Fresh frozen plasma is transfused if APTT is elevated; platelets are transfused if the platelet count is low (<20,000 mm^3); and cryoprecipitate is administered if fibrinogen levels are below normal (<100 mg/dL). Management options for intractable postpartum haemorrhage resulting from DIC include medical management with oxytocin, ergometrine and misoprostol and surgical measures such as uterine compression sutures (discussed in Chapter 17), stepwise devascularization of the uterus (discussed in Chapter 18) and hysterectomy (discussed in Chapter 19). Carboprost is averted due to the risk of bronchospasm. Recombinant factor VIIa is no longer recommended in the handling of coagulopathy because its use has led to vaso-occlusive events and poor outcomes.

Resuscitative Hysterotomy

If AFE occurs beyond 20 weeks in the antepartum period and results in cardiorespiratory arrest, then delivery should be performed immediately, vaginally if feasible or by emergency hysterotomy. Delivery of the fetus within the recommended time period of five minutes improves the success rate of CPR (discussed in Chapter 7). Early delivery improves the neonatal outcome, which is dependent on the time from maternal arrest to delivery.

Close Monitoring

Women who survive may develop multi-organ dysfunction resulting from hypoxia and coagulopathy. Therefore, these women need to be closely monitored. After recovery from the initial insult and subsequently from DIC, measures to reduce the risk of thromboembolism should be instituted, because these women are at an increased risk of venous thromboembolic disease. These measures include early mobilisation, adequate hydration, thromboembolic deterrent stockings and low molecular weight heparin therapy, depending on each individual case.

Recurrence

The risk of recurrence is unknown. Successful pregnancies following AFE have been reported. The recommendation for elective caesarean delivery in successive pregnancies in an attempt to avoid labour is controversial.

Prevention

Although it is said that AFE is largely unpreventable, measures must still be taken to impede trauma to and excessive contractions of the uterus. Trauma to the uterus must be avoided when performing intrauterine manoeuvres such as amniotomy and placement of an intrauterine pressure catheter. Judicious use of oxytocic agents during induction and augmentation of labour is vital in preventing excessively forceful uterine contractions (discussed in Chapter 8).

Future

Serum biomarkers and immunohistochemical staining techniques are currently under development to aid the diagnosis and treatment of AFE. Selective pulmonary vasodilators such as sildenafil and nitric oxide are used in the treatment of severe pulmonary hypertension, and these have shown promise. C1 esterase inhibitors may be a potential therapeutic option. Cell salvage with blood filtration may be used to improve the management of DIC. Plasma exchange has been discovered to be useful in controlling AFE. Intra-aortic balloon pump (IABP) and extracorporeal membrane oxygenation (ECMO) are mechanical supports that are used to maintain circulation and gas exchange as well as increase cardiac output in cardiac and respiratory failure. These may have a more prominent role to play in future cases of AFE.

Key Points

- Amniotic fluid embolism is neither predictable nor preventable.
- The diagnosis of amniotic fluid embolism should be considered in any woman who develops sudden onset cardiorespiratory arrest immediately following delivery or during labour.
- There is no specific test for the diagnosis of AFE.
- Diagnosis of AFE is usually made on clinical grounds after excluding other causes of cardiorespiratory arrest in pregnancy.
- Management is primarily supportive and resuscitative.
- Early diagnosis and multidisciplinary involvement improve the outcome for both the woman and the neonate.

BIBLIOGRAPHY

1. Benson MD. What is new in amniotic fluid embolism?: best articles from the past year. *Obstet Gynecol* 2017;129:941–2.
2. Clark SL, Romero R, Dildy GA, Callaghan WM, Smiley RM, Bracey AW, et al. Proposed diagnostic criteria for the case definition of amniotic fluid embolism in research studies. *Am J Obstet Gynecol* 2016;215:408–12.
3. Clark SL. Amniotic fluid embolism. *Obstet Gynecol* 2014;123:337–48.
4. Knight M, Tuffnell D, Brocklehurst P, Spark P, Kurinczuk JJ, UK Obstetric Surveillance System. Incidence and risk factors for amniotic-fluid embolism. *Obstet Gynecol* 2010;115:910–17.
5. Shamshirsaz AA, Clark SL. Amniotic fluid embolism. *Obstet Gynecol Clin North Am* 2016;43:779–90.
6. Sinicina I, Pankratz H, Bise K, Matevossian E. Forensic aspects of post-mortem histological detection of amniotic fluid embolism. *Int J Legal Med* 2010;124:55–62.
7. Sultan P, Seligman K, Carvalho B. Amniotic fluid embolism: update and review. *Curr Opin Anaesthesiol* 2016;29(3):288–96.

23

Venous Thromboembolism in Pregnancy

Sanjeewa Padumadasa and Aflah Sadikeen

Venous thromboembolism (VTE), a combination of deep vein thrombosis (DVT) and pulmonary embolism (PE), is one of the leading causes of maternal death, particularly in well-resourced countries. The incidence of VTE is 4–5 fold higher in the pregnant than in the non-pregnant population. The majority of VTE events occur in the antenatal period as well as in the first half of pregnancy, but the risk of VTE remains elevated until 12 weeks postpartum. The majority of DVT in pregnancy are left-sided, and the site of origin is ileo-femoral where they are more likely to embolise, as opposed to popliteo-femoral in the non-pregnant population.

Pathophysiology

Pregnancy meets all of the criteria for fulfilling Virchow's triad, i.e. venous stasis, vessel damage and hypercoagulability, which increase the risk of VTE. These are summarised in Figure 23.1.

Risk Factors

In addition to pregnancy itself as a risk factor for the development of VTE, there are additional risk factors that play a role, either individually or in combination, which are listed below.

- History of unprovoked/oestrogen-related VTE event
- Thrombophilias
    - Hereditary – Antithrombin deficiency, Factor V Leiden thrombophilia, prothrombin G20210 variant, protein C deficiency, protein S deficiency
    - Acquired – Antiphospholipid syndrome
- Medical illnesses, e.g. systemic lupus erythematosus, inflammatory conditions, sickle cell disease, nephrotic syndrome, cancer
- Post-surgery, including caesarean delivery
- Age > 35 years
- Obesity
- Multiparity
- Multiple pregnancy
- Gross varicose veins
- Ovarian hyperstimulation syndrome
- Smoking
- Immobility, including long-distance travel (greater than four hours)

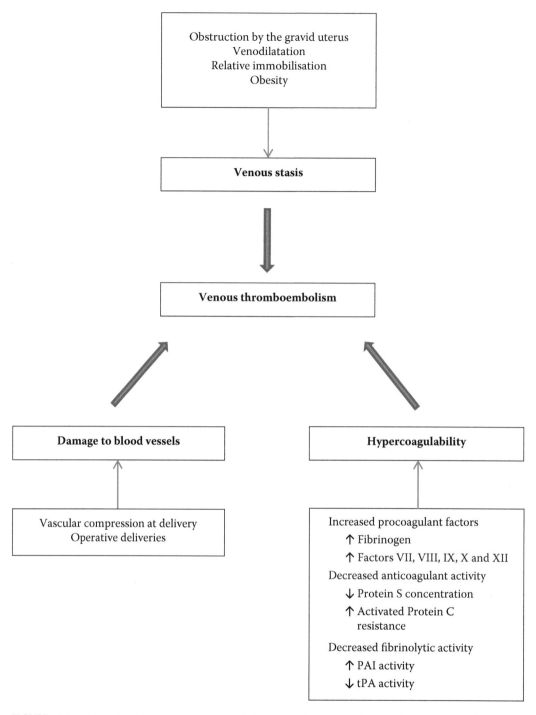

FIGURE 23.1   Virchow's triad (relevant to pregnancy); PAI – plasminogen activator inhibitor, tPA – tissue plasminogen activator.

- Dehydration, e.g. hyperemesis gravidarum
- Intravenous drug use
- Prolonged labour
- Mid-cavity instrumental vaginal delivery

- Postpartum haemorrhage
- Pre-eclampsia
- Sepsis

Prevention

As the risk of VTE increases in the first trimester itself, it is imperative that a risk assessment is made either pre-pregnancy or early in the first trimester, and preventive measures are instituted according to local guidelines and protocols. These preventive measures may vary from simple advice such as avoiding dehydration and long-distance travel, performing simple leg exercises during travel, staying active, using graduated elastic compression stockings up to administering anticoagulants, all depending on the risk level in the woman. If indicated, prophylactic anticoagulation should be continued with low molecular weight heparin (LMWH) throughout the antenatal period and around the time of delivery, and therapy with either LMWH or warfarin should be maintained until at least six weeks postpartum.

If a woman is on warfarin for the prevention of VTE, then it should be discontinued and replaced with LMWH before the sixth week of pregnancy. For women with prosthetic heart valves, finding the delicate balance between adequate anticoagulation of the woman and fetal safety is a challenge. In these women, warfarin should be replaced by LMWH from 6–12 weeks of gestation if the required daily dose of warfarin is more than 5 mg, because there is a considerable risk of teratogenicity. If the required daily dose of warfarin is 5 mg or less, then the risk of teratogenicity is low, and therefore, a changeover to LMWH is unnecessary. However, in these women, warfarin must be replaced by LMWH at 36 weeks of gestation and continued during the peripartum period. Warfarin can be recommenced 24–48 hours after delivery.

Newer anticoagulants which include factor Xa inhibitors (e.g. fondaparinux) and direct thrombin inhibitors (e.g. argatroban, r-hirudin, rivaroxaban) are generally avoided in pregnancy and breast-feeding, because there is a paucity of data regarding their use. However, either these newer anticoagulants or danaparoid sodium may be considered in cases of thrombocytopaenia or allergy due to unfractionated heparin (UH) or LMWH. Aspirin is not advised as a thromboprophylactic agent in pregnancy.

Clinical Features

The typical features of DVT are pain, redness, warmth and swelling of one leg, although these may not be present in all cases. Calf swelling should be measured 10 cm below the tibial tuberosity and is considered significant if it is more than 3 cm when compared with the other calf. There may also be lower abdominal pain which may indicate extension of the thrombus into pelvic vessels.

The general features of PE are sudden shortness of breath, pleuritic type pain or tightness in the chest or upper back, cough and haemoptysis. The other causes of sudden shortness of breath should be considered in the differential diagnosis (Table 23.1). Alternatively, the woman may present in a collapsed state with tachypnoea, tachycardia, hypotension or pulseless cardiac electrical activity. Low-grade fever may also occur in women with VTE.

The diagnosis of DVT and PE in pregnancy is difficult due to the following reasons.

- The clinical features of PE, such as shortness of breath, tachycardia and a feature of DVT which includes leg swelling could be attributable to normal physiological changes that manifest during pregnancy.
- Wells criteria (a pretest probability assessment done to rule out PE using a combination of symptoms and signs) cannot be used in pregnancy because pregnant women were excluded from the analysis.

TABLE 23.1

Causes of sudden shortness of breath in pregnancy

Respiratory causes
  Asthma
  Pneumonia
  Pulmonary embolism
  Amniotic fluid embolism
  Pneumothorax
  Pleurisy
Cardiac causes
  Cardiomyopathy
  Acute myocardial infarction
  Heart failure
  Pericarditis
  Cardiac arrhythmias
  Cardiac tamponade
Other causes
  Choking
  Inhalation of foreign body

- D-dimers begin to rise during the second trimester and remain elevated for 4–6 weeks postpartum as a physiological response to pregnancy.
- Imaging, especially for a diagnosis of PE, involves exposure (although negligible) of the fetus to radiation, and also increases the risk of breast cancer in the woman.

It is important that VTE is accurately diagnosed in pregnancy because it has implications on the mode of delivery and requires long-term treatment during the antenatal and postpartum periods, as well as prophylaxis in successive pregnancies. However, as PE can be rapidly fatal in pregnancy, treatment is usually commenced on clinical suspicion without waiting for the diagnosis to be confirmed.

Investigations

Deep Vein Thrombosis

Compression duplex ultrasound is the primary method of diagnosis of DVT in pregnancy, as it is non-invasive, safe and relatively inexpensive. It is a reliable test used to diagnose lower limb DVT but not pelvic DVT. If it confirms the diagnosis of DVT, then no further tests are necessary even if PE is suspected, since anticoagulant therapy is the same for both conditions. If the test is negative and the clinical suspicion is high, then the test should be repeated after three days, and if necessary, again after seven days after the initial test. Magnetic resonance imaging or conventional venography may be carried out when iliac vein thrombosis is suspected (if back pain, buttock pain or swelling of the entire lower limb is present) or when the clinical suspicion remains high and the compression duplex ultrasound is consistently negative for DVT.

Pulmonary Embolism

Many diagnostic tests and pretest probability tools for the evaluation of suspected PE during pregnancy are neither sensitive nor specific. Although a chest x-ray can be normal in more than 50% of cases of PE, it should be performed mainly to rule out other lung pathologies such as pneumonia or pneumothorax, which not only may present with features that are similar to those of PE, but also determine the appropriate next imaging modality. The chest x-ray may show peripheral wedge-shaped opacities suggestive of pulmonary infarcts or features of basal atelectasis, pulmonary oedema and pleural effusions.

Although the electrocardiogram (ECG) may be normal in more than 50% of cases of PE in pregnancy, it may show sinus tachycardia, T wave inversion, evidence of right heart strain and the classic $S_1Q_3T_3$ pattern. The echocardiogram can appear normal, but it may also reveal right ventricular dilatation in cases of massive PE. However, both ECG and echocardiogram are helpful in excluding alternative diagnoses such as acute myocardial infarction or cardiomyopathy. Similarly, arterial blood gases are not very useful, but hypoxia in the presence of a normal chest x-ray should raise the possibility of PE. Cardiac enzymes are useful in eliminating acute myocardial infarction.

The diagnosis of PE should be confirmed by either computerised tomography pulmonary angiogram (CTPA) or ventilation/perfusion (V/Q) scanning according to a combination of the clinical picture, availability, unit protocols and a discussion with the woman regarding the risks of teratogenicity and breast cancer with each of these tests. Compared to V/Q scanning, CTPA, due to its higher sensitivity and specificity, is usually more effective in cases in which the chest x-ray is abnormal . However, in pregnancy, the sensitivity of CTPA may be lower than in the non-pregnant population due to technical difficulty in interpretation with the hyperdynamic circulation, and it may also disregard peripheral emboli. In addition, the risk of radiation to the breast, which is a risk factor for the development of breast cancer, is higher with CTPA than with V/Q scanning, while the risk of fetal exposure to radiation is higher with V/Q scanning compared to CTPA. Therefore, the current recommendation is to perform V/Q scanning if there is no history of pulmonary disease and the chest x-ray is normal. If there is a history of pulmonary disease or if the chest x-ray is abnormal, then CTPA should be performed. If the V/Q scan is non-diagnostic, then the CTPA must be performed and vice versa. The risk of exposure to radiation of the woman or the fetus from either of these tests is minimal and considered acceptable to diagnose PE which is a rapidly fatal condition.

Investigations should also include full blood count, liver function tests, renal function tests and a coagulation screen. Although the physiologically elevated D-dimer levels during and immediately after pregnancy preclude its use for diagnosing VTE in pregnancy, a low D-dimer level is helpful in ruling out the diagnosis. A thrombophilic screen should not be performed because the results will not influence management to a significant degree and the results are difficult to interpret during pregnancy.

Treatment

Acute Management

Stabilisation of the woman is the priority. This includes addressing the airway, breathing and circulation in an intensive care setting (discussed in Chapter 7). Supplementary oxygen is compulsory in order to maintain the target oxygen saturation of ≥92%. Severe hypoxaemia and respiratory distress may require ventilator support along with haemodynamic stability.

Early involvement of an experienced obstetrician, a radiologist, an emergency medicine physician and a haematologist, is essential. In case of life-threatening PE with haemodynamic compromise, thrombolytic therapy, intravenous UH, percutaneous catheter thrombus fragmentation or surgical embolectomy may be used as a life-saving procedure, depending on the availability of expertise and equipment necessary for these treatment modalities. In these cases, the vascular team should get involved in the management. Thrombolytic therapy is generally considered safe in pregnancy and may be required, as anticoagulant therapy alone may not improve pulmonary circulation.

Anticoagulant Therapy

The aims of anticoagulant therapy are to prevent the clot from propagating and to prevent the formation of new clots. When there is a high suspicion of VTE, anticoagulant treatment should be commenced, unless there is a strong contraindication to its use, and continued for one week. This must be done even if the initial duplex ultrasound and V/Q scan or CTPA are negative, at which point PE should definitely be excluded by appropriate investigations. When there is low suspicion of DVT but no suspicion of PE, anticoagulant therapy can be discontinued if the duplex ultrasound is negative. However, duplex ultrasound should be repeated on days 3 and 7 if clinical suspicion of DVT remains high. Anticoagulant treatment should be recommenced if the repeat duplex ultrasound confirms the diagnosis of DVT.

Low molecular weight heparin has replaced UH as the mainstay of treatment, due to its safety profile and the lower risks of complications such as bleeding, thrombocytopaenia, symptomatic osteoporosis and allergic reactions. As LMWH does not cross the placenta, it does not have adverse effects on the fetus. The dose of LMWH should be based on the woman's booking or early pregnancy weight. It is common practice to use a twice-daily regimen initially and change over to a daily regimen once the acute episode is controlled. However, there is not enough evidence to recommend whether a once-daily or twice-daily regimen should be used. As the risk of heparin-induced thrombocytopaenia is lower with LMWH than with UH, monitoring with regular platelet counts is unnecessary. Monitoring with anti-Xa levels may be required in cases of extremes of body weight, renal impairment and recurrent VTE. A lower dose of LMWH should be used in cases of renal compromise.

For women with potential for bleeding, in whom a delicate balance needs to be achieved between anticoagulation and the risk of bleeding, UH is preferred over LMWH, due to its shorter half-life and the ease of reversibility with protamine sulphate. This applies to women close to term as well, because of the risk of bleeding at delivery. If UH is used, then regular monitoring with activated partial thromboplastin time (APTT) and platelet count should be executed.

General Measures

Traditionally, bed rest and immobilisation have been recommended for women with acute DVT, for fear of dislodging an unstable thrombus and subsequently causing PE. However, recent evidence suggests that neither mobilisation nor leg compression increases the risk of propagation of the thrombus and PE. Therefore, in the initial management of acute DVT, mobilisation should be encouraged, the leg elevated and graduated elastic compression stockings used to reduce swelling and pain. Contrary to earlier belief, recent cases suggest that graduated elastic compression stockings are not effective in preventing the development of post-thrombotic syndrome, which manifests as leg pain, swelling, dermatitis, ulcers and varicosities.

Significance of Temporary Inferior Vena Cava Filter

A temporary inferior vena cava filter may be considered in cases of iliac vein VTE or recurrent PE despite adequate anticoagulation, or when anticoagulation is contraindicated.

Anticoagulant Therapy during the Time of Delivery

Women on LMWH should be advised to not inject any further doses of LMWH if and when they develop signs of labour. Anticoagulant therapy should be discontinued 24 hours before planned caesarean delivery or induction of labour. Regional anaesthesia should be avoided for 24 hours after a therapeutic dose of LMWH has been administered in order to reduce the risk of epidural or spinal haematoma. If the woman has experienced an acute VTE event within one month of delivery, discontinuing anticoagulant treatment for more than 24 hours may be detrimental, and intravenous UH can be used until 4–6 hours prior to the delivery.

Specific Measures during Delivery

In the absence of obstetric indications for caesarean delivery, a careful vaginal delivery that has the potential to cause the least amount of trauma to the woman should be the goal. Selective episiotomy

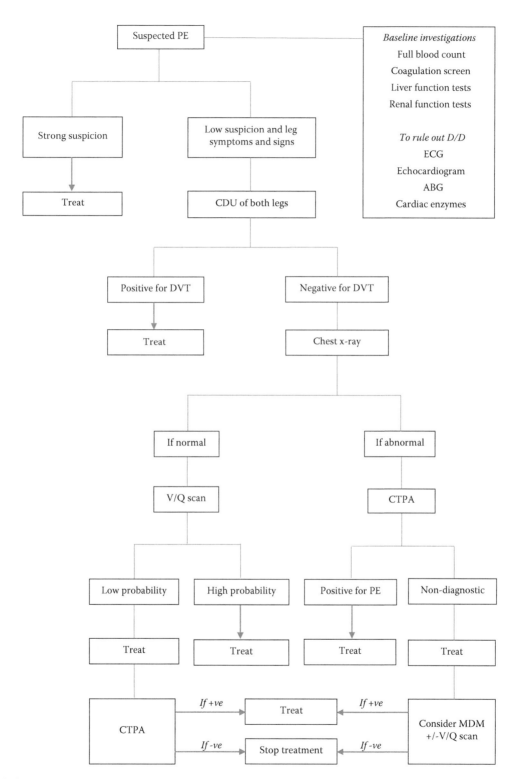

FIGURE 23.2 Summary of diagnostic workup and treatment of venous thromboembolism in pregnancy; PE – pulmonary embolism, CDU – compression duplex ultrasound, ECG – electrocardiogram, ABG - arterial blood gases, DVT – deep vein thrombosis, V/Q scan – ventilation/perfusion scan, CTPA – computerised tomography pulmonary angiogram, MDM – multidisciplinary meeting.

minimises the risk of perineal tears. Instrumental vaginal delivery, if necessary, may be performed carefully (discussed in Chapter 9). In women undergoing caesarean delivery, abdominal and wound drains should be considered, and the skin incision should be closed with interrupted sutures in order to prevent the formation of haematomas.

Management during the Postpartum Period and Follow-up

Delivery, both vaginal and abdominal, is a risk factor for the development of VTE. Following delivery, LMWH should be commenced as soon as possible (i.e. 12 hours after caesarean delivery or 6 hours after vaginal delivery) once bleeding has been excluded and provided no regional anaesthesia had been administered. Low molecular weight heparin should not be recommenced until four hours have elapsed after the administration of spinal anaesthesia or the removal of an epidural catheter. The epidural catheter should not be removed until 12 hours have elapsed after a dose of LMWH.

For women at risk of haemorrhage following delivery, LMWH should be avoided. In these women, mechanical methods such as graduated elastic compression stockings and intermittent pneumatic compression devices should be used as thromboprophylactic measures. Care must also be taken to avoid dehydration which increases the risk of VTE. In women with the potential to bleed, but the risk of VTE also remains high, intravenous UH may be used, as its effects can be easily reversed.

Therapeutic anticoagulation should be continued during the postpartum period for at least six weeks or for a total of three months from the initial episode of VTE, whichever is longer. Either LMWH or warfarin can be used in the postpartum period, and both are safe during breastfeeding. Warfarin can be started between 24–48 hours following delivery, provided that there is no bleeding. As warfarin takes a few days to act, both warfarin and LMWH might need to be continued for a few days until the action of warfarin begins to take effect, by which time the therapeutic level of INR, which is between 2 and 3, would have been reached. Warfarin must not be used in women at an increased risk of secondary postpartum haemorrhage such as those with conservatively managed placenta accreta spectrum disorder.

Women who develop VTE during pregnancy or in the postpartum period should be warned about the risk of recurrence in subsequent pregnancies and with the use of combined oral contraceptives or hormone replacement therapy.

The diagnostic work-up and treatment of VTE in pregnancy are summarised in Figure 23.2.

Key Points

- The risk of VTE increases from the first trimester of pregnancy, and it is imperative that a risk assessment is made at pre-pregnancy or booking visit, and prophylactic measures are instituted.
- Pulmonary embolism should be treated initially on clinical grounds without waiting for investigations.
- Low molecular weight heparin is as effective as UH in the majority of cases of VTE in pregnancy and has a lesser adverse effect profile.
- Embolectomy can make the difference between life and death in a woman with massive PE.

BIBLIOGRAPHY

1. Konstantinides SV, Meyer G, Becattini C, Bueno H, Geersing GJ, et al. 2019 ESC Guidelines for the diagnosis and management of acute pulmonary embolism developed in collaboration with the European Respiratory Society (ERS): The Task Force for the diagnosis and management of acute pulmonary embolism of the European Society of Cardiology (ESC). *Eur Heart J* 2020;41(4):543–603.

2. Amaragiri SV, Lees T. Elastic compression stockings for prevention of deep vein thrombosis. *Cochrane Database Syst Rev* 2000;17(1):CD001484. doi: 10.1002/14651858.
3. Bates SM, Jaeschke R, Stevens SM, et al. Diagnosis of DVT: Antithrombotic Therapy and Prevention of Thrombosis, 9th ed: American College of Chest Physicians Evidence-Based Clinical Practice Guidelines. *Chest* 2012;141(2):e351S–e418S.
4. Bourjeily G, Paidas M, Khalil H, et al. Pulmonary embolism in pregnancy. *Lancet* 2010;375:500–12.
5. Greer IA, Nelson-Piercy C. Low-molecular-weight heparins for thrombo-prophylaxis and treatment of venous thromboembolism in pregnancy: a systematic review of safety and efficacy. *Blood* 2005; 106(2):401–7.
6. Pillny M, Sandmann W, Luther B, et al. Deep venous thrombosis during pregnancy and after delivery: indications for and results of thrombectomy. *J Vasc Surg* 2003;37(3):528–32.
7. Schembri GP, Miller AE, Smart R. Radiation dosimetry and safety issues in the investigation of pulmonary embolism. *Semin Nucl Med* 2010;40:442–54.
8. Van der Mairuhu A, Tromeur C, Couturaud F, Huisman M, Klok F. Use of clinical prediction rules and D-dimer tests in the diagnostic management of pregnant patients with suspected acute pulmonary embolism. *Blood Rev* 2017;31(2):31–6.
9. Wan T, Skeith L, Karovitch A, Rodger M, Le G. Guidance for the diagnosis of pulmonary embolism during pregnancy: consensus and controversies. *Thromb Res* 2017;157:23–8.

24

Obstetric Anal Sphincter Injuries

Ruwan Fernando

Obstetric anal sphincter injuries (OASIS) are defined as perineal trauma involving the anal sphincter complex during childbirth. The reported incidence of OASIS varies between 1.7% and 18% of vaginal births. Over the past decade, there has been an increase in the reported cases of OASIS worldwide. Compared to episiotomy and first and second-degree perineal tears, OASIS are associated with much higher morbidity. These include perineal pain, dyspareunia, wound infection, recto-vaginal fistulae and anal incontinence.

Perineal pain can be very distressing for the mother, may interfere with her ability to breastfeed and cope with the daily tasks of motherhood and could also lead to urinary retention and defaecation problems. In the long term, perineal pain and dyspareunia following OASIS can cause considerable impairment of sexual and social life. A negative body image, anxiety, depression and a feeling of embarrassment and shame are common in women with anal incontinence. Abscess formation, wound breakdown and recto-vaginal fistulae are frequently a result of the failure to recognise the true extent of OASIS at the time of repair, resulting in inadequate sphincter reconstruction. Once occurred, recto-vaginal fistulae are difficult to treat and may require a colostomy. Anal incontinence is considered a problem for at least 1 in 20 women for up to one year after childbirth.

Mismanagement of OASIS is one of the most common causes of litigation. Allegations of negligence include erroneous diagnosis of the true extent and grade of the injury, failure to perform a rectal examination prior to suturing a perineal tear, overlooking consideration to carry out a caesarean delivery or to perform or extend the episiotomy, inability to do the repair and inadequacy of the repair.

Increased awareness of these complications following vaginal birth has led to women requesting elective caesarean delivery without any other clinical indication. However, caesarean delivery is associated with a 16-fold risk of maternal morbidity compared to vaginal birth.

Classification of Perineal Injuries

There is a wide variation in the literature in the classification of OASIS. The classification of perineal injury that is accepted by the International Continence Society, the World Health Organisation and the Royal College of Obstetricians and Gynaecologists is given in Table 24.1 and Figure 24.1.

A rectal buttonhole is described as a tear involving the rectal mucosa above the anal sphincter complex, which is therefore intact, and it is not classified as a fourth-degree tear (Figure 24.2). However, if unrecognised and not repaired, then a buttonhole tear may lead to the formation of a rectovaginal fistula.

Risk Factors for Obstetric Anal Sphincter Injuries

Parity

Nulliparous women have a greater risk of OASIS compared to multipara, due to a relatively inelastic perineum and a higher incidence of instrumental vaginal delivery.

TABLE 24.1

Classification of perineal injury

Injury	Definition
First degree	Injury only to the perineal skin with intact perineal muscles
Second degree	Injury to the perineum involving perineal muscles, but not involving the anal sphincter
Third degree	Injury to the perineum involving the anal sphincter complex (External Anal Sphincter - EAS and Internal Anal Sphincter – IAS) – 3a: Less than 50% of EAS thickness torn, 3b: More than 50% of EAS thickness torn, 3c: IAS torn
Fourth degree	Injury to the perineum involving the anal sphincter complex (EAS and IAS) and rectal mucosa.

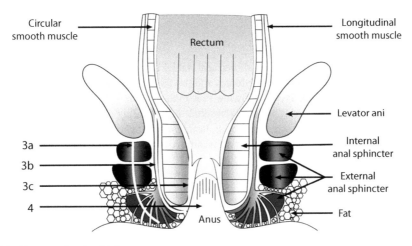

FIGURE 24.1 Degrees of perineal injury.

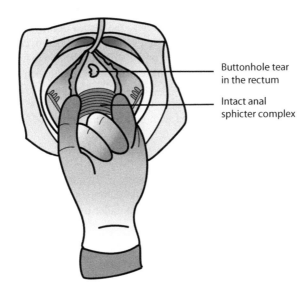

FIGURE 24.2 A rectal buttonhole tear.

Increased Birth Weight

A birth weight that is more than 4 kg is associated with a large head circumference, prolonged labour, a difficult delivery (sometimes with shoulder dystocia) and instrumental vaginal delivery. A large baby is also likely to disrupt the fascial supports of the pelvic floor and cause a stretch injury to the pelvic and pudendal nerves.

Malposition

Occipitoposterior position is associated with incomplete flexion of fetal head, an increase of the presenting diameter and a prolonged second stage of labour. This results in persistent pressure on the perineum leading to oedematous and friable tissues which are more vulnerable to laceration and is also associated with an increased rate of instrumental vaginal deliveries compared to occipitoanterior position. All of these factors contribute to a heightened risk of OASIS.

Duration of Labour

Precipitate labour is associated with cervical, perineal, labial and urethral injury, due to inadequate time for the maternal tissues to adjust to delivery forces and the failure to control delivery with an episiotomy, when necessary. Furthermore, delivery following precipitate labour is more likely to occur under less favourable circumstances, e.g. during transit to hospital, in a standing position and, quite often, without experienced assistance. A second stage of labour lasting more than 60 minutes is associated with an increased incidence of OASIS and increased risk of anal incontinence caused by pudendal neuropathy.

Episiotomy

Compared to routine episiotomy, restrictive episiotomy is associated with less posterior perineal trauma, but with a higher incidence of anterior perineal trauma. There is no significant difference in the occurrence of posterior perineal trauma with a mediolateral versus median episiotomy. The midline episiotomy has a higher risk of OASIS compared to mediolateral episiotomy.

Instrumental Vaginal Delivery

A forceps delivery is more likely to cause injury because the blades occupy almost 10% more space in the pelvis than ventouse, and the shanks of the forceps stretch the perineum, causing injury particularly to the anal sphincter when pulling in the posterolateral direction to encourage flexion of the head. Unlike the ventouse that can detach, the forceps do not have a fail-safe mechanism and therefore, excessive force can be applied, particularly under epidural anaesthesia. The risk of OASIS is 1.5–14.0 times higher with forceps and up to four times higher with ventouse, compared to normal vaginal delivery. The use of sequential instruments is associated with an even higher risk of OASIS.

Combination of Factors

Women with more than one risk factor during the process of labour and delivery have a much higher risk of OASIS as compared to women with a single risk factor, e.g. a large baby leading to prolonged labour, followed by instrumental vaginal delivery and shoulder dystocia.

Prevention of Obstetric Anal Sphincter Injuries

Episiotomy

In a nulliparous woman undergoing vaginal delivery, an accurately performed mediolateral episiotomy could have a role in preventing OASIS and should not be withheld. A 60° episiotomy from the centre of the introitus, resulting in a post-delivery angle of 45° from the midline, is recommended in order to reduce the incidence of OASIS. However, this can be difficult to achieve at 'crowning' when the perineum is fully stretched. The use of specially designed scissors that would ensure an incision angle of 60° when performing episiotomy has been proven to reduce the incidence of OASIS.

Perineal Protection

The introduction of interventions during the second stage of labour for manual perineal protection ('hands-on' techniques) has successfully reduced OASIS rates. Manual perineal protection involves the following steps (Figure 24.3).

- Left hand slowing down the delivery of the head
- Right hand protecting the perineum
- Mother NOT pushing when the fetal head is crowning (communication is paramount)
- Performing an episiotomy and at the correct angle, if needed (high-risk groups)

In addition, the following methods have been documented as effective in reducing perineal injuries.

- Perineal massage with a lubricant during the antenatal period and in the second stage of labour.
- Warm perineal compresses with normal saline when the head is distending the perineum.

However, the exact methods have not been standardised (e.g. frequency and duration, and the temperature of the compresses). Therefore, these necessitate further evaluation.

Management of Obstetric Anal Sphincter Injuries

All women undergoing vaginal birth are at risk of sustaining an OASIS or buttonhole tear. Therefore, they should be examined systematically, and this includes a digital rectal examination to assess the severity of damage, particularly prior to suturing. Before assessing for perineal trauma, healthcare professionals should adhere to the following steps.

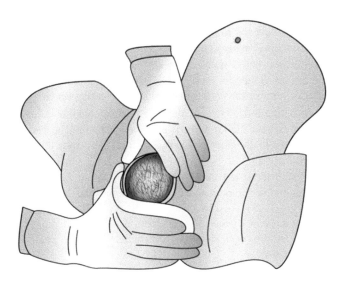

FIGURE 24.3 Manual perineal protection.

- Explain to the woman the exact plan and corresponding reasons
- Offer analgesia if currently not under regional analgesia
- Ensure good lighting
- Position the woman prioritising both her comfort and the visibility of genital structures

Examination

The examination should be performed delicately and preferably immediately after the delivery. If perineal trauma is identified following birth, then a further systematic assessment should be carried out, including a rectal examination. Systematic assessment of genital trauma should be carried out as listed below.

- Further explanation of which the healthcare professional plans to do and why.
- Confirmation that effective local or regional analgesia is in place.
- Visual assessment of the extent of perineal trauma including all of the structures involved, the apex of the injury and assessment of bleeding.
- Careful examination of the labia, clitoris and urethra in order to identify any injuries, as these structures need repair prior to the perineal repair.
- A rectal examination to assess whether there has been any damage to the external or internal anal sphincter, if there is any suspicion that the perineal muscles are damaged.
- Reviewing the extent of the trauma by a more experienced healthcare professional, if uncertainty exists as to the nature or extent of the sustained trauma.
- Complete and preferably pictorial documentation of the systematic assessment and its results.

Repair

- Immediate repair of the perineal injury is advisable, because immediate repair will reduce the bleeding and pain associated with the injury, which may in turn affect early breastfeeding and bonding. Prompt repair also prevents the development of oedema, which may affect the subsequent recognition of structures involved and also reduces the risk of infection.
- Repair should be performed only by a healthcare professional experienced in OASIS repair or by a trainee, under direct supervision.
- The repair should be conducted in the operating theatre where there is access to good lighting, appropriate equipment and aseptic conditions.
- Regional or general anaesthesia is an important prerequisite because the inherent tone in the sphincter muscle can cause the torn muscle ends to retract within its sheath. Muscle relaxation is necessary in order to retrieve the ends and overlap without tension.
- In the presence of a fourth-degree tear, the torn anal epithelium is repaired with interrupted 3/0 Polyglactin sutures with the knots tied in the anal lumen. The use of PDS sutures is not recommended for repair of the anorectal mucosa since these take longer to dissolve and may cause discomfort and irritation in the anal canal.
- The internal anal sphincter (IAS) must be identified. The internal anal sphincter is the continuation of the longitudinal smooth muscle of the large intestine and appears paler than the external anal sphincter (EAS). Any IAS tear must be repaired separately from EAS with either interrupted or mattress sutures using 3/0 PDS with a mindful attempt to not overlap. Primary surgical repair of the IAS has been shown to be beneficial in 3c perineal tears and leads to a less incidence of anal incontinence.
- The external anal sphincter should be repaired with either 3/0 PDS or 2/0 Polyglactin sutures with either end-to-end (Figure 24.4) or overlapping technique (Figure 24.5). The overlap technique can

be used for 3c tears, whereas an end-to-end technique should be used for all 3a and some 3b tears. A Cochrane review has demonstrated that there is no difference in outcomes between an end-to-end and an overlap repair and therefore, the end-to-end technique can be used for all external sphincter tears.

- Great caution should be exercised when reconstructing the perineal muscles in order to provide support to the sphincter repair and maintain the vagino-anal distance.
- Burying surgical knots beneath the superficial perineal muscles is recommended to be able to minimise the risk of knot and suture migration to the skin.
- A vaginal and rectal examination must be performed, and swab and needle count must also be taken.

Postoperative Care

- The use of broad-spectrum antibiotics is recommended following repair of OASIS in order to reduce the risk of postoperative infections and wound dehiscence. Intravenous antibiotics should be commenced intraoperatively and continued orally for one week.
- Laxatives are recommended to reduce the risk of wound dehiscence and pain caused by the passage of a large bolus of hard stools. A stool softener, such as Lactulose 10 mL, is recommended for at least two weeks postoperatively. However, the patient should be advised to reduce or stop the dose of stool softeners completely if stool becomes too loose. Bulking agents should not be given routinely with laxatives. Local guidelines should be followed regarding the use of antibiotics and laxatives.
- A comprehensive record should be documented together with a diagram in order to demonstrate the injury. This is vital for audit and risk management purposes (Figure 24.6).

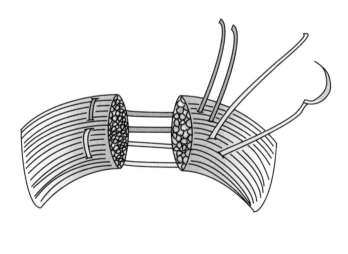

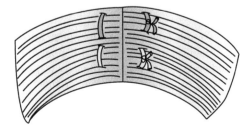

FIGURE 24.4   End-to-end technique of repair of the external anal sphincter.

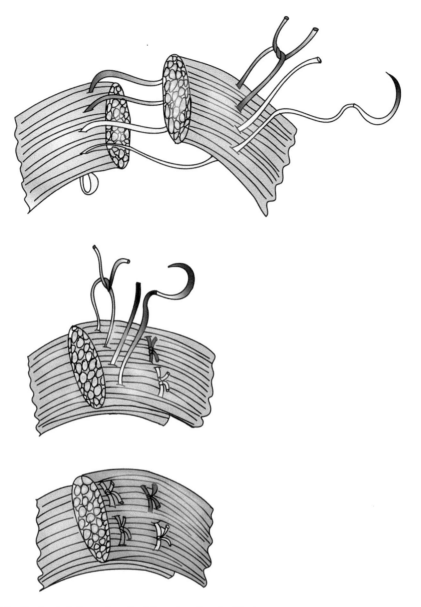

FIGURE 24.5   Overlap technique of repair of the external anal sphincter.

Follow-up after the Repair

At present, there are scant studies to guide how a woman should be followed up with after OASIS. It has been recommended that all women should be warned of the possible sequelae of anal sphincter disruption and ideally, they should be assessed at approximately 6–12 weeks postpartum, with anal manometry and endoanal ultrasound to assess anal sphincter function and anatomical integrity. Symptoms should be assessed using a validated bladder and bowel symptom questionnaire. This would enable the evaluation of the symptoms in an objective manner and is also useful for audit purposes.

Record of Perineal Trauma / Repair

* "All perineal trauma including reasons for episiotomy, type of repair and suture material used is recorded"
* "outcome of perineal trauma whether sutured or not, should be recorded"
(Ref. Effective procedures suitable For Audit, RCOG Clinical Audit June 1997)

Full Name:_____ Hospital Number:_____

Address label

Definitions of spontaneous Tears

Degree	Trauma	Please Tick √
First	Injury to the skin **only**	
Second	Injury to the perineum involving perineal muscles but **not** involving the anal sphincter	
Third	Injury to perineum involving the **anal sphincter complex**:	
3a	Less than 50% of EAS thickness torn	
3b	More than 50% of EAS thickness torn	
3c	Both EAS and IAS torn	
Forth	Injury to perineum involving the anal sphincter complex (EAS & IAS) and **anal epithelium**	

Episiotomy: ☐ (if episiotomy please state reason) ....

Extent of Trauma: (please Tick √ all appropriate boxes& use the diagram)

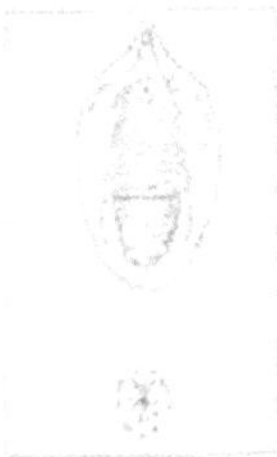

PR as part of initial assessment of trauma- Yes:☐ No:☐
Labial Involvement:☐
Unilateral vaginal tear:☐   Bilateral vaginal tear:☐
Straight skin edges:☐   Ragged skin edges:☐
Perineal skin edges down to anal margin:☐
Other (please describe): ....

Perineal Trauma Sutured:☐ Not Sutured:☐

Anaesthetic: None:☐ Lignocaine (1%):☐ Total amount:.........mls Epidural ☐ Spinal ☐ Other:.........

	Method of Repair	Suture material
Vagina	Continuous / Interrupted / non-locking / locking	VicrylRapide / Vicryl / Other ....
Perineal muscle	Continuous / Interrupted / non-locking / locking	VicrylRapide / Vicryl / Other ....
Perineal skin	Subcutaneous / Continuous / Interrupted	VicrylRapide / Vicryl / Other ....
EAS	Overlap / End-to-end / Other	PDS/Vicryl/Other:...............
IAS	Continuous / Interrupted / Other	PDS/Vicryl/Other:...............
Anal epithelium	Continuous / Interrupted / Other	Vicryl / Other:...................

Additional Information: ....

Antibiotics:No ☐ Yes ☐ **Type**.................... Dose .... IV/Oral Duration: Single dose / .....Days
Laxatives: No ☐ Yes ☐ **Type**.................... Dose ....   Duration: ....Days
Analgesics: No ☐ Yes ☐ **Type**.................... Dose ....   Duration: ....Days

PR: Yes ☐ No ☐   PV: Yes ☐ No☐
Indwelling catheter: Yes ☐   No☐
Sutured in unsupported Lithotomy: Yes☐   No☐   Supported Lithotomy Yes☐ No☐
Tampon: Used ☐ Not Used ☐

Checked By (print name):
Number Of Needles:.....................   1 ....
Number of Swabs: ....   2 ....
Estimated Blood Loss: After Delivery: .... mls   After Suturing: ....mls Total Blood Loss: ....mls

Time suturing commenced: ...../....hrs/mins
Was there more than a 60min delay in commencing the repair: Yes☐ No☐
If **YES** please state the reason: ....

Advice Re: Hygiene ☐   Pain Relief☐   Pelvic Floor exercises ☐   Diet ☐
Full explanation given to women re: Extent of trauma ☐   Type of repair ☐

Follow-up appointment in Pelvic Floor Clinic - **Yes** ☐ No ☐   Other clinics .... **Yes** ☐ No ☐

Repaired by (print name): ....   Designation:...............................
Signature:..................................   Date &Time: ....

FIGURE 24.6 Record of perineal trauma.

Endoanal Ultrasound Scan

The endoanal ultrasound scan using a 360° rotating transducer is the gold standard for assessing anal sphincter anatomy. This enables the identification of any defects in the anal sphincter complex (Figures 24.7–24.10).

Anal Manometry

Anal manometry assesses the resting and squeeze pressures of the anal sphincter complex (Figures 24.11–24.13). The IAS generates most of the resting pressure, whereas the EAS produces most

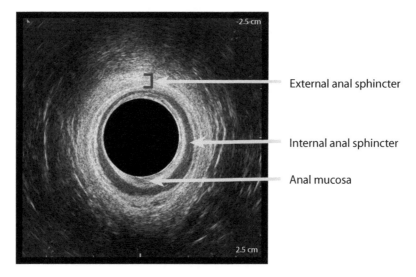

FIGURE 24.7   Endoanal ultrasound showing normal anal sphincter complex.

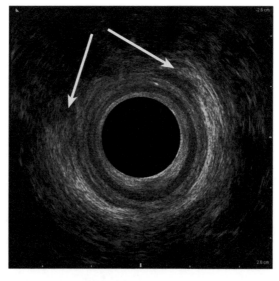

FIGURE 24.8   Defect in external anal sphincter with intact internal anal sphincter.

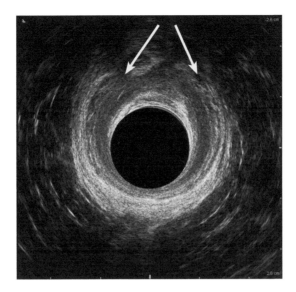

FIGURE 24.9 Endoanal ultrasound showing defects in both anal sphincters.

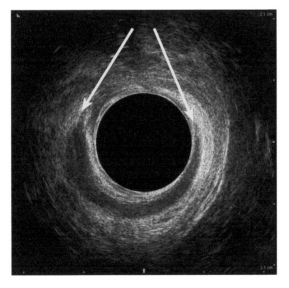

FIGURE 24.10 Endoanal ultrasound showing isolated internal anal sphincter defect with an intact external anal sphincter.

of the squeeze pressure. The normal squeeze pressure varies between 70–140 mmHg depending on the system, whereas the normal resting pressure fluctuates between 35–75 mmHg.

Management of Subsequent Pregnancy Following Obstetric Anal Sphincter Injuries

The incidence of OASIS in a subsequent delivery in women who had previously sustained OASIS during their first vaginal delivery is reported to be approximately 7.2%, compared with a rate of about

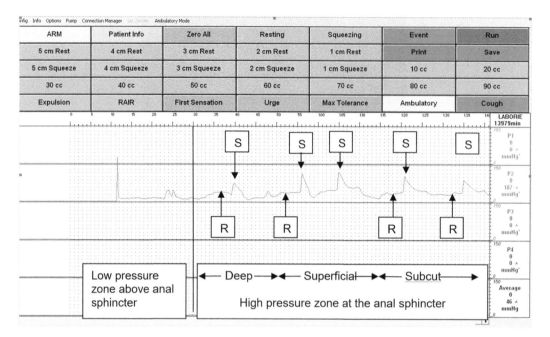

FIGURE 24.11   Normal anal manometry trace; R – resting pressure, S – squeeze pressure.

1.3% in women who did not. There are no randomised studies that address the effectiveness of interventions in a subsequent pregnancy. Several descriptive studies have shown that women who were asymptomatic with normal anal manometry and normal endoanal ultrasound scan underwent a vaginal birth without any deterioration of anorectal function. Those who were symptomatic or had abnormal anal manometry and endoanal ultrasound scan and had an elective caesarean delivery also did not show any deterioration of anorectal function.

Asymptomatic women with low squeeze pressures and a defect of greater than one quadrant are at an increased risk of developing anal incontinence following another vaginal delivery and therefore, counselling should include the option of caesarean delivery. If manometry and anal ultrasound facilities are unavailable locally, then all symptomatic women should be referred to a specialist centre for these investigations. If no such facilities are available, then counselling regarding the mode of delivery should be based on symptoms and clinical examination. An experienced midwife or doctor can perform vaginal delivery on symptomatic women with no clinical evidence of a deficient perineum or low anal sphincter tone. As there is no evidence that an elective prophylactic episiotomy will prevent another tear, an episiotomy should be performed only if clinically indicated, i.e. if the perineum is thick and inelastic and if the episiotomy will prevent multiple radial tears.

Symptomatic women with severe injuries should be offered a secondary sphincter repair, and elective caesarean delivery should be performed in subsequent pregnancies. Women with mild symptoms should be provided with dietary advice to avoid gas-producing foods, regulation of bowel action, bulking agents, constipating agents such as loperamide and codeine phosphate and biofeedback. This group of women are at risk of deterioration with a subsequent vaginal delivery and therefore, should be granted with the option of undergoing caesarean delivery.

Management of subsequent pregnancy following OASIS is summarised in Figure 24.14.

Key points

- Anal sphincter injury following childbirth is associated with significant maternal morbidity.

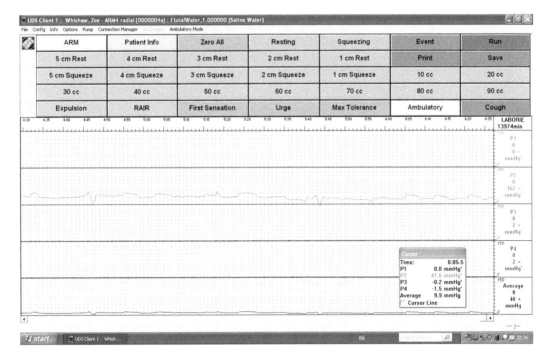

FIGURE 24.12 Low resting pressure and low squeeze pressure in a patient who had both external and internal sphincter defects.

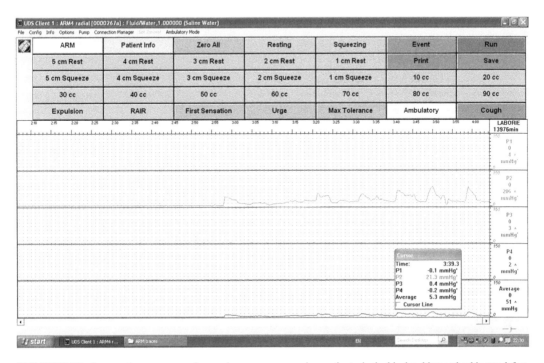

FIGURE 24.13 Low resting pressure and normal squeeze pressure in a patient who had isolated internal sphincter defect.

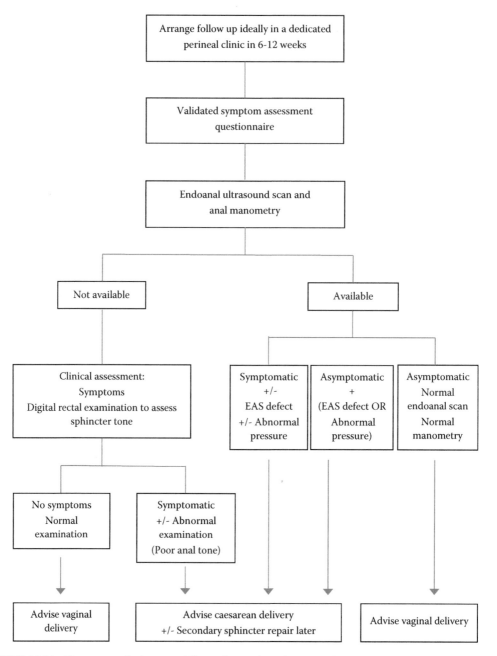

FIGURE 24.14 Management of subsequent delivery after previous obstetric anal sphincter injuries; EAS – external anal sphincter.

- Guidelines based on current evidence should be followed in order to prevent morbidity associated with OASIS.
- All women should be adequately examined for possible OASIS (with a digital rectal examination, if considered necessary) as soon as practical after vaginal birth.
- A digital rectal examination to exclude fourth-degree and buttonhole tears should be carried out.

- The EAS and IAS must be identified individually and sutured separately using the appropriate technique and suture material.
- Detailed documentation of OASIS and its management is needed, ideally on a proforma.
- Antibiotics, laxatives and pain relief are necessary following the procedure.
- Debriefing the woman and following up in ideally around 6–12 weeks in a dedicated clinic with a validated bowel symptom questionnaire, endoanal ultrasound and anal manometry, are recommended.
- Counselling the mode of subsequent delivery based on symptoms, clinical examination, endoanal scan and anal manometry findings, is important.

BIBLIOGRAPHY

1. Gurol-Urganci I, Cromwell D, Edozien L, Mahmood T, Adams E, Richmond D, et al. Third- and fourth-degree perineal tears among primiparous women in England between 2000 and 2012: time trends and risk factors. *BJOG* 2013;120:1516–25.
2. National Health Service Litigation Authority. *Ten Years of Maternity Claims. An Analysis of NHS Litigation Authority Data*. London: National Health Service Litigation Authority;2012.
3. Fernando RJ, Sultan AH, Radley S, Jones PW, Johanson RB. Management of obstetric anal sphincter injury: a systematic review and national practice survey. *Biomed Central Health Services Res*. 2002;2(1):9. doi: 10.1186/1472-6963-2-9.
4. Royal College of Obstetricians and Gynaecologists. RCOG Green Top Guideline 29: Management of Third and Fourth Degree Perineal Tears Following Vaginal Delivery. Fernando RJ, Sultan AH, Freeman RM, Williams A, Adams E. London: Royal College of Obstetricians and Gynaecologists;2015.
5. Verghese TS, Champaneria R, Kapoor DS, Latthe PM. Obstetric anal sphincter injuries after episiotomy: systematic review and meta-analysis. *Int Urogynecol J* 2016;27:1459–67.
6. National Institute for Health and Clinical Excellence. *Intrapartum care: care of healthy women and their babies during childbirth. NICE Clinical Guideline 55*. Manchester: National Institute for Health and Clinical Excellence;2007
7. Sultan AH, Thakar R. Lower genital tract and anal sphincter trauma. *Best Pract Res Clin Obstet Gynaecol* 2002;16:99–115
8. Fernando RJ, Sultan AH, Kettle C, Thakar R. Methods of repair for obstetric anal sphincter injury. *Cochrane Database Syst Rev* 2013;12:CD002866. doi: 10.1002/14651858.CD002866.pub3.
9. Karmarkar R, Bhide A, Digesu A, Khullar V, Fernando R. Mode of delivery after obstetric anal sphincter injury. *Eur J Obstet Gynecol Reprod Biol* 2015;194:7–10.

25

Assisted Vaginal Breech Delivery

Sanjeewa Padumadasa and Malik Goonewardene

In breech presentation, the buttocks or one foot or both feet of the fetus instead of the head are present at the maternal pelvis. It is the most common malpresentation, with an incidence of 3–4% of all the deliveries at term. External cephalic version is recommended after 36 weeks of gestation in order to reduce the number of breech presentations at term (discussed in Chapter 27). Since the publication of the 'Term Breech Trial' back in the dawn of the 21st century, many obstetricians worldwide have opted to deliver 'breech babies' using the scalpel rather than trusting their skills and choosing to vaginally deliver these babies instead. This has deskilled the modern-day obstetrician to such an extent that he/she may be incapable of performing even the most straightforward assisted vaginal breech delivery (AVBD), if and when the need arises. There has been concern regarding the conduct, interpretation and applicability of the 'Term Breech Trial', and in addition, there is evidence that supports AVBD as a safe method in delivering certain 'breech babies' after careful selection of cases. Therefore, AVBD continues to be performed safely and frequently in many centres around the world. Furthermore, due to poor antenatal clinic attendance or rarely even misdiagnosis as a cephalic presentation antenatally, a woman in advanced labour may be detected to have a previously undiagnosed breech presentation, at which point it may be too late and risky to perform a caesarean delivery. In addition, some women, especially multigravida, make an informed choice to deliver their 'breech babies' vaginally. Therefore, the skill of performing an AVBD is an essential one to possess.

Almost all of the principles of AVBD apply when performing a caesarean delivery for a breech presentation. However, there is one fundamental difference: traction should not be applied during an AVBD. On the other hand, delivery is not possible during a caesarean delivery unless traction is applied.

Types of Breech

The main types of breech are frank (extended), complete (flexed) and footling (Figure 25.1). Knee presentation is a rare type of breech (Figure 25.2).

- Frank (Extended): Fetal thighs are flexed, but the legs are extended at the knees and lie alongside the trunk, with the feet positioned near the fetal head. This is the most common type and accounts for approximately 65% of breech presentations at term.
- Complete (Flexed): Fetal thighs and knees are flexed, with the feet above or at the level of the buttocks.
- Footling: One or both feet present below the fetal buttocks, with the hips and knees partially flexed. This type is more probable when the fetus is preterm.
- Knee presentation: In this rare type of breech, one or both knees present below the fetal buttocks, with one or both hips extended and the knees flexed.

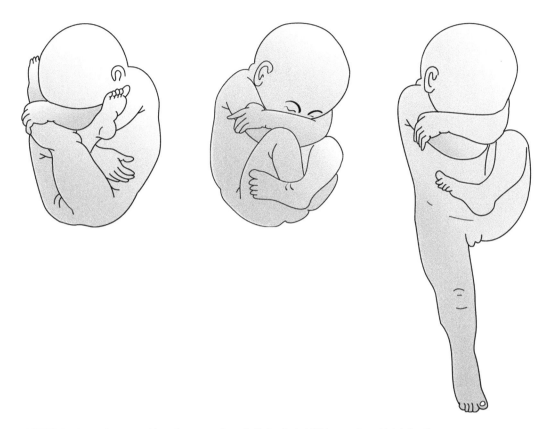

FIGURE 25.1   Main types of breech presentation: (left) frank, (middle) complete, (right) footling.

Predisposing Factors for Breech Presentation

Breech presentation may occur in any pregnancy, but could be associated with the following factors.

- Multiparity
- Preterm
- Multiple pregnancy
- Placenta praevia
- Uterine malformations
- Fibroids in the lower segment of the uterus
- Polyhydramnios / oligohydramnios
- Fetal abnormalities, such as CNS malformations, neck masses and aneuploidy

Fetal Risks in Breech Presentation

As a group, fetuses in a breech presentation have a higher risk of prematurity and intrinsic abnormalities compared to those in cephalic presentation, and this may also account for the worse outcome for these babies, irrespective of the mode of delivery. However, during labour and delivery, a fetus in breech presentation is also at a higher risk of birth asphyxia and trauma.

Birth asphyxia during delivery may occur due to cord prolapse or cord entanglement, the risk of which is higher in a footling breech compared to other types of breech. Therefore, women with viable

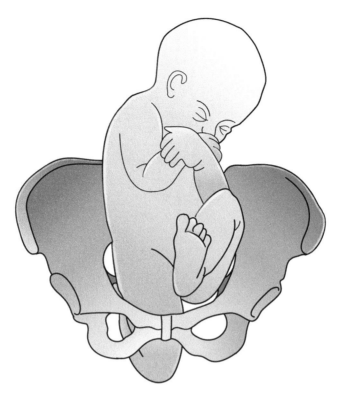

FIGURE 25.2   Knee presentation.

fetuses in a footling breech presentation will usually undergo an elective caesarean delivery. It is also possible for the cord to get compressed from the time the aftercoming head descends below the pelvic brim, as externally marked by the appearance of the lower border of the scapula, up to the time of delivery of the fetus. This can lead to asphyxia if there is an undue delay in delivery of the fetal head.

Damage to intra-abdominal organs, especially the liver and spleen, may occur if the operator places his/her hands on the fetal abdomen rather than on the hip when assisting delivery. Fetal limbs can get injured, especially in the case of extended or nuchal arms. Injuries to the brachial plexus, cervical spine and even the fetal skull due to the application of undue traction or twisting of the fetal body, have also been reported.

Although the fetal buttocks and trunk may pass through an incompletely dilated cervix, the fetal head can get entrapped behind this if an AVBD has been initiated without ensuring that the cervix is fully dilated. This is particularly important in the preterm or in growth-restricted fetus, as the difference in the diameters of the fetal head and the trunk is significantly marked than in the term, normally grown fetus. Also, the fetal arms can get entrapped behind an incompletely dilated cervix. Sudden decompression of the fetal head at the point of delivery can cause tentorial tears and intracranial haemorrhage, if delivery of the head is not controlled.

Prerequisites for an Assisted Vaginal Breech Delivery

Assisted vaginal breech delivery should be undertaken only by an experienced obstetrician who is skilled in performing AVBD and managing complications that may arise during delivery in a centre with facilities for emergency caesarean delivery. All of the contraindications for vaginal delivery should be excluded. As there is an increased risk of scar dehiscence during the manoeuvres used during delivery, a scarred uterus is considered a contraindication for AVBD. In a twin pregnancy, cephalic presentation of the first twin is the main determinant of vaginal delivery, irrespective of the presentation of the second twin. Caesarean delivery is performed, if the first twin is in breech presentation (discussed in Chapter 26).

The following are considered as favourable factors for a safe and successful AVBD.

- Frank or complete breech
- Estimated fetal weight between 2,500 g and 3,500 g
- Adequate maternal pelvis
- Non-compromised fetus
- Flexed fetal neck, as indicated on ultrasound

Candidates for AVBD should be selected on a case-by-case basis after offering the alternative option of caesarean delivery. Informed written consent, highlighting the risks associated with AVBD, should be obtained from the woman.

Management of Labour

If a decision has been made to proceed with an AVBD, then spontaneous onset of labour should be anticipated up to 40 weeks of gestation. Induction or augmentation of labour should be avoided as much as possible, because fetopelvic disproportion may be masked and may possibly lead to complications at the delivery of the fetus. Poor progress of labour may be a sign of fetopelvic disproportion, and this is an indication for caesarean delivery. The neonatal team should be alerted in case the neonate needs to be resuscitated. The fetus must be continuously monitored during labour by cardiotocography. The fetal membranes should be left intact for as long as possible, and the high risk of cord prolapse which could occur with spontaneous rupture of membranes or with amniotomy should be kept in mind (discussed in Chapter 2).

Analgesia in the form of narcotic and inhalational analgesia during labour, combined with local anaesthetic infiltration of the perineum at the time of delivery, provides the woman with adequate analgesia and also with the ability to effectively bear down during the second stage of labour. On the other hand, epidural analgesia has the advantage of preventing the woman from prematurely bearing down during the late first stage of labour before full dilatation of cervix, thus minimising the risk of head entrapment. However, epidural analgesia can abolish the woman's urge to push during the active phase of the second stage of labour, thereby compromising maternal bearing down efforts which are essential in conducting an AVBD. A selective type of epidural analgesia that prevents the urge to push during the late first stage of labour but allows motor function to be retained so that full maternal effort can be utilised during the bearing down stage would be ideal.

The Technique for Assisted Vaginal Breech Delivery

Although a 'hands off the breech' policy is usually recommended, delivery needs to be assisted at various points in order to ensure safe delivery of the fetus. These points where assistance is provided are referred to as landmarks on the journey of an AVBD.

If the woman starts bearing down, and the cervix is not fully dilated, then she should be placed in the left lateral position and advised to breathe deeply and avoid bearing down. When the breech is visible after ensuring that the cervix is fully dilated, the woman should be placed in lithotomy position, as this facilitates the performing of manoeuvres needed to assist a vaginal breech delivery (Figure 25.3). The operator should place himself / herself in a seated position between the maternal thighs. The perineum should be cleaned and draped, and the bladder must be emptied. If epidural analgesia has not already been administered, then the perineum should be infiltrated with a local anaesthetic agent.

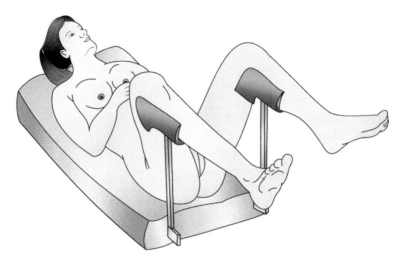

FIGURE 25.3   Lithotomy position.

Delivery of the Breech and Legs

The woman should be encouraged to strain in a synchronous manner with uterine contractions. In a frank or flexed breech, the first landmark is the point at which the breech climbs the perineum, does not recede between uterine contractions, and the fetal anus is visible. Frequently, an epsiotomy is then performed while taking care to avoid damage to the soft tissues of the fetus, including the genitalia. The bitrochanteric diameter of the fetus, which is the widest part of the breech, will usually orient itself in the anteroposterior direction because the anteroposterior diameter is the widest part of the maternal pelvic outlet (Figure 25.4). At this stage, the fetus should not be rotated to the sacroanterior position, because this will be moving against the natural birth mechanisms of a fetus presenting by breech and will complicate the delivery. If the fetus shows any tendency to rotate into the sacroposterior position, then this should be prevented. The fetus may pass meconium when the breech is squeezed through the birth canal, but this is not an indication of acute fetal compromise.

The breech should be allowed to descend with the aid of uterine contractions and maternal effort. Traction should not be applied, as this may cause deflexion and extension of the upper limbs and the head of the fetus, thereby making delivery difficult (Figure 25.5). The diameters of the fetal head at the birth canal increase with progressive deflexion of the fetal head, and the importance of cranial flexion is emphasised in Figure 25.6.

In a case of a flexed breech, the delivery of the legs is not much of a problem. Assistance is required to deliver extended legs in the case of a frank breech. When the popliteal fossa (i.e. second landmark) is visible, the thigh should be abducted and the knee flexed by placing the thumb on the popliteal fossa, and the index and middle fingers on the leg below the knee. Each leg should be delivered in turn by sweeping it out of the vagina through the space between the two thighs of the fetus. The posterior leg is usually at a lower level than the anterior leg. Therefore, it is easier to deliver the posterior leg and subsequently the anterior one, rather than the other way around (Figure 25.7).

Delivery of fetal abdomen

The fetus should be allowed to deliver spontaneously up to the level of the lower abdomen with solely maternal effort. The third landmark is the fetal umbilicus. When the fetal umbilicus is visible, a loop of umbilical cord should be gently hooked down in order to relieve tension on the umbilical cord. Excessive handling of the umbilical cord should be avoided, as this may cause spasms of umbilical vessels, which may in turn lead to fetal hypoxia.

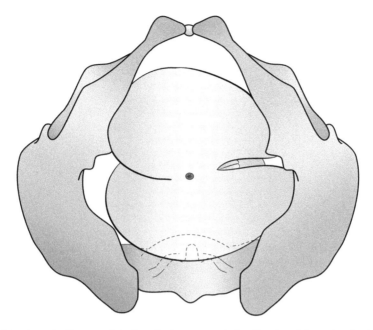

FIGURE 25.4   Bitrochanteric diameter of the fetus in the anteroposterior diameter of the maternal pelvis.

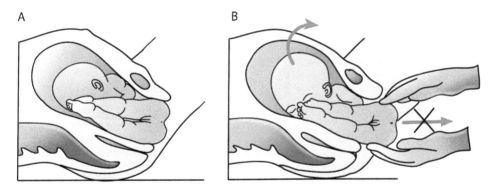

FIGURE 25.5   A - allow the breech to descend with the aid of uterine contractions and maternal effort, B - avoid traction.

Again, it is important to let the fetus deliver with its back in an anterolateral direction, along the wider anteroposterior diameter of the pelvic outlet (Figure 25.8). This will allow natural birth mechanisms to take place, thus leading to the safe delivery of the fetus. If the fetus shows any tendency to rotate to sacroposterior position, then this should be managed.

The fetal body should be wrapped in a warm, sterile towel to prevent hypothermia and to obtain a firm grip, but the importance of identifying the inferior border of the scapula as the landmark for delivery of the shoulders and arms should be kept in mind.

Delivery of the Shoulders and Arms

The fourth landmark is when the lower border of the scapula comes into view below the pubic arch. At this point, the fetal head is entering the maternal pelvis, and the umbilical cord is partially or completely occluded. Therefore, delivery should be completed within the next 2–3 minutes. Although it may not be apparent, 2–3 minutes is adequate to complete the delivery of the fetus, and excessive haste which may

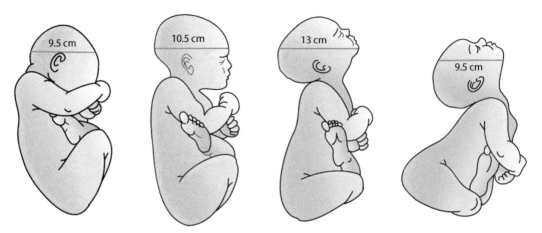

FIGURE 25.6 The diameters at the birth canal with deflexion of the fetal head: A - flexed head and B, C, D - the change of diameters with progressive deflexion of the fetal head.

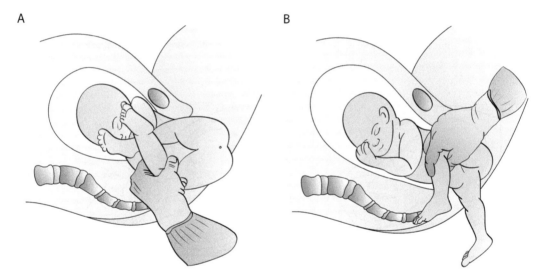

FIGURE 25.7 Delivery of extended legs: A - delivery of the posterior Leg, B - delivery of the anterior leg.

lead to birth trauma should be avoided. At the same time, an undue delay should be avoided, as this may cause birth asphyxia.

Delivery of Flexed Arms

By passing the index and middle fingers over the ventral aspect of the fetus, the position of the fetal arms should be examined for. If the arms are flexed and the forearms are palpable, then their delivery should be assisted by applying gentle traction on the medial side of the anterior forearm just near the elbow (Figure 25.9A), in order to extend it and sweep it across the fetal chest (Figure 25.9B). Thereafter, the posterior arm should be delivered in the same manner and is aided by lifting the body of the fetus slightly upwards (Figure 25.10). Alternatively, the body of the fetus can be rotated by 180° in order to bring the posterior arm into view beneath the pubic symphysis. It is important to maintain sacroanterior position midway during this rotation.

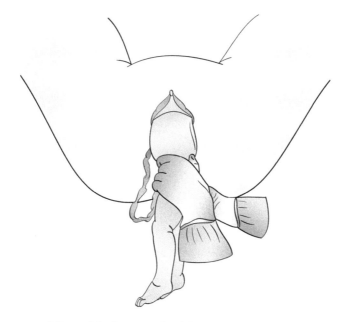

FIGURE 25.8 Spontaneous delivery of the fetus up to the abdomen.

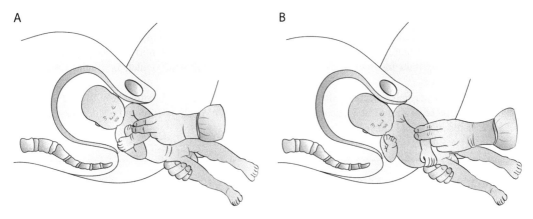

FIGURE 25.9 Delivery of the flexed anterior arm.

Delivery of Extended Arms

Upon passing the index and middle fingers over the ventral aspect of the fetus, if the fetal arms are discovered to be extended, then Lovset's manoeuvre should be performed. The posterior fetal shoulder enters the maternal pelvic cavity before the anterior shoulder, and therefore, will usually be lower down in the sacral hollow, while the anterior shoulder will be above the pubic symphysis. Both hands of the operator should be placed around the hips of the fetus with the thumbs on the sacrum and the fingers over the iliac crests. This avoids trauma to intra-abdominal organs. The fetal body should be slightly lifted in order to cause lateral flexion of the fetal body, thereby facilitating further descent of the posterior shoulder along the sacral curve (Figure 25.11A).

The body of the fetus should then be rotated by 180° while maintaining a sacroanterior position midway during this movement and lowering the fetal body during the latter part (Figure 25.11B). The posterior shoulder which was below the pelvic brim will then come to lie anteriorly below the pubic symphysis (Figure 25.11C), and by inserting the index and middle fingers above the upper arm, the arm can be delivered by sweeping it across the fetal chest (Figure 25.11D).

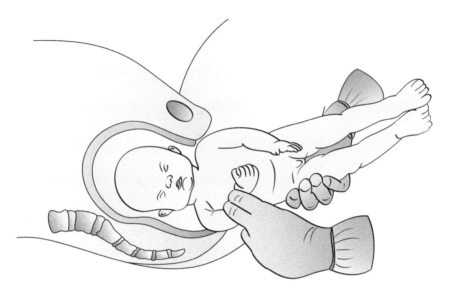

FIGURE 25.10   Delivery of the flexed posterior arm.

The body of the fetus should again be lifted anteriorly, as described above, and rotated back through 180° in the opposite direction while maintaining a sacroanterior position midway during this movement and lowering the fetal body during the latter part. This is done in order to bring the former anterior shoulder, which is currently posterior, again anteriorly, below the pubic symphysis, thereby enabling the delivery of the arm (Figure 25.11E). Maintaining a sacroanterior position midway during these rotatory movements is important in order to promote flexion of the fetal head, which is crucial for the safe delivery of the fetus.

Extended arms may also occur if the trunk has passed through an incompletely dilated cervix, in which case an incision should be made on the cervix at the 2 o'clock position to be able to facilitate the delivery of the arms, and subsequently, the head.

Delivery of a Nuchal Arm

A nuchal arm is a rare situation in which the fetal shoulder is extended with the elbow flexed and the forearm trapped behind the occiput (Figure 25.12). Inappropriate traction on the fetal body and performing rotational manoeuvres earlier than necessary may lead to this situation.

When a nuchal arm is encountered, the fetal trunk should be rotated by 90° in the direction where the hand is pointing in order to free the forearm from behind the occiput (Figure 25.13A). The occiput then rotates past the arm, and with further rotation, the fetal arm and shoulder are then freed. When this occurs, the arm can be delivered by sweeping it across the chest (Figure 25.13B).

In the extremely rare event of bilateral nuchal arms, the rotation of the fetus in one direction will assist the release of one arm, but will correspondingly aggravate the entrapment of the other arm. In this situation, a gentle rotation should be attempted in either direction in order to find out which arm can be easily released first. This should be followed by a rotation of the fetus in the opposite direction in order to deliver the other arm.

Delivery of the Head

The key elements for the delivery of the head are flexion and descent of the head, protection of the cervical spine from undue traction or hyperextension, and safety of the fetal brain from compression and

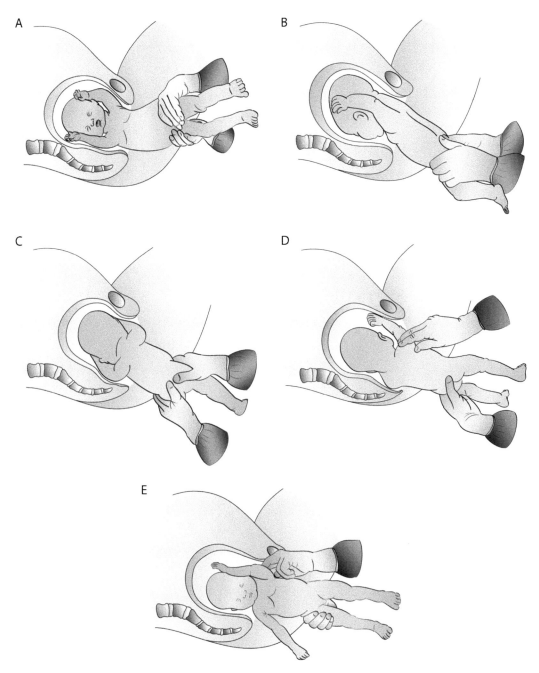

FIGURE 25.11 Lovset's manoeuvre.

sudden decompression forces at the time of delivery over the maternal perineum. After the delivery of the arms, the fetus should be rotated to the sacroanterior position and suspended vertically with partial support from the operator's hands (Figure 25.14). The fetus should not be allowed to hang by its own weight, because this may lead to an extension of the head, thereby making delivery of the head difficult.

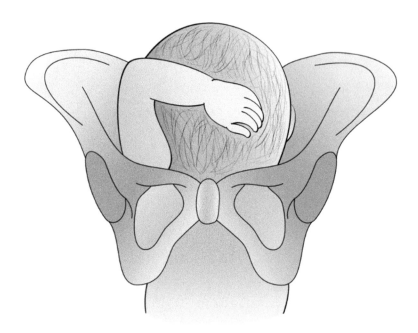

FIGURE 25.12   Nuchal arm.

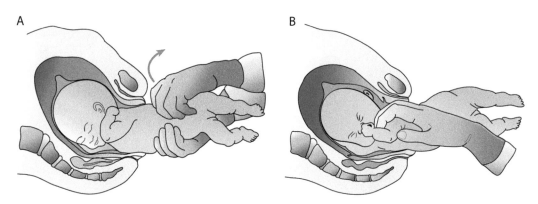

FIGURE 25.13   Delivery of the nuchal arm.

In addition, a small fetus may deliver completely uncontrolled if not supported at this stage. An assistant could apply suprapubic pressure which aids flexion and descent of the fetal head.

When the hairline on the back of the head (i.e. the nape) is visible (the fifth landmark), the whole fetal head is within the pelvic cavity and is ready for delivery at this point. The delivery of the fetal head should be controlled, as the sudden decompression of the fetal head at the point of delivery can cause tentorial tears and intracranial haemorrhage. Out of the many manoeuvres used to deliver the aftercoming head of the breech, the application of forceps and the Mauriceau-Smellie-Veit (MSV) manoeuvre are the most commonly used today. After delivery, the baby should be handed over to the neonatal team.

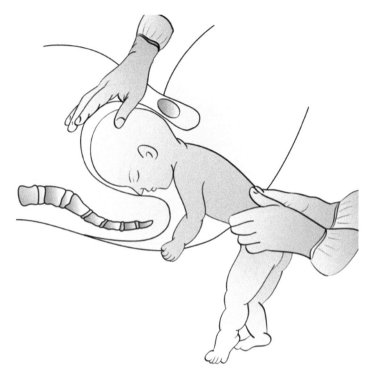

FIGURE 25.14 Supporting the baby after delivery of the arms.

Forceps to the Aftercoming Head

Forceps provide the greatest degree of control and protection to the fetal head due to its cradling effect, and it is also the safest method in applying mild traction that may become necessary in order to complete delivery of the fetal head. Although Piper forceps were especially designed for the delivery of the aftercoming head of the breech, it is now considered obsolete, and any long-handled forceps such as the Simpson forceps would suffice. However, Wrigley forceps are not suitable because in this case, the body of the fetus would hinder its proper application.

While an assistant holds the fetal body at an angle of approximately 45° above the horizontal plane, the blades of forceps should be applied along the sides of the fetal head. Although the fetal body is already delivered, and the blades are applied from the direction of the neck, the technique of application is similar to that in a direct occipitoanterior position in a vertex presentation (Figure 25.15). A second assistant may be required to hold the left blade during the application of the right blade. It is important to avoid lifting the fetal body excessively, as this may cause hyperextension of the fetal head, thereby making delivery difficult, and may also cause injuries to the cervical spine.

When applying forceps for delivery of the aftercoming head of a breech, horizontal traction until the chin and mouth are visible, followed by upward traction, are applied in order to complete delivery (Figure 25.16). The direction of traction should promote flexion of the fetal head, which reduces its diameter and aids delivery. Downward traction on forceps leads to extension and larger anteroposterior diameters of the aftercoming fetal head, which would make delivery difficult.

Mauriceau-Smellie-Veit Manoeuvre

The Mauriceau-Smellie-Veit manoeuvre is useful in controlling the delivery of the fetal head when delivery occurs rapidly, and the application of forceps may not be feasible. This method is also useful if there is no assistant to hold the fetal body in order to apply forceps.

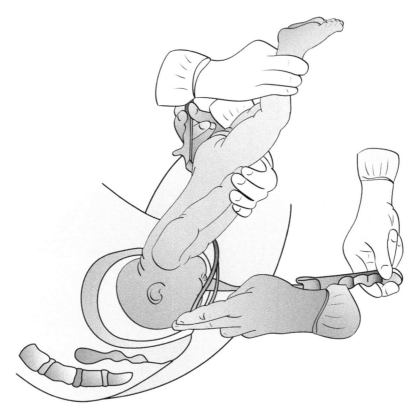

FIGURE 25.15 Application of blades of forceps to the aftercoming head.

The operator should place his/her dominant hand under the fetal body which should be maintained in a neutral position with fetal legs on either side. The index and middle fingers should be placed on the maxilla beside the nose to promote flexion of the fetal head. The other (non-dominant) hand should be placed on the fetal back with the middle finger of the operator's arm on the occiput, which could be used to cause flexion of the fetal head, and the other fingers resting on the fetal shoulders (Figure 25.17). Placing the non-dominant hand on the fetal body prevents the operator from applying undue traction on the fetal body. An assistant may apply suprapubic pressure in order to further aid flexion and delivery of the fetal head. As the fetal head is delivered, the operator should rise from the seat.

Originally, the MSV manoeuvre involved 'jaw flexion' by inserting a finger into the mouth of the fetus, to promote flexion of the head, followed by 'shoulder traction'. This led to complications, mainly the dislocation of the lower jaw. Therefore, the technique was modified so that the head was flexed by using pressure on the maxillae. The aim of this manoeuvre is to control the delivery of the fetal head and to avoid sudden decompression in case of a rapid delivery where the application of forceps is not feasible. In this case, traction is minimal.

Burns-Marshall Technique

The feet of the fetus are grasped, and with gentle traction, swept over the woman's abdomen. This usually leads to flexion of the fetal head and delivery (Figure 25.18). The procedure may lead to hyperextension of the fetal head, making delivery difficult, and also damage to the cervical spine of the fetus, if not carried out properly (Figure 25.19).

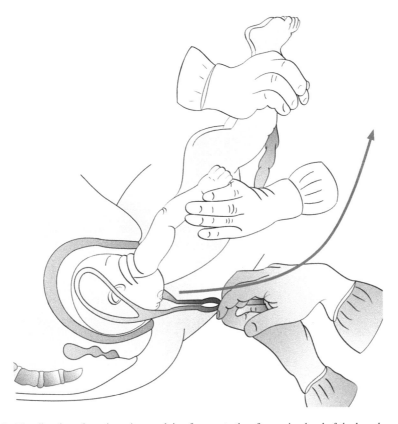

FIGURE 25.16 The direction of traction when applying forceps to the aftercoming head of the breech.

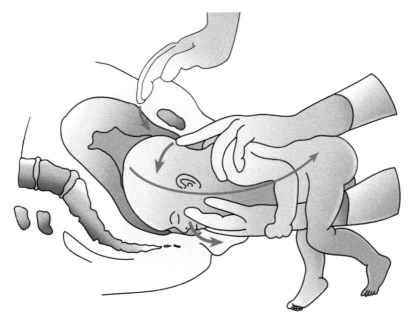

FIGURE 25.17 Mauriceau-smellie-veit manoeuvre.

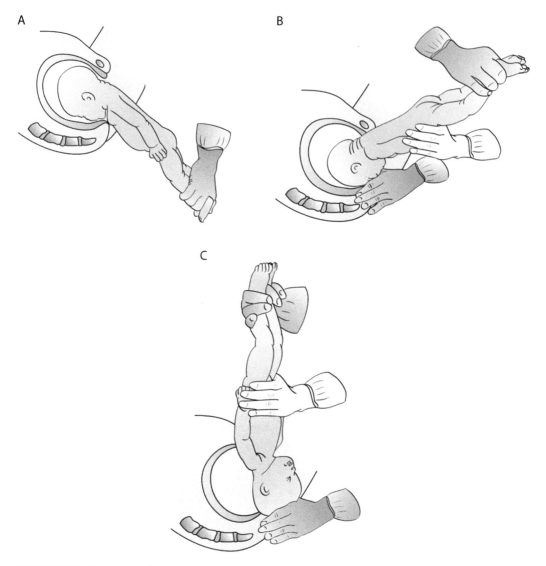

FIGURE 25.18 Burns-marshall manoeuvre.

PROCEDURE – ASSISTED VAGINAL BREECH DELIVERY

General Considerations

- Ensure that the cervix is fully dilated.
- Place the woman in lithotomy position.
- Sit between the maternal thighs.
- Clean and drape. Empty the bladder.

Delivery of the breech, legs and abdomen

- Consider administration of an epsiotomy.

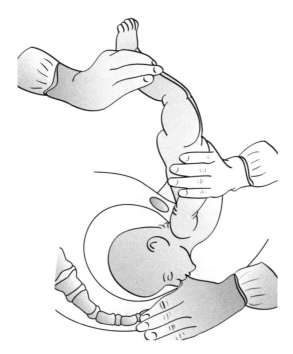

FIGURE 25.19 Excessive elevation of the fetal body over the maternal abdomen causing hyperextension of the fetal head.

- Avoid traction.
- Allow the breech to deliver with its bitrochanteric diameter in the anteroposterior diameter of the maternal pelvic outlet.
- If the legs are flexed, deliver each leg in turn out of the vagina. If the legs are extended, abduct the fetal thigh, flex the knee and deliver each leg in turn by sweeping it out of the vagina through the space between the fetal thighs.
- Allow spontaneous delivery of the abdomen with the back orientated along the anteroposterior diameter of the maternal pelvic outlet. Support the baby by holding from the hip bones.
- Release a loop of the umbilical cord.

Delivery of the Arms

- Insert the index and middle fingers over the ventral aspect of the fetal body and try to palpate the forearm.
- If the arms are flexed and the forearms are palpable, then extend the anterior elbow and sweep the anterior arm across the fetal chest. Repeat the process for the posterior arm.
- If the arms are extended, then grasp the fetal body from the hip bones and lift slightly anteriorly to facilitate the descent of the posterior shoulder along the sacral curve.
- Rotate the fetal body by 180° while maintaining the sacroanterior position to bring the former posterior shoulder anteriorly underneath the pubic symphysis, and deliver that arm

by inserting the index and middle fingers above the upper arm and sweeping it across the fetal chest.

- Again, lift the fetal body slightly anteriorly and rotate in the opposite direction to deliver the other arm.

Delivery of the Head

- When the arms of the fetus have been delivered, rotate to a sacroanterior position and partially support the body, without allowing the fetus to hang on its own, until the hairline is visible underneath the pubic symphysis.
- Suprapubic pressure could be applied by an assistant.

Forceps to the Aftercoming Head

- Request an assistant to hold the fetus at an angle between the horizontal and vertical planes.
- Apply long-handled forceps along the sides of the head.
- Apply horizontal traction followed by upward traction.

Mauriceau-Smellie-Veit Manoeuvre

- Place the dominant hand under the fetal body with index and middle fingers on the maxilla and the other hand on the fetal back with middle finger on the occiput and the remaining fingers on the shoulders.
- Flex the fetal head.
- An assistant may apply suprapubic pressure to further aid flexion and delivery of the fetal head.
- Control the delivery of the aftercoming head of the breech.

Difficulties Encountered during the Delivery of the Aftercoming Head of the Breech

Rarely, the following complications may be encountered during the delivery of the aftercoming head of the breech.

- Extension of the fetal head
- Entrapment of the fetal head
- Aftercoming head of the breech in the occipitoposterior (OP) position
- Head stuck inside the pelvis

However, these complications are extremely rare after the proper selection of cases and when skilled assistance is available at delivery.

Extension of the fetal head

This could happen if rapid, spontaneous delivery occurs before the availability of a skilled person to conduct the delivery or an unskilled person has applied traction after the fetal body has been delivered, and the fetal head has become extended. An assistant should apply suprapubic pressure in order to aid flexion and descent of the fetal head, while the operator performs the MSV manoeuvre to deliver the fetal head or bring it down sufficiently for the application of long-bladed forceps.

Entrapment of the Fetal head

Entrapment of the aftercoming head of the breech typically occurs in a preterm or growth-restricted fetus when the fetal breech and trunk, which are smaller in diameter as compared with the head, pass through an incompletely dilated cervix. This is the reason why it is essential to ensure that the cervix is fully dilated before attempting the delivery of a fetus presenting by breech.

An incision, referred to as Duhrssen's incision, should be made on the cervix at the 2 o'clock position, and if necessary, also at the 10 and 6 o'clock positions, in order to deliver the entrapped head (Figure 25.20). Some advise to incise the cervix at the 4 and 7 o'clock positions. The principle behind the placement of the incisions at these positions is to avoid the uterine vessels which lie laterally on the cervix.

Aftercoming Head of the Breech in the Occipitoposterior Position

This complication should not occur if delivery has been assisted, and any tendency of the fetal back to rotate posteriorly has been avoided. However, this situation may occur if the fetal trunk has been delivered before skilled assistance is available.

Firstly, hold the fetus as when performing the MSV manoeuvre, and attempt to rotate it to an occipitoanterior (OA) position. It is extremely important to rotate both the head and the trunk at the same time in order to avoid twisting the neck. After the fetus has been rotated to the OA position, the delivery of the fetal head can be accomplished by applying forceps or by performing the MSV manoeuvre.

If rotation of the fetus to the OA position is not possible, then the fetal head can be delivered in the OP position using forceps. The other method used to deliver the head in OP position is exerting gentle

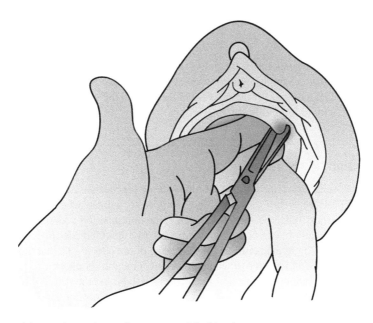

FIGURE 25.20 Incision on the cervix to relieve entrapped fetal head.

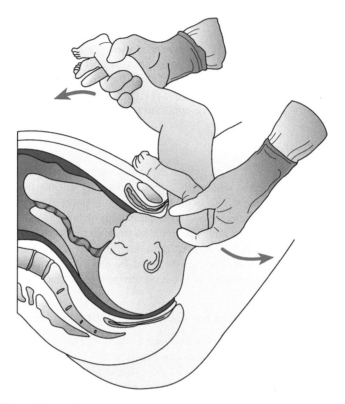

FIGURE 25.21 Delivery of the head in the occipitoposterior position.

traction downwards and backwards on the fetal shoulders with one hand, while the other hand lifts and flexes the fetus similar to a 'reversed Burns Marshall' manoeuvre (Figure 25.21).

Head Stuck Inside the Pelvis

The fetal head could become stuck inside the pelvis due to fetopelvic disproportion, if a proper selection of cases has not been made. Symphysiotomy (described in Chapter 10) and caesarean delivery have been described as possible methods for the delivery of the fetus in this case. However, these methods are associated with considerable morbidity for the woman.

Breech Extraction

Breech extraction of a singleton fetus has no place in obstetric practice today, except in fetal demise, and in the case of cord prolapse at full dilatation in a multiparous woman when there is a delay in performing caesarean delivery. When performing breech extraction, traction is applied to one or both feet in case of a flexed breech, and to one or both groins in case of a frank breech (Figure 25.22). Care must be exercised to position the umbilical cord on the outer side of the operator so that the cord does not get entangled during the process of bringing down the fetal legs. Traction should be exerted downwards and backwards in line with the longitudinal axis of the maternal pelvis, and the delivery of the fetus must be completed using the manoeuvres pertinent to an AVBD. As breech extraction involves applying traction on the fetus, the arms and head will usually be extended.

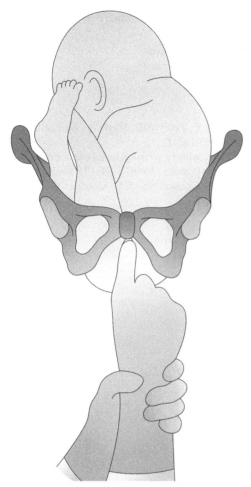

FIGURE 25.22 Traction on the groin in a frank breech during breech extraction.

Acquisition of Necessary Skills in Conducting an Assisted Vaginal Breech Delivery

It is imperative that every obstetrician is competent with the technique of AVBD, because there will be instances when this procedure will have to be carried out even in centres that strongly recommend a policy of elective caesarean delivery for all women with breech presentation. Practising on manikins as well as rehearsing the manoeuvres during caesarean delivery for fetuses presenting by breech are useful in acquiring the basic skills in preparation for gaining hands-on experience of AVBD in clinical practice.

Key Points

- Traction should not be applied when performing an AVBD.
- Assistance is given at several points, which are referred to as landmarks.
- The fetus should have its transverse diameter in the anteroposterior diameter of the maternal pelvis, up to the point of delivery of the abdomen.

- The sacroanterior position should be maintained midway during rotation when delivering the fetal arms, as well as before and during delivery of the fetal head.
- The aftercoming head is usually delivered with long-handled forceps.

BIBLIOGRAPHY

1. Alarab M, Regan C, O'Connell MP, Keane DP, O'Herlihy C, Foley ME. Singleton vaginal breech delivery at term: still a safe option. *Obstet Gynecol* 2004;103:407–12.
2. Berhan Y, Haileamlak A. The risks of planned vaginal breech delivery versus planned caesarean section for term breech birth: a meta-analysis including observational studies. *BJOG* 2016;123:49–57.
3. Mode of term singleton breech delivery. ACOG Committee Opinion No. 745. American College of Obstetricians and Gynecologists. *Obstet Gynecol* 2018;132:e60–e63.

26

Twin Delivery

Sanjeewa Padumadasa and Malik Goonewardene

The advent of assisted reproductive technology has led to an increased incidence of twin and higher-order multiple pregnancies. The perinatal morbidity and mortality of twin pregnancies are 5–10 times higher and even greater in higher-order multiple pregnancies compared to that in singleton pregnancies. Prematurity, fetal growth restriction, congenital malformations, twin-to-twin transfusion syndrome, cord accidents, intrapartum hypoxia and birth trauma contribute to the increased perinatal morbidity and mortality rates in multiple pregnancies. The woman is also at greater risk compared to a woman with a singleton pregnancy, and this is due to anaemia, hypertensive disorders of pregnancy, diabetes mellitus, postpartum haemorrhage (PPH) and venous thromboembolic disease.

Factors that Influence the Mode of Delivery

In the absence of other complications, the presentation of the first twin is the main determinant of the mode of delivery. The presentation of the first twin is cephalic in 75%–80% of cases at term, and in such situations, vaginal delivery is possible. Elective caesarean delivery is considered the norm if the first twin is in a non-cephalic presentation, as well as in viable, higher-order multiple pregnancies which carry a higher risk of maternal and perinatal morbidity and mortality compared to singleton and twin pregnancies. The other fetal factors that are taken into consideration in deciding the mode of delivery are extremes of weight (less than 1.5 kg or more than 3.5 kg), a discrepancy of weight between the twins, especially a larger second twin, and fetal compromise due to growth restriction or twin-to-twin transfusion syndrome. The presence of these factors tilts the balance towards favouring an elective caesarean delivery. The rare occurrence of conjoined twins also necessitates elective caesarean delivery.

At term, when the first twin is in cephalic presentation, then the second twin is in a transverse lie or breech presentation in 20–25% of cases. Furthermore, the second twin could alter its presentation following the delivery of the first twin in up to 20% of the cases. The decision as to the mode of delivery in a non-cephalic second twin depends on the experience of the obstetrician. In the hands of an experienced obstetrician, safe vaginal delivery is possible for a non-cephalic second twin.

The maternal factors that are taken into consideration in deciding the mode of delivery include age, parity, history of subfertility and the presence of placenta praevia or a scarred uterus. In a woman with a twin pregnancy who had undergone a previous caesarean delivery, the usual practice is to perform a repeat caesarean delivery due to the fear of possible scar rupture because of overdistension of the uterus which would, in turn, be contracting during labour and also because of the possible need for manipulations, such as external cephalic version (ECV), internal podalic version and breech extraction. It is recommended that uncomplicated monochorionic monoamniotic twins, who account for about 1% of all twin pregnancies, are delivered by elective caesarean delivery at 34 weeks of gestation after a course of antenatal corticosteroids has been considered, due to the risk of cord prolapse, cord entanglement and separation of the placenta following the delivery of the first twin.

Vaginal delivery remains a safe option for the majority of twins in the hands of the experienced. It is important that every trainee is competent with the vaginal delivery of twins. The availability of expertise in performing obstetric manoeuvres such as ECV or internal podalic version and breech extraction, which may be necessary to deliver the second twin, is a key factor in determining the mode of delivery for twin pregnancies in a given maternity unit.

Timing of Delivery

Many women with multiple pregnancy will deliver preterm, and therefore, corticosteroids should be administered after 24 weeks of gestation to improve the lung maturity of the fetus, which is threatened by preterm labour. If not, induction of labour is commonly practised with an uncomplicated dichorionic twin pregnancy at 37 weeks of gestation, and with an uncomplicated monochorionic diamniotic twin pregnancy at 36 weeks after a course of antenatal corticosteroids has been considered, due to the increased risk of intrauterine fetal demise beyond these gestations. Similar procedures for labour induction as used in a singleton pregnancy, such as insertion of vaginal prostaglandins or transcervical Foley catheter and amniotomy followed by oxytocin infusion can be used depending on the modified Bishop's score.

Management of Labour

Women with a twin pregnancy undergoing vaginal delivery should be informed about the possible need for obstetric manoeuvres, including caesarean delivery, and consent must be obtained in order to proceed with any such procedures, if the need arises. The vaginal delivery of twins should be conducted by an experienced obstetrician. Two neonatal teams, which include two neonatologists, nurses and an anaesthesiologist, must also be involved. Cardiotocography with twin probes and on-site ultrasound, if feasible, should likewise be made available. Round-the-clock access to the operating theatre is also a prerequisite for the safe vaginal delivery of twins.

First Stage of Labour

The neonatal teams should be informed when labour has begun.

There is much to be gained from epidural analgesia, as it offers adequate analgesia during labour as well as for internal podalic version and breech extraction or caesarean delivery, which may be deemed necessary for the delivery of the second twin.

Intravenous access should be obtained by inserting a cannula, and an infusion should be commenced. One unit of packed red cells needs to be crossmatched in case the need for transfusion arises, if PPH were to occur. Both fetuses should be monitored using cardiotocography with twin probes. As there is a possibility that the same fetus is monitored while the other fetus remains undetected, some experts advocate applying a fetal scalp electrode on the first twin as early as possible and externally monitoring the second twin (Figure 26.1). Whichever method is used, it is important that two distinct heart rate tracings are obtained in order to ensure that both fetuses are monitored simultaneously. During the first stage of labour, the rest of management, including augmentation with oxytocin, is similar to that of a singleton pregnancy. Caesarean delivery may be indicated in case of arrest of labour or fetal compromise of either fetus.

Second Stage of Labour

Vaginal delivery should be anticipated, or if the need arises, instrumental vaginal delivery may be performed to deliver the first twin. If instrumental vaginal delivery is performed, then the same prerequisites as for a singleton pregnancy should be fulfilled. An episiotomy should be performed for the usual indications, but this may not be needed because the twin fetuses are usually smaller than in a singleton pregnancy. The bolus dose of an oxytocic agent should not be administered as prophylaxis against PPH at the time of delivery of the first twin, because this may cause premature separation of the

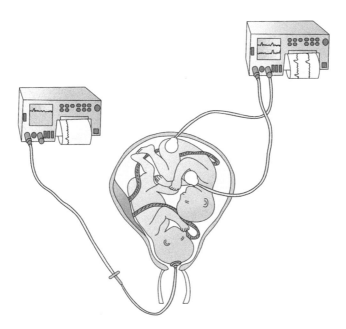

FIGURE 26.1 Intrapartum fetal monitoring in twin pregnancy.

placenta before the delivery of the second twin. When the first twin is delivered, the cord should be immediately divided between two secure clamps. Cord clamping should not be delayed. Abdominal and if necessary, a vaginal examination should be performed to determine the lie and presentation of the second twin. An ultrasound scan may be used when there is unclear information about the lie or presentation of the fetus. The fetal heart rate of the second twin should be constantly monitored.

If the presentation of the second twin is cephalic, then vaginal delivery should be anticipated. Usually, there is a cessation of uterine contractions temporarily following the delivery of the first twin. Therefore, it is advisable to start an oxytocin infusion (or increase the rate if an infusion is already running) to initiate uterine contractions at this stage, as the lack of uterine contractions for a prolonged period may cause a subsequent delay in the delivery of the second twin and is associated with fetal hypoxia and emergency delivery. Ideally, the membranes should not be ruptured if the presenting part is high, because this increases the risk of cord prolapse. When uterine contractions are established and the fetal head has descended, the membranes should be ruptured. If the presenting part remains high despite adequate uterine contractions, then a controlled amniotomy should be carried out after excluding cord presentation, and the liquor must be released slowly while an assistant stabilises the fetal head over the pelvic brim. Although there is no consensus as to how long one can wait until the delivery of the second twin once the first twin is delivered, one must use clinical judgement in order to achieve a balance between too early and rapid intervention which may possibly lead to a potentially traumatic delivery and excessive delay which may cause fetal hypoxia due to partial separation of the placenta resulting in reduced blood flow to the intervillous space. An intertwin delivery interval of not more than 20 minutes is reasonable. Instrumental vaginal delivery, with the same prerequisites as for a singleton pregnancy, may be performed in case of delay or fetal distress (Figure 26.2).

Assisted vaginal breech delivery could be safely carried out by an experienced obstetrician if the second twin is in a breech presentation (described in Chapter 25). Similar to a case where the second twin is in cephalic presentation, membranes may be ruptured only when uterine contractions are established and the presenting part has engaged. In seldom cases, even breech extraction may be carried out by an experienced obstetrician, in case of delay or fetal distress. The options for the delivery of the second twin lying transversely after delivery of the first twin are attempting an ECV (described in Chapter 27) or emergency

A   B

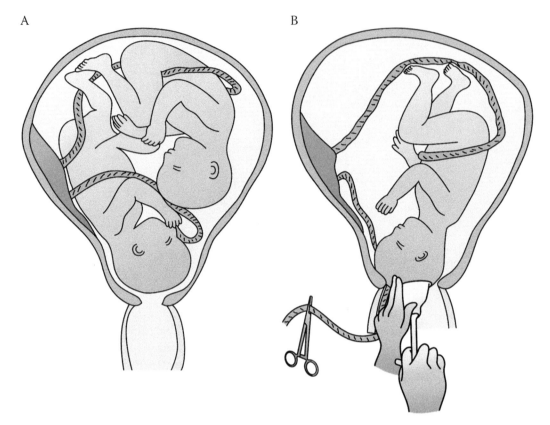

FIGURE 26.2   Instrumental vaginal delivery of the second twin: A, Prior to delivery of first of twin; B, Vacuum delivery of second twin.

caesarean delivery. If the ECV is successful, then management should proceed as described earlier. If the ECV fails, then an internal podalic version followed by breech extraction (described in Chapter 28) which would avoid a potentially serious second-stage caesarean delivery may be possible in the hands of an experienced obstetrician. The success rate of an internal podalic version and breech extraction could be as high as 97%, as compared to 40%–50% with ECV. In addition, many women with multiple pregnancy may prefer to avoid emergency caesarean delivery for delivery of the second twin once the first twin has been delivered vaginally. However, the increasing trend of performing a caesarean delivery for the delivery of the second twin once the first twin has been delivered vaginally suggests that present-day obstetricians feel more confident in the abdominal than in the vaginal route. The findings of the 'term breech trial' may possibly have an influence on decision-making in this instance, although the trial addressed singleton breech presentations instead of those in multiple pregnancy.

Following the delivery of twins, ideally, cord blood gases should be obtained. The cords should be marked (e.g. one clamp for cord of first twin and two clamps for cord of second twin) for easy identification.

Third Stage of Labour

The risk of PPH is higher than that for singleton pregnancies due to uterine atony resulting from overdistension of the uterus. Active management of the third stage, which includes administration of oxytocics with the delivery of the second twin, delivery of the placenta by controlled cord traction and oxytocin infusion, should be instituted as preventive measures against PPH. The placenta should be examined in order to confirm chorionicity and amnionicity.

The management of labour in twins (when the first twin is cephalic) is summarised in Figure 26.3.

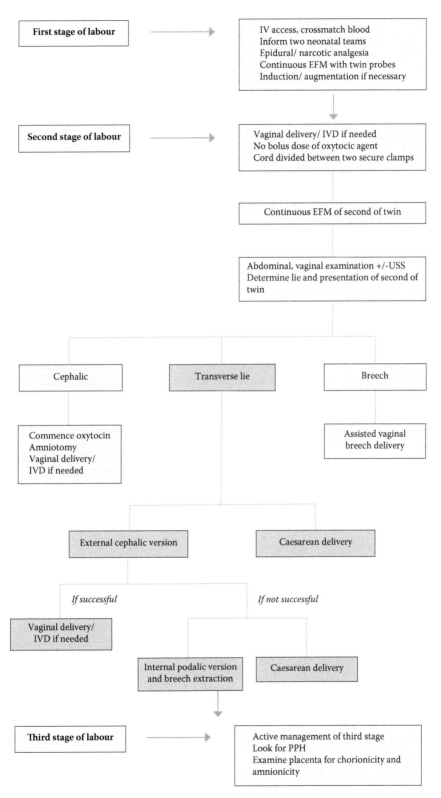

FIGURE 26.3 Management of labour in twins (when the first of twin is cephalic); IV – Intravenous, EFM - Electronic fetal monitoring, IVD – Instrumental vaginal delivery, USS – Ultrasound scan, PPH – Postpartum haemorrhage.

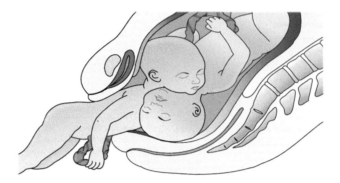

FIGURE 26.4 Locked twins.

Locked Twins

The rare complication of locked twins usually occurs when the first twin is in breech presentation, and its trunk is delivered, but its aftercoming head is locked with the head of the second twin, which is in cephalic presentation (Figure 26.4). However, other fetal and maternal factors have also been reported to give rise to this extremely rare complication. The incidence of locked twins is exceedingly low, occurring in less than 0.1% of twin deliveries, and it has dwindled further in the recent past because a caesarean delivery is commonly performed when the first twin is in a breech presentation. The first twin is at risk of hypoxia, trauma and even death. Moreover, the second twin may be compromised as well.

Management of Locked Twins

Under general anaesthesia and uterine relaxation, the body of the first twin should be elevated in order to facilitate the disimpaction of the head of the second twin from the pelvis. Next, breech extraction of the first twin should be conducted, and the second twin must be delivered in the usual manner.

The alternative is performing an emergency caesarean delivery. A generous incision should be made on the uterus. Reverse extraction of the first twin should be performed followed by delivery of the second twin.

Prevention of Locked Twins

Routinely performing a caesarean delivery when the first twin is breech and the second twin cephalic, should prevent this extremely rare complication. The possibility of interlocking twins may be suspected when there is failure of descent of the first twin in the presence of adequate uterine contractions and an adequate pelvis. However, the majority of cases are diagnosed during the second stage when there is difficulty in the delivery of the first twin.

Key Points

- In most instances, the first twin is in cephalic presentation, and in the absence of other maternal or fetal complications, both fetuses could be safely delivered vaginally, irrespective of the antepartum presentation of the second twin.
- Ideally, both fetuses should be monitored with continuous electronic fetal monitoring.
- Two neonatal teams must be in attendance at the delivery.

- The method adopted (e.g. ECV, internal podalic version and breech extraction or emergency caesarean delivery) for the delivery of the non-cephalic second twin following the vaginal delivery of the first twin, depends on the skill and experience of the attending obstetrician.
- Elective caesarean delivery is indicated for monochorionic monoamniotic and conjoined twins.
- Twin pregnancies carry a higher risk of PPH as compared to singleton pregnancies.

BIBLIOGRAPHY

1. American College of Obstetricians and Gynaecologists Committee on Practice Bulletins-Obstetrics; Society for Maternal-fetal Medicine; ACOG Joint Editorial Committee. ACOG Practice Bulletin 356: Multiple gestation: complicated twin, triplet, and high-order multiple pregnancy. *Obstet Gynecol* 2004;104:869–83.
2. Barrett J., Aztaloz E., Wilian A., et al. The twin birth study: a multicentre RCT of planned CS and planned VB for twin pregnancies. *Am J Obstet Gynecol* 2013;208(1):S4.
3. Barrett J.F.. Twin delivery: method, timing and conduct. *Best Prac Res Clin Obstet Gynaecol* 2014;28(2):327–38.
4. Breathnach F.M., McAuliffe F.M., Geary M., Daly S., Higgins J.R., Dornan J., Perinatal Ireland Research Consortium. Optimum timing for planned delivery of uncomplicated monochorionic and dichorionic twin pregnancies. *Obstet Gynecol* 2012;119:50–59.
5. Houlihan, C., Knuppel, R.A.. Intrapartum management of multiple gestations. *Clin Perinatol* 1996;23:91–116.
6. National Guideline Alliance (UK). *Twin and Triplet Pregnancy*. London: National Institute for Health and Care Excellence (UK);2019.

27

External Cephalic Version

Malik Goonewardene and Sanjeewa Padumadasa

External cephalic version (ECV), which was apparently first described by Aristotle (384–322 BC), involves the manipulation of the fetus through the maternal abdomen in order to rotate the fetus into a cephalic presentation. It is currently performed mainly for a singleton breech presentation in order to avoid caesarean delivery. It is recommended for ECV to be performed at or after 36 weeks of gestation, allowing for a spontaneous version to a cephalic presentation until this period. Reversion to a breech presentation is also likely if ECV is performed before 36 weeks of gestation. If attempted at later gestations, then ECV may be unsuccessful due to relative reduction of liquor. It is also carried out as an elective procedure for a singleton transverse or oblique lie, as well as an emergency procedure for a transverse or oblique lie of the second twin after the vaginal delivery of the first twin.

Procedure

Absolute contraindications for ECV, such as placenta praevia, placental abruption, antepartum haemorrhage, severe pre-eclampsia, abnormal cardiotocography (CTG), Rhesus isoimmunisation, ruptured membranes and significant oligohydramnios, should be excluded. On the other hand, a history of one uncomplicated lower segment transverse caesarean delivery is not a contraindication for a careful ECV. External cephalic version should be conducted only when facilities for CTG and emergency caesarean delivery are available. However, as the risk for an emergency caesarean delivery is low, the woman does not have to undergo fasting, and a light snack may be offered about two hours prior to the procedure. Intravenous access is not necessary. Informed written consent should be obtained prior to initiating the procedure. Tocolytics (e.g. subcutaneous terbutaline 0.25 mg) may be useful when there is good uterine tone, when the uterus is irritable and contracts when palpated, and especially for a repeat attempt at ECV following one failed attempt without tocolytics. Furthermore, analgesia is not necessary.

An ultrasound scan should be done to confirm the fetal lie, presentation and position and location of the placenta, and CTG must be performed in order to confirm fetal well-being. Additional gel should be applied or the gel can be replaced with talcum powder on the maternal abdomen, depending on the preference of the obstetrician. Maintaining eye contact, communicating with the woman and requesting her to concentrate on breathing in and out are important to prevent her from tightening the anterior abdominal wall muscles. The breech may be engaged, especially in the case of a frank breech, and if so, should be dislodged from the pelvis (Figure 27.1). This is achieved by pushing both hands downwards between the fetal breech and the maternal pelvis, cradling the breech and lifting it towards the abdomen. The fetus should be rotated to a cephalic presentation, by a forward somersault (which is preferable as it flexes the fetal head) or a backward somersault by using both hands in unison in order to apply pressure on both fetal poles, maintaining flexion of the fetal body (Figures 27.2 and 27.3). During the procedure, the hands should be interchanged after the halfway mark when the fetus is lying transversely to facilitate pushing the head to the lower pole (Figure 27.4). An assistant should hold the fetus while the hands are being switched. The procedure could be attempted up to a maximum of three times and over a period of ten minutes. The fetal heart should be observed intermittently, every 1–2 minutes during the procedure. Following a successful version, the fetal attitude should be maintained for a few minutes. An ultrasound

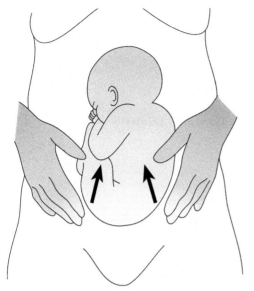

FIGURE 27.1 Disengagement of the fetal breech.

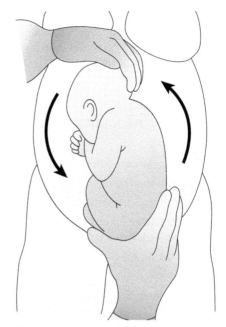

FIGURE 27.2 Forward somersault.

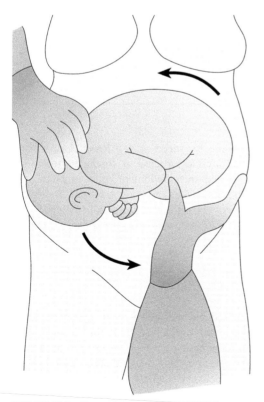

FIGURE 27.3 Forward somersault (Continued).

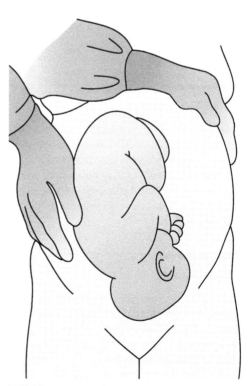

FIGURE 27.4 Completion of ECV.

scan should be performed to confirm a successful version. A repeat CTG for at least 30 minutes should be done to confirm fetal well-being. Abdominal pain, vaginal bleeding or leakage of liquor, should be looked for. Anti-D should be administered if the woman is Rhesus negative, and the dose could be guided by performing a Kliehauer Test. Following the ECV, the woman can be discharged in the absence of any complications.

PROCEDURE – EXTERNAL CEPHALIC VERSION

- Exclude contraindications for ECV.
- Obtain informed written consent.
- Consider tocolysis, especially prior to a repeat attempt.
- Confirm fetal lie, presentation and position, the location of the placenta by ultrasound scan and fetal well-being by CTG.
- Apply additional gel or replace gel with talcum powder on the maternal abdomen.
- Maintain eye contact, talk to the woman and advise her to take deep breaths.
- Dislodge breech, if engaged.
- Rotate the fetus to a cephalic presentation, by a forward (preferred) or backward somersault while maintaining flexion of the fetal body.
- Do not attempt the procedure for more than three times over a period of ten minutes.
- Following a successful version, maintain fetal attitude for a few minutes.
- Confirm successful version by ultrasound scan as well as fetal well-being by CTG.
- Look out for abdominal pain, vaginal bleeding or leakage of liquor.
- Administer Anti-D, if the woman is Rhesus negative.
- Discharge the woman in the absence of any complications.

Factors for Success

The success rate of ECV is higher with multiparity. Meanwhile, the success rate is lower closer to or at term, with maternal obesity, firm anterior abdominal wall muscles, a tense or contractile uterus, an anteriorly located placenta and decreased amniotic fluid volume. Increased liquor volume increases the likelihood of success, but may possibly be associated with spontaneous reversion to breech. The risk of failure is higher when the breech is engaged as compared to when it is not. The risk of failure is also higher in a frank breech (with splinting of the fetal body with the extended legs) rather than a complete or footling breech.

Complications

The complications of ECV are rare and can easily be diagnosed and managed with emergency caesarean delivery. The most common complication is temporary fetal bradycardia (usually lasting less than three minutes), which is actually a physiological phenomenon representing the fetal response to head compression, and it resolves on its own. The woman should be placed in the left lateral position and oxygen should be administered if this occurs. Emergency caesarean delivery is advised if the fetal bradycardia remains unresolved within ten minutes, or if the CTG becomes pathological.

Umbilical cord entanglement may occur and could result in a pathological CTG. Although turning the fetus back to its original malpresentation may resolve the fetal hypoxia, an emergency caesarean delivery may be indicated. However, the need for emergency caesarean delivery following ECV is low. Rupture of membranes and even cord prolapse could infrequently occur. Placental abruption, significant feto-maternal haemorrhage and uterine rupture are extremely rare following ECV. Withdrawing from the procedure rather than persisting, in case of difficulty or pain experienced by the woman, would prevent these complications and ensure the safety of both the fetus and the woman.

Key Points

- External cephalic version is currently performed at or after 36 weeks of gestation mainly for a singleton breech presentation, but also for a singleton transverse or oblique lie and transverse or oblique lie of the second twin following the vaginal delivery of the first twin.
- This should be performed by an experienced operator or by a trainee, under direct supervision, and only if facilities for CTG and emergency caesarean delivery are available.
- Complications are rare, the most notable being fetal bradycardia, which is usually transient and resolves on its own.

BIBLIOGRAPHY

1. American College of Obstetricians and Gynecologists. Practice Bulletin No.161: external cephalic version. *Obstet Gynecol* 2016;127:e54–61.
2. Cluver C, Gyte GM, Sinclair M, Dowswell T, Hofmeyr GJ. Interventions for helping to turn breech babies to head first presentation when using external cephalic version. *Cochrane Database Syst Rev* 2015;2:CD000184.
3. Hofmeyr GJ, Kulier R, West HM. External cephalic version for breech presentation at term. *Cochrane Database Syst Rev* 2015;4:CD000083.
4. Hutton EK, Hofmeyr GJ, Dowswell T. External cephalic version for breech presentation before term. *Cochrane Database Syst Rev* 2015;7:CD000084.
5. Impey LWM, Murphy DJ, Griffiths M, Penna LK on behalf of Royal College of Obstetricians and Gynecologists. External cephalic version and reducing the incidence of term breech presentation. *BJOG* 2017;124:e178–92.
6. Qureshi H, Massey E, Kirwan D, Davies T, Robson S, White J, et al. British Society for Haematology. BCSH guideline for the use of anti-D immunoglobulin for the prevention of haemolytic disease of the fetus and newborn. *Transfus Med* 2014;24:8–20.

28

Internal Podalic Version and Breech Extraction

Sanjeewa Padumadasa and Malik Goonewardene

Internal podalic version, which was apparently first described by Hippocrates (460–370 BC), is a procedure where a series of manoeuvres are performed with one hand inside the uterus, with the aim of bringing one or both feet through a fully dilated cervix. This is followed by breech extraction, i.e. the application of traction on the fetus in order to complete the delivery. The safety of caesarean delivery and the gradual loss of traditional obstetric skills have almost placed this manoeuvre on the verge of becoming defunct in the field of obstetrics.

In skilled hands, internal podalic version and breech extraction continues to have a place in modern obstetrics, for the delivery of the second twin lying transversely, especially when external cephalic version (ECV) has been attempted and failed. However, in many centres, this has largely been replaced by caesarean delivery, probably due to lack of expertise compounded by the publication of the 'term breech trial'. Internal podalic version and breech extraction for the second twin has a higher success rate than ECV and avoids a potentially unnecessary and dangerous second-stage caesarean delivery. The uterus is distended, and the uterine contractions usually cease immediately following delivery of the first twin. The second twin is usually small in size, although this is not always the case. These factors create the ideal conditions for the procedure of internal podalic version and breech extraction.

Internal podalic version and breech extraction has also been described as an alternative to emergency caesarean delivery in a multigravid woman with a singleton fetus lying transversely, under exceptional circumstances such as profound bradycardia and there is delay in performing surgery or when the fetus is already dead. However in these circumstances, because of the higher rates of complications as compared with its use during delivery of the second twin, the procedure is currently not recommended.

Procedure for Internal Podalic Version and Breech Extraction

Internal podalic version and breech extraction should not be performed in the presence of fetal macrosomia or possible fetopelvic disproportion. An experienced obstetrician should perform the procedure in the operating room, which provides the advantage of being able to resort to emergency caesarean delivery in case the procedure fails. Adequate analgesia in the form of epidural or spinal anaesthesia should be provided. Otherwise, the woman can possibly go into shock. Although general anaesthesia may be used, the lack of maternal straining during breech extraction may hinder delivery. Acute tocolysis (e.g. subcutaneous terbutaline 0.25 mg) may be necessary in order to relax the uterus. The neonatal team should be in attendance and ready for resuscitation of the newborn. The fetus should be monitored by continuous cardiotocography.

The woman should be placed in lithotomy position, cleaned and draped and her bladder should be emptied. Vaginal examination should be performed to be able to ensure full dilatation of cervix. While wearing a long, well-lubricated glove, one hand should be inserted through the vagina continuing into the uterus, and the fetal parts must be identified through the intact membranes (Figure 28.1). Both feet of the fetus, or if that is not possible then at least one foot (preferably the anterior), should be grasped (Figure 28.2). If both feet are grasped, then the ankles should be held with the middle finger of the operator lying between them. Proper care must be taken to make sure that a fetal hand is not mistaken for a foot. The toes are shorter, somewhat equal in length and in the same plane as the big toe which is not separated from the other toes. The fingers are longer, unequal in length and the separation between the thumb and the rest of the fingers is pronounced. Furthermore, the foot is longer and a heel is palpable in contrast to the hand.

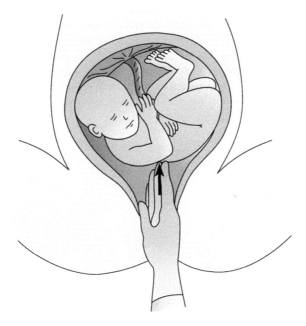

FIGURE 28.1   Insertion of the hand through the intact membranes into the uterus.

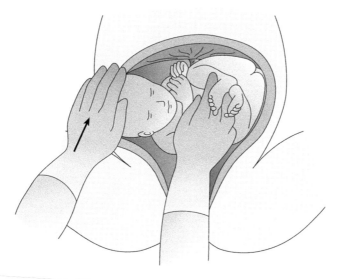

FIGURE 28.2   Grasping of the fetal feet.

Traction should be applied downwards and backwards in line with the longitudinal axis of the maternal pelvis in order to bring both feet or one foot into the vagina. The distended, relaxed uterus will enable the fetus to convert from a transverse lie into a breech presentation. This process can be aided by manipulating the fetus to a longitudinal lie by using the external hand (Figure 28.3). Although the amniotic fluid is expected to protect the fetus from trauma during its journey through the uterine cavity and the vagina, the membranes will usually rupture during the procedure. With gentle traction, the feet are brought through the introitus (Figure 28.4). If only one leg has been grasped, the operator should continue to apply traction until the popliteal fossa of the other leg appears at the introitus. The other leg must then be delivered by abducting the thigh and flexing the leg by applying slight pressure over the popliteal fossa and hooking the index and middle fingers over the leg. As the legs emerge through the vulva, these should be wrapped in a sterile towel to obtain a firm grip, as the vernix caseosa makes them slippery. The calves, and then the thighs are grasped and traction continued with both hands. Once the hips are delivered, the thumbs are placed over the sacrum and the fingers over the iliac crests. The rest of the delivery should subsequently be performed as in the case

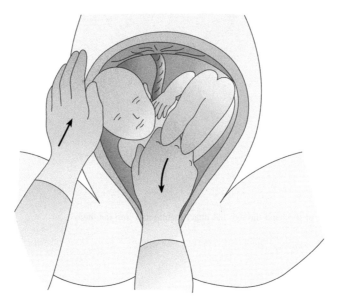

FIGURE 28.3   Traction along the axis of the maternal pelvis.

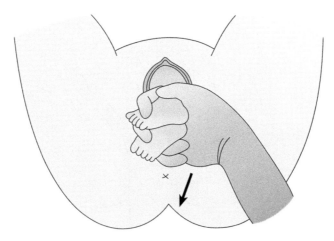

FIGURE 28.4   Bringing the feet through the introitus. Note the grip on the feet.

of an assisted vaginal breech delivery (described in Chapter 25). However, the difference is that traction is applied in this case (breech extraction). An episiotomy is often performed during delivery of the fetal buttocks, but this may be avoided if the fetus is small. The fetal body should be maintained in a sacrolateral position during traction, which enables the wider anteroposterior diameter of the maternal pelvic outlet to accommodate the wider transverse diameter of the fetal body.

Lovset's manoeuvre must usually be performed, as the fetal arms will be extended as a result of applying traction on the fetus. The fetal head could also become extended as traction has been applied during delivery of the fetal body. Application of suprapubic pressure by an assistant helps in flexing the head and promotes its descent into the pelvis. When the head has flexed and descended, it can be delivered with forceps. If the head remains extended, then the Mauriceau-Smellie-Veit manoeuvre is required to deliver the head. Following delivery, the woman should be observed for vaginal bleeding, and the uterus, cervix and vagina should be examined carefully for any lacerations.

PROCEDURE – INTERNAL PODALIC VERSION AND BREECH EXTRACTION

- Obtain informed verbal consent.
- An experienced obstetrician should perform the procedure in the operating theatre with adequate analgesia and uterine relaxation.
- The neonatal team should be in attendance.
- Monitor the fetus with continuous cardiotocography.
- Place the woman in lithotomy position, clean and drape and empty the bladder.
- Insert the hand through the vagina and the fully dilated cervix, into the uterus and through the fetal membranes.
- Grasp preferably both feet, or the anterior foot, and ensure that a fetal hand is not mistaken for a foot.
- Apply traction downwards and backwards in line with the longitudinal axis of the maternal pelvis, assisted by manipulations using the external hand to rotate the fetus to a breech presentation.
- If considered necessary, perform an episiotomy when delivering the fetal buttocks.
- Complete the delivery of the fetus as in an assisted vaginal breech delivery, the only difference being the application of traction.
- Perform Lovset's manoeuvre to deliver extended arms.
- Deliver the head using forceps or the Mauriceau-Smellie-Veit manoeuvre, following suprapubic pressure applied by an assistant.
- Observe for vaginal bleeding and examine the uterus, cervix and vagina for any lacerations.

Possible Difficulties during the Procedure

The fetal arm and hand may prolapse during the manoeuvre, and it is difficult as well as traumatic to replace them. If this occurs, then it should be ignored, and the feet (or one foot) should be grasped and traction continued in order to accomplish delivery of the fetus.

If it is the posterior foot that has been brought down, then there is a possibility of the anterior foot getting arrested at the pubic symphysis (Figure 28.5). In order to prevent this, the posterior leg should be rotated by 180° in a wide arc during traction and subsequently brought anteriorly.

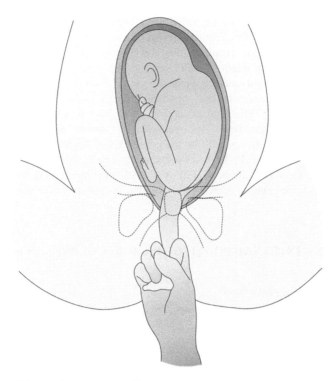

FIGURE 28.5   Arrest of the anterior foot at the pubic symphysis, when the posterior foot has been brought down.

Nuchal arms (unilateral or bilateral) should be anticipated. Management of nuchal arms is described in Chapter 25.

Complications

Complications of internal podalic version and breech extraction are rare and have largely been reported following the procedure in singleton pregnancies. As a result, the method has become obsolete in the management of singleton pregnancies.

It is generally a safe procedure when used during the delivery of the second twin. Fetal complications reported include cord prolapse, shoulder presentation with prolapsed arm, injury to the femur, humerus, skull and intra-abdominal organs, hypoxic injury and death. Maternal complications such as uterine rupture, vaginal and perineal lacerations, placental abruption, postpartum haemorrhage and infection of the uterus have been infrequently reported.

Key Points

- Internal podalic version and breech extraction is a safe and effective option for a skilled obstetrician in delivering the second twin in transverse lie, following vaginal delivery of the first twin.
- The dwindling rates of internal podalic version and breech extraction over the years have resulted in the lack of opportunities for trainees to practise the art. It is vital that trainees initially practise on manikins and, then, perform the procedure on actual patients under the direct supervision of an experienced consultant before carrying out the procedure on their own.

BIBLIOGRAPHY

1. Barrett JFR, Knox Ritchie W. Twin delivery. *Best Pract Res Clin Obstet Gynaecol* 2002;16:43–56.
2. Chauhan AR, Singhal TT, Raut VS. Is internal podalic version a lost art? Optimum mode of delivery in transverse lie. *J Postgrad Med* 2001;47:15–18.
3. Chauhan SP, Roberts WE, McLaren RA, Roach H, Morrison JC, Martin JN Jr. Delivery of the non-vertex second twin: breech extraction versus external cephalic version. *Am J Obstet Gynecol* 1995;173:1015–20.
4. Hirnle P, Franz HB, Sulkarnejewa E, Pfeiffer KH, Kiesel L. Caesarean section for the second twin after vaginal delivery of first. *J Obstet Gynaecol* 2000;20:329–95.
5. Jonsdottir F, Henriksen L, Secher NJ, Maaloe N. Does internal podalic version of the non-vertex second twin still have a place in obstetrics? A Danish national retrospective cohort study. *Acta Obstet Gynecol Scand* 2015;94(1):59–64.
6. Rabinovici J, Barkai G, Reichman B, Serr DM, Mashiach S. Internal podalic version with unruptured membranes for the second twin in transverse lie. *Obstet Gynecol* 1988;71:428–30.
7. Webster SNE, Loughney AD. Internal podalic version and breech extraction. *TOG* 2011;13:7–14.

29

Non-Reassuring Fetal Status

Tiran Dias, Amarnath Bhide, and Austin Ugwumadu

Antepartum and/or intrapartum fetal hypoxaemia, acidosis, acidaemia, fetal host inflammatory response to ascending or vertical intrauterine infection, and other disease states such as fetal hypoglycaemia may present with fetal heart rate (FHR) abnormalities, which were previously captured under the ill-defined terminology 'fetal distress' but more recently termed 'non-reassuring fetal status'. It is defined as progressive fetal asphyxia (i.e. insufficiency or absence of the exchange of the respiratory gases) that will result in decompensation of the physiologic responses if not corrected and cause permanent central nervous system and other organ damage or death. Non-reassuring fetal status may be suspected during the antenatal period on the basis of reduced fetal movements, abnormal FHR patterns on cardiotocography (CTG), ultrasound scan/Doppler waveform analyses, and during the intrapartum period, by fetal scalp blood sampling (FBS) or electrocardiography (ECG). However, no single test is sufficiently sensitive and/or specific to separate out entirely normal fetal state and varying degrees of asphyxia.

Intrapartum Non-Reassuring Fetal Status

Although fetal monitoring using intermittent auscultation (IA) is adequate in low-risk pregnancies during labour, continuous electronic fetal monitoring is recommended for high-risk pregnancies such as fetal growth restriction (FGR), pre-eclampsia, and multiple pregnancy.

Pathophysiology

Usually, placental transfer is adequate in meeting the needs of the fetus throughout pregnancy and helps it to adapt to modest degrees of hypoxic ischaemic insults during labour. Non-reassuring fetal status may occur due to high demand during the latter part of pregnancy, failing placental functional capacity or reduced oxygen delivery. Non-reassuring fetal status is associated with emergency operative delivery, short-term morbidity such as neonatal acidaemia, intensive care admission, hypoxic ischaemic encephalopathy (HIE), perinatal death, neurodevelopmental disability, and cerebral palsy.

Intrapartum uterine contractions reduce uteroplacental perfusion. In a healthy, well-grown, term fetus, no significant hypoxia or damage results from these contractions. However, in the growth restricted fetus or the appropriately grown fetus exposed to uterine tachysystole, there is a risk of fetal hypoxaemia and hypoxia, which, in turn, activates the peripheral chemoreflex. The aim of the chemoreflex activation is to centralise the circulation and prioritise the blood and oxygen supply to central organs such as the heart, brain, and the adrenals, at the expense of the non-essential organs such as the skin, skeletal muscles, gastrointestinal organs, and the kidneys. If this adaptation is sustained for too long and/or fails, the fetus is at increased risk of central hypotension, hypoperfusion of essential organs, and reperfusion injuries.

Identification

Cardiotocography

Although there is controversy around the evidence for the benefits of admission cardiotocography (CTG) in low-risk women, this is standard practice in many centres. A normal intrapartum CTG in a term or near-term fetus would exhibit the features listed below.

- Stable baseline FHR between 110 and 160 bpm without significant decelerations
- Normal FHR variability between 5 and 25 bpm above and below the stable baseline FHR
- Periods of reduced FHR variability, which alternate with periods of increased FHR variability with or without accelerations (i.e. 'fetal cycling activity')

A normal CTG indicates normal fetal behavioural state, neurological integrity, and the absence of significant hypoxia or acidosis. Unlike during the antenatal period, where accelerations are required to define a normal CTG, the absence of spontaneous accelerations during labour is of unknown clinical significance, provided that the other features of fetal well-being are present. 'Fetal cycling activity' may be absent in chronic hypoxia, meconium aspiration syndrome, intraamniotic infection, exposure to drugs (e.g. oxytocin, sedatives, narcotics, atropine), complete heart block, fetal cerebral haemorrhage or brain malformations. Cardiotocography in twin pregnancies should be performed with dual-channel monitors that enables simultaneous monitoring of both fetuses.

Fetal Heart Rate Decelerations

Fetal heart rate decelerations refer to a parasympathetic-mediated chemoreflex of the cardiovascular system in response to a brief period of fetal oxygen deprivation. Morphologically, FHR decelerations are characterised by transient episodes of slowing of the fetal heart rate of more than 15 bpm and lasting longer than 15 seconds. These are believed to reduce the myocardial workload and oxygen demand. These are classified in relation to uterine contractions and are described below.

- Variable decelerations – These vary in shape, form and timing, in relation to uterine contractions, and are considered to occur due to compression of the cord.
- Early decelerations – These are synchronous with uterine contractions (mirror image of the contraction) and are assumed to occur with head compression in the late first stage or second stage.
- Late decelerations – These lag behind the uterine contractions and are caused by impaired oxygen transfer across the placenta. The nadir is observed after the peak uterine contraction, and the baseline is not reached at least 20 seconds after the contraction wanes.

Fetal Heart Rate Variability

This is the random fluctuation of the baseline FHR. This could be irregular in amplitude and frequency. A healthy fetus needs the coordination of the cerebral cortex, midbrain, vagus nerve and cardiac conductive tissues in order to exhibit normal FHR variability.

Patterns of variability are described below.

- Reduced variability – Reduction or absence of FHR variability is an important indicator of fetal hypoxia and evolving acidaemia in both term and preterm fetuses.
- Increased variability (saltatory pattern) – A bandwidth value exceeding 25 bpm and lasting for more than 30 minutes is thought to be caused by fetal hyperactivity or autonomic instability. Although it may be observed with recurrent decelerations, a pattern lasting for more than 30 minutes may indicate hypoxia even without decelerations.

- Sinusoidal pattern – A regular, smooth, undulating signal resembling a sine wave with an amplitude of 5–15 bpm and a frequency of 3–5 cycles per minute occurs in association with severe fetal anaemia that is caused by anti-D alloimmunisation, feto-maternal haemorrhage, twin-to-twin transfusion syndrome, and ruptured vasa praevia. It has also been described in cases of acute fetal hypoxia, infection, cardiac malformations, hydrocephalus, and gastroschisis.

Intrapartum Cardiotocograph Patterns Associated with Fetal Hypoxia and Neurological Injury

Depending on the nature and severity, the CTG would show abnormalities which are reliable predictors of progressive fetal asphyxiation and risk of neurological injury. There are four recognisable patterns of intrapartum fetal hypoxia.

1. *Slowly Evolving Hypoxia*

    Oxygen deprivation results in the appearance of FHR decelerations associated with uterine contractions (Figures 29.1A, B). The amplitude and duration of the deceleration depend on the hypoxic insult. This could be caused by cord compression or injudicious use of oxytocin during labour. If the insult persists, then it will manifest as an increase in the FHR of usually up to 160–180 bpm (Figure 29.1C), as the fetus increases its cardiac output via an adrenaline surge in order to compensate for the stressful stimuli. Therefore, a continuous fetal tachycardia preceded by repetitive decelerations with uterine contractions is indicative of a compensatory increase in fetal cardiac output. The critical factor in slowly evolving hypoxia is the availability of time for the fetus to produce metabolic and cardiovascular system adjustments. In the absence of acidaemia, the fetus can sustain its protective circulatory adaptations almost indefinitely (Figure 29.1D).

    If hypoxia continues, then the fetal myocardial glycogen may become exhausted and results in a fall in FHR towards bradycardia (Figures 29.1E, F). A well-grown, healthy, term fetus in spontaneous labour with clear liquor and previously normal CTG would take at least an hour to exhibit these changes.

2. *Subacute Hypoxia*

    Subacute hypoxia is characterised by high amplitude decelerations of 60 bpm or more and lasting for 90 seconds or longer, and on recovery spends less than 60 seconds at the baseline before the onset of the next deceleration (Figures 29.2A–D).

3. *Acute Hypoxia*

    Acute hypoxia presents as a prolonged deceleration lasting for longer than five minutes (Figure 29.3A) or for more than three minutes if associated with reduced variability within the deceleration (Figure 29.3B).

    The causes of acute hypoxia are categorised into two groups.

    - Sentinel events: umbilical cord prolapse, placental abruption, uterine rupture
    - Iatrogenic: maternal hypotension (usually secondary to supine hypotension or epidural top-up) and uterine hyperstimulation (caused by oxytocin or prostaglandins, or spontaneous increased activity)

4. *Preexisting Hypoxia or Neurological Injury*

    The heart rate pattern in fetuses with preexisting hypoxia or neurological injury is characterised by a relatively fixed baseline rate but low variability that does not exhibit fetal cycling activity (Figures 29.4A and B). In some cases, fetal tachycardia may occur (Figure 29.4C).

Infection, Inflammation and Fetal Heart Rate Abnormalities

The current intrapartum electronic FHR monitoring technology lacks sufficient sensitivity to detect placental inflammation or fetal systemic inflammatory response or to predict neonatal sepsis. Tachycardia, reduced variability or the lack of cycling may occur, but these changes are inconsistent.

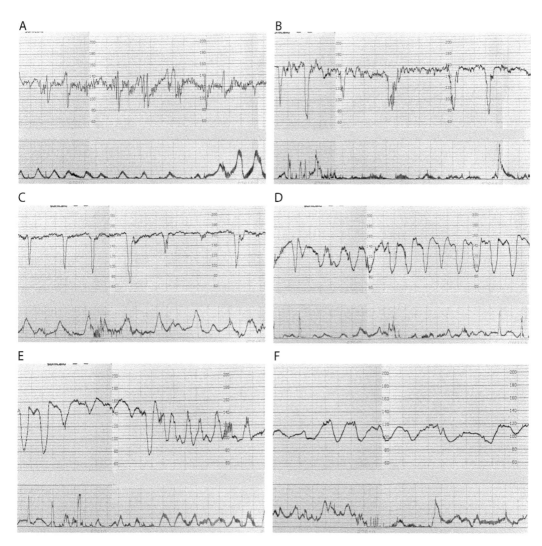

FIGURE 29.1 Cardiotocograph changes in slowly evolving hypoxia.

There should be a high degree of suspicion as the risk of fetal infection is high, if fetal tachycardia is associated with meconium-stained liquor in early labour.

Inadvertent Monitoring of Maternal Heart Rate

During the active phase of the second stage of the labour, the maternal heart rate could easily be mistaken for the FHR, because the FHR could collapse and the CTG machine may pick up pulsations from a maternal abdominal or pelvic vessel. Seemingly immense and broad accelerations coinciding with the peak of uterine contractions and maternal bearing down efforts help to differentiate the maternal heart rate from the FHR (Figure 29.5).

Fetal pH and Lactate Levels

These are revealed by fetal blood sampling, and require a capillary blood gas (ABG) analysis. Fetal blood sampling should be carried out only if the CTG trace remains pathological. A sample of blood is

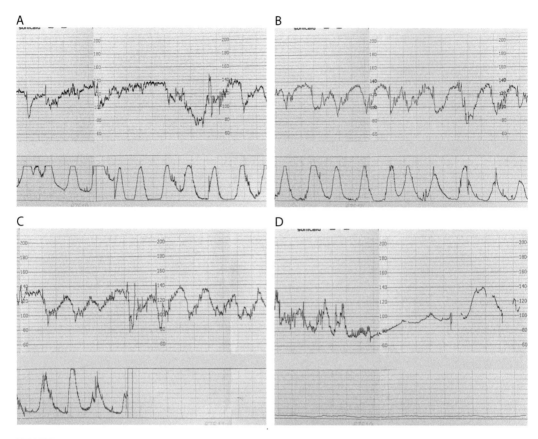

FIGURE 29.2 Cardiotocograph changes in subacute hypoxia.

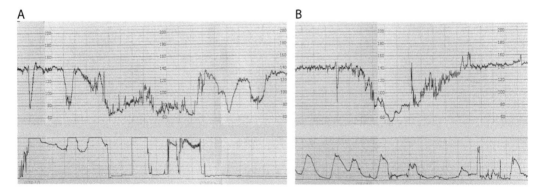

FIGURE 29.3 Cardiotocograph changes in acute hypoxia.

drawn from the fetal scalp by making a small laceration. However, this should not be performed during or immediately after a pathological deceleration. These results should be interpreted while taking into consideration previous measurements and clinical circumstances.

Fetal scalp pH levels are classified as:

- Normal – 7.25 or more
- Borderline – 7.21 to 7.24

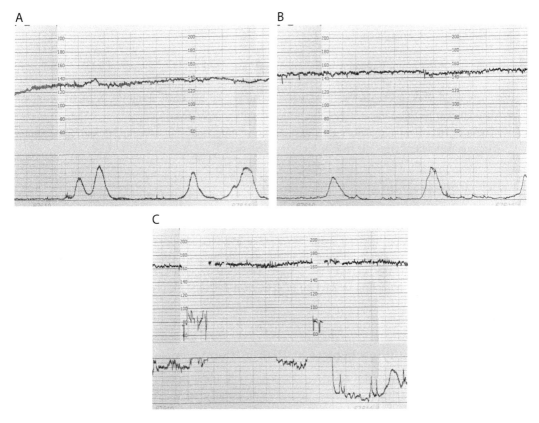

FIGURE 29.4 Cardiotocograph changes in preexisting hypoxia or neurological injury.

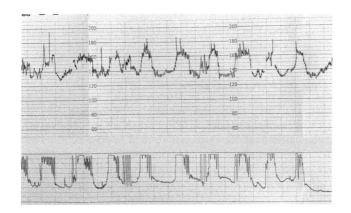

FIGURE 29.5 Maternal heart rate.

- Abnormal – 7.20 or less

Lactate levels are classified as:

- Normal – 4.1 mmol/L or less

- Borderline – 4.2 to 4.8 mmol/L
- Abnormal – 4.9 mmol/L or more

Fetal blood sampling is not indicated in the situations described below.

- There is an acute event such as cord prolapse, suspected placental abruption or uterine rupture.
- The clinical picture indicates that the birth should be expedited.
- There is risk of maternal to fetal transmission of infection, e.g. hepatitis B and C or human immunodeficiency virus, or risk of bleeding disorder.

Fetal Electrocardiogram

Fetal electrocardiogram is performed in order to supplement the CTG when there is a need to continuously monitor the fetus. It should be done only after the rupture of membranes, as it requires the application of electrodes on the fetal scalp. Myocardial hypoxia induces changes in ventricular depolarisation–repolarisation sequence leading to significant alterations in the morphology of the ST segment of the fetal ECG and the height of the T wave. However, fetal ECG complementing conventional CTG does not lead to a reduction in the rate of caesarean delivery for presumed fetal compromise or metabolic acidosis.

Techniques in Identifying Fetuses at Risk of Compromise in Labour

Since there have been many false positives associated with intrapartum CTG monitoring, identifying pregnancies at risk of fetal compromise would help identify those who require continuous CTG monitoring during labour. Various techniques are employed in this context.

Doppler Ultrasound Velocimetry

Doppler Ultrasound Velocimetry is usually performed in growth-restricted fetuses, as FGR is associated with brain sparing effect characterised by reduced resistance in the middle cerebral artery (MCA) and cerebral redistribution of blood flow. The type of Doppler ultrasound velocimetry carried out is determined by the period of gestation.

Umbilical Artery Doppler Velocimetry

Umbilical artery doppler velocimetry is the screening test used to identify FGR secondary to suboptimal placentation in small for gestational age fetuses. Increased values of umbilical artery resistance indices are associated with pathological fetal heart rate patterns and adverse neonatal outcomes.

When comparing with other techniques, the addition of umbilical artery Doppler velocimetry to the admission CTG has not shown a positive correlation with improved neonatal outcomes. Umbilical artery Doppler velocimetry alone is a poor predictor of adverse perinatal outcomes.

Middle Cerebral Artery Doppler Velocimetry

Doppler velocimetry of the middle cerebral artery (MCA) plays a major role in the identification of FGR and fetal anaemia and is currently being used to risk stratify pregnancies prior to labour. Abnormal MCA Doppler velocimetry has been proven to be useful in predicting meconium-stained liquor in post-term pregnancies and identifying those at increased risk of caesarean delivery for non-reassuring fetal status in small for gestational age fetuses.

Cerebro-Placental Ratio

The cerebro-placental ratio assesses both the umbilical artery and middle cerebral artery resistance indices, and it represents the ratios of the MCA pulsatility index (PI) to the umbilical artery PI. It is considered as the most accurate method in identifying a brain sparing fetal circulation. The cerebro-placental ratio, when measured in early labour, has been reported to be significantly low in fetuses who require emergency delivery due to presumed compromise, whereas a high cerebro-placental ratio appears to be protective against fetal compromise during labour, with a negative predictive value of almost 100%. Assessment of the cerebro-placental ratio is less time-consuming than CTG or biophysical profile. Although associations have been shown, this is not in standard use for clinical decision-making.

Umbilical Venous Flow

Although mainly used in the assessment of growth-restricted fetuses, umbilical venous flow can identify fetuses who are at risk of fetal compromise and require emergency delivery, even in uncomplicated pregnancies. Pulsatile umbilical venous flow is indicative of significant fetal circulatory resistance and afterload and requires delivery before decompensated fetal cardiac failure.

Other Antenatal Assessments

Clinical risk factor evaluation, mid-trimester uterine artery Doppler velocimetry in high-risk women and serial measurement of symphysio-fundal height are used in identifying fetuses at risk of growth restriction. Although routine monitoring of fetal movements has been found to increase maternal anxiety and subsequent unnecessary admissions, it is an extremely useful tool used to assess fetal well-being in high-risk pregnancies, especially in resource-poor settings. The assessment of short-term variability on computerised CTG is helpful in deciding on delivery in preterm FGR. The biophysical profile has regained its place in the evaluation of a growth-restricted fetus, and a score of 4 or below is an indication for delivery.

Treatment

In situations such as umbilical cord prolapse, the fetus should be delivered immediately after confirmation of viability without fetal monitoring. If emergency delivery is required, then a caesarean delivery is usually performed, unless a straightforward instrumental vaginal delivery is feasible or when normal vaginal delivery is imminent. In case of fetal distress, it is important that the least stressful method is used for delivery. The timing of delivery depends on the severity of the abnormality. Prolonged bradycardia or repetitive late decelerations without variability requires delivery within 30 minutes, while recurrent variable decelerations or late decelerations with minimal variability necessitate delivery within an hour. Communication with the neonatal team is vital in order to ensure optimisation of resuscitation of the newborn.

There are options other than delivery for management of non-reassuring fetal status.

- Stopping or reducing the dose of oxytocin, removal of vaginal prostaglandin and if these measures fail to correct the abnormality, administration of a tocolytic agent, e.g. terbutaline 0.25 mg subcutaneously, in case of uterine hyperstimulation
- Turning the woman into left lateral position in supine hypotension
- Rapid administration of fluids and/or application of an intravenous ephedrine bolus in hypotension following epidural or spinal anaesthesia

Administration of oxygen in women with adequate oxygenation and administration of fluids in normotensive women have not been proven to be effective in the management of non-reassuring fetal status.

Key Points

- Interpretation of cardiotocographs depends mainly on pattern recognition.
- Abnormalities detected during fetal monitoring should be interpreted in the clinical context.
- Good clinical judgement is necessary for timely intervention and for the avoidance of unnecessary interference.
- Emergency delivery is the mainstay of treatment for non-reassuring fetal status, but conservative measures may be adopted, provided that the abnormality is corrected.

BIBLIOGRAPHY

1. Lees CC, Stampalija T, Baschat AA, da Silva Costa F, Ferrazzi F, Figueras F, et al. ISUOG Practice Guidelines diagnosis and management of small-for-gestational-age fetus and fetal growth restriction. *Ultrasound Obstet Gynecol* 2020;56:298–312.
2. American College of Obstetricians and Gynecologists. Practice bulletin no. 116: management of intrapartum fetal heart rate tracings. *Obstet Gynecol.* 2010;116:1232–40.

30

Resuscitation of the Newborn

Amit Gupta and Anshuman Paria

Background

Birth asphyxia accounts for a quarter of neonatal deaths worldwide. However, for the majority of newborn infants, the transition to extrauterine life is smooth, and only 10% require some assistance in establishing regular respiration at birth. Less than 1% require chest compressions; about 0.2% require intubation and ventilation; while adrenaline is needed in about 0.6%. Profound hypoxia is generally a problem of term babies. Successful resuscitation at birth requires rigorous training, preparation, strict adherence to evidence-based guidelines that are appropriately adapted to suit different settings, and access to suitable equipment.

Initiation of Breathing at Birth

The increase of cortisol, thyroid hormones and catecholamines immediately prior to labour leads to the inhibition of the production of lung fluid and the removal of lung fluid from the airways. The absence of these mechanisms during an antepartum caesarean delivery explains the increased risk of transient tachypnoea in the newborn following an antepartum caesarean delivery, compared to following vaginal delivery. The mechanisms of initiation of respiration at birth are complex. It is postulated that the decreased oxygen concentration, increased amount of carbon dioxide, and the decrease in pH, which occur at birth when the fetus is no longer dependent on the umbilical cord, may stimulate the aortic and carotid chemoreceptors, thus triggering the respiratory centre in the medulla to commence respiration. In preterm infants, as immature pneumocytes do not secrete adequate amounts of surfactant, there is heightened surface tension in the alveolar – air interface, which prevents normal alveolar expansion at birth and leads to the collapse of alveoli during expiration, hence giving rise to respiratory distress syndrome.

Pathophysiology of Apnoea and Gasping

Although fetal breathing movements, which are essential for normal lung development and their maturation, are inhibited at the onset of labour owing to the action of increased circulating prostaglandins, these are reinitiated by significant hypoxia. Following this episode of rapid and shallow breathing, the breathing movements stop (primary apnoea). During this period, the blood supply to the brain, heart, and adrenal glands is prioritised. If intrauterine hypoxia continues further, then shuddering, agonal gasps (whole-body respiratory gasps of approximately 12 per minute) occur. The gasping abruptly stops as it is only a primitive reflex, but it may lead to aspiration of meconium, if present (described later in this chapter). The fetus then moves into the second period of apnoea (terminal apnoea), the cardiac compromise worsens, and without adequate resuscitation, the term neonate will usually die within 20 minutes. If delivery occurs during primary apnoea, then the neonate can be stimulated to restart breathing. In contrast, positive pressure ventilation at the very least is necessary in the case of terminal apnoea. However, as it is practically impossible to differentiate between primary and terminal apnoea at birth, it is advisable to automatically commence positive pressure ventilation in all babies who are not breathing at birth.

Prerequisites for Resuscitation of the Newborn

Each institutional birth should be attended by a person who is capable of performing the initial steps of resuscitation. When significant perinatal risk factors are present (e.g. meconium, bleeding, infections, prematurity, fetal growth restriction, multiple pregnancy), the probability of needing extensive resuscitation is increased, and therefore, additional personnel with advanced resuscitation skills, which include the ability to perform chest compressions, endotracheal intubation and umbilical vein catheter insertion, should be available on-site. However, the abovementioned skills may occasionally be required in babies without risk factors. Hence, each institution should have a system in place for the rapid deployment of a team with complete newborn resuscitation skills. Each resuscitation team should have a designated leader who should conduct a pre-resuscitation briefing whenever possible, during which challenges are identified, likely interventions prioritised and specific tasks allocated to team members based on their skills. Resuscitation is more likely to be successful if effective leadership, teamwork and communication can be ensured. Each institution should follow a standardised checklist, which ensures the proper functioning of the equipment and the availability of necessary supplies (Table 30.1). In case of extreme prematurity, a plastic bag or exothermic mattress for effective thermoregulation, a small mask and endotracheal tube for respiratory support and surfactant may have to be available.

Cord Clamping

Delayed cord clamping and resuscitation with an intact umbilical cord result in higher oxygen saturations and APGAR scores compared to early cord clamping in babies who require resuscitation at birth. Therefore, the newborn resuscitation trolley should be by the bedside both in the labour room as well as in the operating room. However, immediate cord clamping will be necessary if the newborn is grossly compromised at birth and requires intubation and ventilation.

TABLE 30.1

Necessary equipment and consumables for resuscitation of the newborn

Equipment	Consumables
• Radiant warmer with timer	• Umbilical clamp
• Self-inflating bag of 450 mL OR a T-piece resuscitation device (Neopuff)	• Umbilical catheter or feeding tubes of sizes 3.5, 4.0 and 5.0 French gauge (FG)
• Three different sizes of transparent masks 00, 0 and 0/1	• 5 cc, 2 cc and 10 cc syringes and needles
• Laryngoscope with size 00, 0 and 1 straight blades	• Adrenaline 1:10,000 solution
• Endotracheal (ET) tubes of three different sizes 2.5, 3.0 and 3.5 mm	• 0.9% sodium chloride (normal saline)
• Oro-pharyngeal airways of different sizes- 00, 0 and 1	• 10% dextrose
• Gases – wall/cylinder O_2 and compressed air	• 4.2% (or 8.4%) sodium bicarbonate
• Blender, which is already present in some of the T-piece devices	• Adhesive tapes
• Suction apparatus	• Suction catheters (large-bore)
• Stethoscope	• 24G peripheral intravenous cannula
• Set of cord scissors	• Sterile gauze
• Clock	• Local record sheet
	• Umbilical venous catheter (UVC) insertion set
	• Surgical blade with scalpel blade handle
	• Toothed forceps
	• Uncrossmatched O negative packed cells (refrigerated)
	• Warm dry towels

Steps of Resuscitation

Initial steps

Once the baby is born, the clock on the resuscitaire should be started, and for term babies, the baby should be quickly dried and completely wrapped in a dry, warm cloth (except for the face and upper chest). Next, an assessment of colour, tone, breathing and heart rate should be carried out and repeated every 30 seconds, if necessary. A baby with pink lips and tongue, good tone, regular breathing and a heart rate >100 bpm, does not need resuscitation, while a floppy baby with blue or pale lips, no observable breathing and a heart rate <100 bpm, requires resuscitation. The baby should be placed in a neutral position, i.e. face parallel to the surface, and not flexed nor extended (Figure 30.1).

Temperature Maintenance

Temperature maintenance is one of the basic requirements of newborn resuscitation. Hypothermia has been directly implicated in neonatal death, with each 1°C decrease below 36.5°C being associated with a 28% increase in mortality in low birth weight infants. Special precautions must be taken for preterm babies, such as wrapping in polyethylene bags without drying, the use of a hat, mittens, exothermic mattress, radiant heater and pre-warming the delivery room (ambient temperature 26°C). Hyperthermia (>37.5°C) should be avoided as well. Likewise, it is essential to reduce the heater output from radiant warmer in case of concurrent use of exothermic mattresses, in order to prevent hyperthermia.

Inflation Breaths

It is recommended that five sustained inflation breaths, each lasting 2–3 seconds are given initially, by slowly squeezing the bag in order to facilitate the opening of the infant's lungs and repeated, if necessary. The mask should be of the right size, form a good seal over the baby's mouth and nose, and should not press on the eyes or overhang the chin. The baby's chest movements should be observed with each inflation breath, and the bag must be allowed to reinflate after each breath. Counting out loud, 1-2-3, 2-2-3, 3-2-3, 4-2-3 and 5-2-3 helps to maintain an accurate rhythm. Recommended pressures are 30 cm of H_2O for term babies and 20–25 cm H_2O for babies born ≤30 weeks. In most cases, placing the baby in a neutral position and giving inflation breaths are all that is necessary for the baby to establish regular breathing.

Ventilation Breaths

Following a set of inflation breaths which result in good chest movement but fail to initiate spontaneous breathing, or where the heart rate remains below 60 bpm, ventilation breaths (with a pressure of approximately 20 cm H_2O, each inspiratory time ≤1 second, about 30 breaths per minute) are started. Adequacy of lung aeration is evident by a heart rate that is above 100 bpm and can also be checked with saturation in the pulse oximeter, which should reach at least 60% at two minutes of age. If a heart rate of

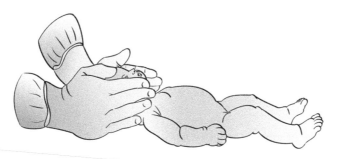

FIGURE 30.1 Neutral position.

>100 bpm is not achieved after 30 seconds of ventilation breaths, then reassessment of airway position and ventilation technique is mandatory. Jaw thrust (Figure 30.2) or insertion of an oropharyngeal airway is needed if initial aeration is not successful. Initial resuscitation of term babies should be performed on-air, and that of preterm babies in low concentrations of oxygen (21%–30%). Pulse oximetry attached to the right wrist should guide subsequent titration of oxygen.

Chest Compression

Heart rate slower than 60/minute or absent after five effective inflation breaths and 30 seconds of adequate ventilation breaths is an indication for commencing chest compressions. In addition, it is vital to ensure that the chest is moving in response to ventilation before commencing chest compressions, as chest compressions are ineffective if the airway is not open or if the lungs are not inflated. Chest compressions should be performed at 90/minute along with ventilation breaths of 30/minute at a ratio of 3:1, for a total of 120 events/minute. This should be done in a coordinated manner, to avoid simultaneous delivery of chest compressions and ventilation breaths. However, if the newborn is intubated, both chest compressions and ventilation breaths can be performed synchronously. The hand encircling technique with overlapping thumbs on the lower third of the sternum, compressing one-third of the depth of the chest while allowing for adequate relaxation, is recommended (Figure 30.3). When one person is resuscitating the newborn, a two-finger chest compression manoeuvre should be used (Figure 30.4). Adequate relaxation between chest compressions is important as perfusion of coronary arteries, which is a vital step in the restoration of cardiac activity, is achieved only during diastole. The heart rate should be reassessed every 30 seconds (usually after 15 cycles of 3:1). Chest compressions should be continued until the heart rate is consistently at >60/min and rising.

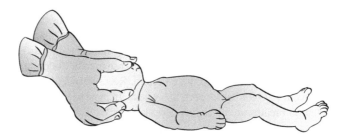

FIGURE 30.2   Jaw thrust.

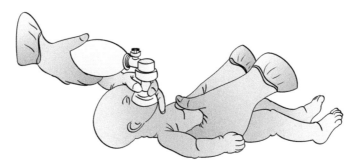

FIGURE 30.3   Hand encircling technique for chest compression.

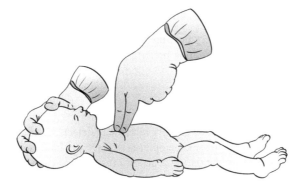

FIGURE 30.4 Two-finger chest compression manoeuvre.

TABLE 30.2

Medication used in newborn resuscitation

DRUGS	Dose
Adrenaline (UVC/IV)*	Intra-tracheal:1 mL/kg of 1:10,000 Umbilical: 0.1 mL/kg of 1:10,000 as the first dose, subsequent doses at 0.3 mL/kg of 1:10,000 dilution. Each dose must be flushed with 1–2 mL of 0.9% NaCl.
Sodium chloride (UVC/IV)	10 mL/kg of 0.9% sodium chloride if hypovolaemia is suspected because of placental abruption or fetal blood loss (10 mL/kg of uncrossmatched O Rhesus negative blood is a better option in this scenario).
Sodium bicarbonate (UVC/IV)	If there is no response to two doses of adrenaline, consider sodium bicarbonate 4.2 (or 8.4) % intravenously in a dose of 2 mmol per Kg slowly over a minute.
Dextrose (UVC/IV)	3 mL/kg of 10% dextrose if hypoglycaemia is evident on cord blood analysis

Note:
* UVC – umbilical vein catheter, IV - intravenous

Drugs

If the heart rate fails to improve beyond 60 bpm after 30 seconds of performing cardiac compressions, then the administration of medication should be considered (Table 30.2). Up to three doses of adrenaline should be administered, with one dose of sodium bicarbonate given before the third dose, depending on the response. Insertion of an umbilical venous catheter (UVC) is the quickest method to gain access to the circulatory system in a collapsed newborn. Insertion of a UVC to a depth of 4–5 cm in a sterile manner is required for the successful administration of drugs.

Intubation

Rarely, intubation may be required for babies who fail to establish spontaneous respiration following a reasonable duration of approximately 30 minutes of ventilation breaths, or where chest movements could not be initiated even with a two-person technique (i.e. one performing jaw thrust, while the other performs hand ventilation using the bag and mask). Laryngeal mask airway can be considered in babies >2 kg and >34 weeks when intubation is not successful. Intubation should be confirmed with colour change capnography, if available. However, the colour change may not occur in babies with reduced cardiac output despite proper lung aeration.

Delivery Room Continuous Positive Airway Pressure (CPAP)

Delivery room continuous positive airway pressure may be used during the transition and subsequent respiratory support of spontaneously breathing preterm infants at ≤30 weeks of gestation.

Stopping Resuscitation

Resuscitation can be stopped if the cardiac activity remains undetectable after ten minutes of adequate resuscitation. However, it is essential to seek the opinion of a senior clinician as well as discuss with the parents before calling off the resuscitation. A decision on a case-to-case basis has to be taken with regard to discontinuing resuscitation, if the heart rate has not improved beyond 60/min after 20 minutes of resuscitation.

Debriefing

It is essential to debrief the parents, following resuscitation of the newborn. Resuscitation can be complicated and emotionally draining for the team involved, and it is important to debrief the staff involved as well.

The steps of resuscitation of a newborn are summarised in Figure 30.5.

Challenging Scenarios Requiring Resuscitation

With the improvement in antenatal scanning, a vast majority of congenital malformations are diagnosed antenatally. However, from time to time, the attending team will be faced with undiagnosed and challenging conditions. Some of these conditions are medical emergencies, while a few may require surgical attention. The key management strategies for these and for feto-maternal haemorrhage are outlined in Table 30.3.

Meconium Staining versus Meconium Aspiration

Passage of meconium (i.e. dark green, sterile faecal material) may normally occur at term. It may also happen in response to hypoxia, as a result of a vagal response with increased peristalsis and a relaxed anal sphincter. Meconium aspiration may arise when the fetus gasps (with an open glottis due to poor tone) in-utero, or when meconium, which is present in the upper airway, enters the lungs during breathing after birth. Meconium aspiration primarily affects infants born after 34 weeks of gestation, because meconium is rarely found in the amniotic fluid prior to this gestation. Meconium aspiration syndrome causes hypoxia due to airway obstruction, surfactant dysfunction, chemical pneumonitis and pulmonary hypertension and also predisposes to pulmonary infection. Understanding the exact relationship among passage of meconium, its aspiration and its corresponding consequences, has remained an enigma since it was first described by the Greek philosopher, Aristotle.

If the baby is vigorous, then it is likely that only meconium staining is present, and he/she does not require resuscitation. On the other hand, if the baby is compromised at birth, meconium aspiration is likely, and he/she requires resuscitation. Suctioning is not necessary if the baby is vigorous. Even if the airway is obstructed with meconium, intubation and ventilation should be the priority, as meconium may be present even in the distal airway which is not accessible for suctioning. If suctioning must be performed, then it should be carried out as explained below.

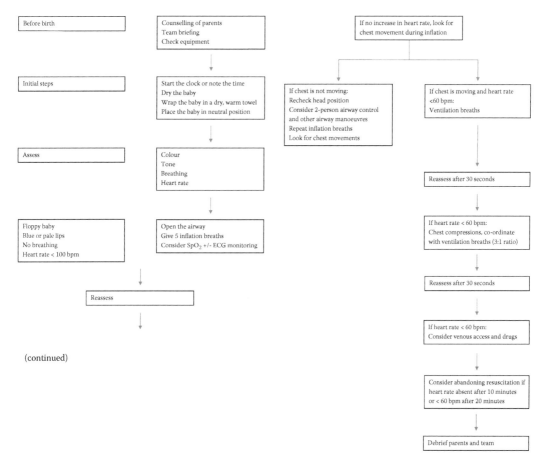

FIGURE 30.5 Summary of resuscitation of a newborn: SpO_2 – oxygen saturation, ECG – electrocardiogram.

- Gentle suctioning of the oral cavity should be performed before any attempts at suctioning of the nostrils are made, as suctioning of the nostrils may stimulate the baby to breathe and lead to aspiration of meconium present inside the mouth.
- If pharyngeal suctioning is required to remove meconium obstructing the airway, then it should be performed promptly by an experienced clinician, using a large-bore suction catheter and under direct vision (e.g. using a laryngoscope) before giving any respiratory support or stimulating the baby to breathe.

Palliative Care on the Delivery Suite – Managing End of Life in Life-Limiting Situations

The cut-off gestation at which resuscitation is provided will vary depending on the setting. However, the survival rate of babies born around the threshold of viability remains quite low, and due to the high mortality rate and poor neurodevelopmental outcomes in these babies, providing palliative care is a sensible option. Life-sustaining therapy can be offered based on individual assessment and informed parental choice in babies <24 weeks of gestation. However, if additional risk factors, such as severe growth restriction or congenital malformations are present, providing palliative care is a feasible option. Furthermore, providing palliative care is the most appropriate option in babies with congenital

TABLE 30.3

Key management strategies for challenging scenarios

Condition	Challenge	Management Strategies
Tracheo-oesophageal fistula and oesophageal atresia	Possibility of choking and difficulty in passing a nasogastric tube	Confirm diagnosis with a chest x-ray following the insertion of a large nasogastric tube, and refer for surgery
Exomphalos and gastroschisis	Risk of bowel necrosis and dehydration	Cover the bowels in normal saline-soaked gauze and cling film, and refer for surgery
Congenital diaphragmatic hernia	Severe respiratory distress and poor oxygen saturation	Prompt intubation, insertion of a nasogastric tube, and ventilation at <30 mmHg pressure
Congenital cystic adenomatoid malformation, pleuropulmonary blastoma, large tumours in the neck (e.g. teratoma)	Severe airway obstruction	EXIT (ex utero intrapartum treatment) procedure, i.e. the establishment of airway access while the baby continues to receive oxygen through the umbilical cord with only the head and shoulders delivered
Spina bifida and meningomyelocele	Difficult positioning and risk of infection	Lateral positioning, cover the lesion with normal saline-soaked gauze, and refer to neurosurgeon
Antenatally diagnosed duct dependent cardiac lesions	Keeping the ductus arteriosus open	Administer prostaglandins
Hydrops fetalis	Pleural effusion and ascites making ventilation difficult	Insert chest drain and high-pressure ventilation
Feto-maternal haemorrhage	Possibility of early-onset heart failure and ARDS	Early transfusion of O negative blood

anomalies (e.g. anencephaly) and chromosomal abnormalities (e.g. trisomy 13) which are incompatible with life. However, all such decisions should be made at a consultation between the neonatologist and the parents before birth. During the meeting, parents' prior knowledge should be explored, balanced verbal and written information shared and risk of mortality in the delivery room and later, along with the risk of severe disability, conveyed unambiguously yet sympathetically. When the consensus is to follow a palliative pathway, then the focus should be on family-centred care. The emphasis is on alleviating any pain, prevention of any separation between the parents and baby and providing the parents with the opportunity to cherish the limited time they have with their baby.

Key Points

- Effective resuscitation at birth can prevent the majority of deaths due to birth asphyxia.
- As the requirement for the resuscitation of the newborn may be unpredictable, it is important that every birth practitioner is conversant with basic newborn resuscitation skills.
- In newborn resuscitation, after placing the baby in a neutral position, inflation breaths, ventilation breaths and chest compressions should be performed in sequence. It is important to proceed to the next if regular breathing and a heart rate > 60 bpm are not established within 30 seconds.
- Rarely, medication (adrenaline and sodium bicarbonate) and/or intubation may be necessary.
- The prevention of hypothermia is vital during the resuscitation of a newborn.

BIBLIOGRAPHY

1. Australian and New Zealand Committee on resuscitation. ANZCOR Guideline 13.4. Airway management and mask ventilation of the newborn infant. ANZCOR, April 2016.
2. Bruschettini M, O'Donnell CPF, Davis PG, Morley CJ, Moja L, Calevo MG. Sustained versus standard inflations during neonatal resuscitation to prevent mortality and improve respiratory outcomes. *Cochrane Database of Syst Rev* 2020;3(3). Art. No.: CD004953. DOI: 10.1002/14651858.CD004953.pub4.
3. Katheria A, Poeltler D, Durham J, Steen J, Rich W, Arnell K, et al. Neonatal resuscitation with an intact cord: a randomized clinical trial. *J Pediatr* 2016;178:75–80.e3. doi: 10.1016/j.jpeds.2016.07.053
4. McCall EM, Alderdice F, Halliday HL, Jenkins JG, Vohra S. Interventions to prevent hypothermia at birth in preterm and/or low birthweight infants. *Cochrane Database Syst Rev* 2010;2018(3):CD004210.
5. Wyllie J, Perlman JM, Kattwinkel J, Atkins DL, Chameides L, Goldsmith JP, Guinsburg R, Hazinski MF, Morley C, Richmond S, Simon WM, Singhal N, Szyld E, Tamura M, Velaphi S. Neonatal Resuscitation Chapter Collaborators Part 11: neonatal resuscitation: 2010 international consensus on cardiopulmonary resuscitation and emergency cardiovascular care science with treatment recommendations. *Resuscitation* 2010;81(1):e260–87. doi: 10.1016/j.resuscitation.2010.08.029.
6. Wyllie J, Perlman JM, Kattwinkel J, et al. Part 7: Neonatal resuscitation: 2015 International Consensus on Cardiopulmonary Resuscitation and Emergency Cardiovascular Care Science with Treatment Recommendations. *Resuscitation* 2015;95:e169–201.

31

Simulation in Obstetric Emergencies

Sanjeewa Padumadasa and Sabaratnam Arulkumaran

'I hear and I forget. I see and I remember. I do and I understand', the frequently quoted words of Confucius (551–479 BC) explain the basis of simulation in a nutshell. Simulation is defined as a 'technique that replaces or amplifies real-life experiences with artificially contrived guided experiences'. Simulation in medicine has several advantages. Rare clinical events and emergencies could be mimicked at a convenient and predetermined time and place, thus enabling healthcare teams to acquire expertise in managing these events. This facilitates a training and feedback method in which learners perform tasks and practise procedures in lifelike scenarios in a controlled, non-threatening environment. It can enhance patient safety by removing the patient from the trainee's learning curve. While enabling a large number of trainees to undergo the training in batches, it also allows individual trainees to practise performing specific tasks as frequently as they wish and at their own pace and convenience. It also permits frequent and regular practise in order to prevent or minimise deskilling which invariably occurs with time.

The Evolution of Simulation-Based Training in Obstetric Emergencies

The idea of practising on manikins before performing a certain task on actual patients dates back to antiquity. As early as the 9th century, wax and wooden figures have been in use, and antique obstetric simulators known as 'phantoms' were employed as way back as the 17th century in order to teach midwives how to manage difficult deliveries. In the 1970s, there was a transition from birthing pelvises to life-size interactive birthing simulators. However, it was not until the early part of the 21st century when simulation-based training (SBT) in obstetric emergencies was recommended to reduce the adverse maternal and perinatal outcomes, that it emerged in the field of obstetrics. Today, not only has SBT in obstetric emergencies been incorporated into several medical curricula, but it has also become an integral part of several evaluation and credentialing programmes.

The Concept of 'Team Training'

The concept of 'team training' originated in the aviation industry. The work environments of aviation and healthcare share more or less similar characteristics such as complexity, stress, time sensitivity, the involvement of multiple personnel and the requirement to work consistently in a highly charged environment. 'Crew resource management' is a term that originated in a National Aeronautics and Space Administration Workshop in the late 1970s, and this focused on anticipating and planning, teamwork, communication, leadership, mobilisation of resources and decision-making of flight crews. Consequently, this concept has been introduced to the field of obstetrics.

The Relevance of Simulation-Based Training in Obstetric Emergencies

The relatively low frequency and the unpredictability of obstetric emergencies make SBT the ideal method for healthcare providers to achieve and maintain competence in managing these events. The management of even the rarest of emergencies such as maternal cardiac arrest can be rehearsed through simulation. In addition, a reduction in the number of working hours compounded by an increase in the number of trainees has resulted in less exposure of trainees to obstetric emergencies, and simulation is an avenue for the trainees to acquire the necessary skills in managing these emergencies. Simulation in the field of obstetrics brings together various healthcare professionals including doctors, nurses, midwives, other supporting staff and other healthcare providers such as anaesthesiologists and intensivists and provides the platform for all of them to work as one team.

Today, patients are increasingly concerned that they are being used as study material or 'guinea pigs'. Simulation provides a safe arena to practise procedures and tasks as many times as one requires, without causing harm to patients. From a simple adjunct to learning for novices, simulation has evolved into an educational tool for experienced professionals to learn new procedures and widen their scope of knowledge and skills.

Research into simulation has proven that it leads to improvements in the confidence and competence of learners. Studies have found that simulation resulted in a reduction in neonatal brachial plexus injury following management of shoulder dystocia, as well as a reduction in maternal trauma resulting from forceps delivery, and an improvement in the management of postpartum haemorrhage as well as efficiency in performing emergency caesarean delivery. Some obstetric manoeuvres, such as internal podalic version and breech extraction, which have been extensively utilised in the past, are seldom used today. Simulation is the ideal method to impart these procedures on the future generations of obstetricians, thus equipping them with the essential skills necessary for providing care to women, since most of these techniques are under threat of becoming defunct in the specialty.

In several countries, there are well-established multi-professional SBT programmes in obstetric emergencies. Simulation-based training in obstetric emergencies differs according to the setting, fidelity and the resources used.

Setting

It has been proven that multi-professional training conducted locally at the unit level rather than training conducted at distant simulation centres is more effective in improving maternal and neonatal outcomes. This may be because learning to use guidelines and protocols that are developed locally and engaging in teamwork are more important than the acquisition of new skills. Maternal cardiorespiratory arrest, eclampsia and postpartum haemorrhage are some of the areas where multi-professional local training is particularly important. Local training also exposes system errors that can impede care during emergencies. In addition, a locally run course is cheaper and provides the opportunity to train greater numbers of staff as compared to a distantly conducted course. However, workload and lack of local expertise are barriers in conducting such training courses at the institutional level.

Fidelity

Simulation-based training is an active event in which participants, as well as facilitators, are immersed in a realistic clinical environment and having an environment similar to that of a real-life scenario is an essential component in any simulation programme. Simulation can be categorised into high, medium and low fidelity, according to the degree to which it is true to reality. 'Low fidelity' simulators (e.g. various birthing simulators and locally produced models for manual removal of the placenta) are available for initial training of skills, especially in low-resource settings, while computer assisted 'high fidelity' birthing simulators with sensors, which are considered to be more realistic, are available in well-resourced settings. Fidelity in simulation is also classified as conceptual, physical, psychological and sociological fidelity.

- Conceptual fidelity: the degree to which the simulator replicates the behaviour of what it is supposed to mimic., e.g. labelled medicine bottles, properly equipped birth instrument trays, red gelatin clots for simulated haemorrhage, participants wearing scrubs, patients wearing gowns.
- Physical fidelity: the degree to which the simulator replicates the physical characteristics of the actual task.
- Psychological fidelity: the degree to which the trainee perceives the simulation to be close to reality.
- Sociological fidelity: the ability of a simulation programme to enhance communication and inter-professional teamwork.

Resources

Standardised patients (SPs), manikins and interactive computer-based delivery systems (i.e. virtual reality trainers) are currently used in SBT. In terms of obtaining informed consent for obstetric procedures and providing culturally sensitive medical education, SPs have made a great impact on SBT. However, the inability to perform invasive manoeuvres is a disadvantage when SPs are used. The manikins range from low-cost pelvises to expensive, whole-body simulators with different specifications that determine their uses. A well-designed curriculum coupled with competent trainers can make even a low fidelity SBT programme invaluable in the teaching-learning process.

The pairing of a simulator with another simulator or a human creates a 'hybrid simulator', which provides an easy-to-use, portable, practical simulation tool that can achieve realism at very little cost. The hybrid patient provides the opportunity to practise scenarios such as shoulder dystocia, assisted vaginal breech delivery, instrumental vaginal delivery and management of postpartum haemorrhage, without causing harm to the patient, but at the same time allowing interaction between the patient and the learner.

Virtual reality simulators recreate a three-dimensional environment on a computer screen display. Virtual reality simulators may be equipped with haptics that provide sensory and tactile stimuli in addition to visual stimuli in order to resemble the actual environment as closely as possible. This concept can be adopted to enhance realism when using manikins as well. One such example is to place a waterproof fetal manikin in a thin plastic bag filled with water. When such a manikin was used along with a waterproof pelvic model for practising internal podalic version and breech extraction, it was discovered to enhance realistic sensations which made the experience both enjoyable and memorable.

Important Aspects of a Simulation-Based Training Programme

Initial Design

Initial designing of an SBT programme can be a daunting task, but it is time well spent. Designing a successful SBT programme is started by an initial assessment of the needs for the programme. Areas of importance that are specific to the particular unit may be identified through risk management, root cause analysis and the review of sentinel events and near misses. The more relevant the training is, the more engaged the participants would be. Furthermore, a SWOT analysis with regard to Strengths, Weaknesses, Opportunities and Threats of conducting an SBT programme is helpful. The duration, target group and the number of participants per programme should be determined. The venue should be identified, which could possibly be a dedicated simulation laboratory or a vacant room in the labour suite. A simulation laboratory provides an environment that is similar to that in real life, but without distractions as apparent in a ward.

A crucial factor in designing an SBT workshop is prudently selecting the facilitators. Enthusiasm and commitment of the facilitators are crucial to the successful running of any training programme. In addition to facilitators, SPs and other key support workers such as clerks, timekeepers and staff to videotape stations should be selected as required. A 'pre-brief' discussion among the facilitators is important to ensure that all have a clear understanding of their roles and responsibilities. Currently recommended guidelines and protocols, modified if necessary according to the local context, should be adhered to. There should be a script in place describing a clinical scenario in detail with utmost attention paid to timelines. An essential feature of scenario building is a good story with the ability to captivate the learner. A script can be developed for any type of emergency and should be tailor-fit to the particular setting in which the healthcare providers work. If SPs are used, then both the actress and the facilitator should be thorough with the script. There should be separate instructions for the participants. The equipment that would be used should be identified depending on the specific learning objectives. Task trainers (e.g. pelvis) may be more suited for training procedural skills, while whole-body high-fidelity simulators may be more appropriate for training soft skills.

Pilot sessions should be conducted in order to identify practical problems that may arise when running the programme. Sharing the outline of the programme with the participants prior to the session may be helpful. Moreover, a budget has to be prepared and funds obtained. Logistics need to be considered and prior approvals from relevant authorities obtained. Leadership and support by the institution are important in ensuring the sustainability of any institution-based SBT programme.

Providing an Environment Conducive to Learning

The role of the facilitator, as the term implies, is to facilitate learning among the participants and not to engage in formal classroom-type teaching. It is important that the facilitator conducts the programme in such a manner that the trainees do not feel threatened, embarrassed or belittled at any time. In addition, providing a learner-centred, interactive and collaborative environment facilitates learning. There is no 'right way' that a simulation would proceed. Therefore, the facilitator should be prepared to handle a variety of circumstances similar to those in real life. Scheduling regular breaks is important to maintain the focus of the participants.

Pretest

A pretest at the beginning of the workshop can be used to identify the spectrum of knowledge and skills of the participants. An online Kahoot Quiz can be used for this purpose, and it will also serve as an 'ice-breaker' for participants who are not known to one another.

Demonstration of Manoeuvres

Before the participants practise on manikins, a facilitator usually demonstrates the procedure after a brief description, emphasising the practical aspects rather than theory. This is where experience, not only in performing the procedure but also in teaching, counts. A blended method of training may be used with the incorporation of interactive lectures at the beginning of the programme.

Areas Covered

Eclampsia, shoulder dystocia, postpartum haemorrhage, assisted vaginal breech delivery, cord prolapse, instrumental vaginal deliveries, neonatal resuscitation and maternal cardiorespiratory arrest are some of the areas that are frequently covered in SBT in obstetric emergencies. It is important that scenarios are pitched at the right level, depending on the participants. Simulated scenarios can include low-frequency emergencies such as acute inversion of the uterus as well as situations that are not usually covered in training programmes but require great skill to manage, such as second stage caesarean delivery with the fetal head impacted within the pelvis. Simulation programmes can also be expanded to encompass areas of importance that may have surfaced recently, such as maternal sepsis.

Soft Skills

Acquisition of knowledge alone does not directly transform into one's ability to apply it into clinical practice, especially when working in stressful and unpredictable circumstances. 'Train together those who work together' is a concept of inter-professional training. In an SBT programme, it is important to emphasise non-technical skills such as communication, leadership, situation awareness, critical and strategic thinking, decision-making, conflict management, teamwork and professionalism, which cannot be acquired from traditional classroom teaching.

Debriefing

Debriefing, where the magic of learning takes place, is the most critical part of the simulation. It is the discussion that takes place between the facilitator and participants after the encounter, where events that occurred during simulation are reflected upon and constructive feedback is given and taken. An effective debriefing session would usually take twice the time as the actual simulation and requires considerable skill and expertise on the part of the facilitator.

First, the 'good' (what was done well) must be acknowledged and appreciated by the facilitator. Participants are bound to make mistakes when managing emergency obstetric scenarios. Therefore, it is essential that the facilitator diffuses emotions and provides reassurance for the participants to engage in the debriefing process in a meaningful manner. Issues with regard to hierarchy and intergroup differences have to be ironed out to provide a tension-free environment for all of the participants to get involved in the discussion. The focus should be on events instead of individuals. If something goes wrong, then there needs to be an in-depth discussion on what went wrong, why did it happen and how it could have been avoided. How certain tasks could have been done better should be discussed, and 'take home messages' must be emphasised. During debriefing, the facilitators provide structured feedback using global rating scales and checklists made up of tasks that the learner must complete in order to satisfy learning objectives. A video-assisted debriefing can be a compelling teaching tool and provides an opportunity to review in detail what went well and what needs to be improved or changed. However, the limitations of this method include financial and logistical considerations, as well as time spent on playback.

When the session is on team training and involves a multitude of professionals, then it is better to have a member from each discipline provide expertise on the subject matter. Team debriefing can also build camaraderie and team cohesiveness. Lessons learned during the process of debriefing will be what the participant takes back into his/her practice, and skilled feedback slows the rate of deterioration of skills acquired through SBT.

Evaluation of Training Courses

Historically, the evaluation of SBT has focused on the satisfaction and confidence of participants. Next, through evaluation of participant learning (e.g. changes in knowledge, skills and attitudes) and application of what was learned into the clinical environment, it has evolved into an evaluation of patient, organisational and system outcomes. The input of education specialists will be invaluable in the evaluation of an SBT programme. In addition to an assessment of the learners, it may be worthwhile to conduct an appraisal of the facilitators as well.

Frequency of Simulation-Based Training

Simulation-based training should be conducted at a frequency that is appropriate for the sustenance of the clinical skills of participants. This may range from once every three months to once a year and may differ depending on the need, the participants and the simulated scenarios. The first drill can be used to identify deficiencies both within the individuals and those of the team and implement corrective measures. Subsequent drills can be used to evaluate the effectiveness of any corrective measures and improve on identified weaknesses.

Review of the SBT Programme

Irrespective of the type of SBT, it is imperative that the curriculum, content delivery and evaluation process are reviewed frequently so that the programme can be consistently improved according to the needs that may arise in the future.

The important aspects of SBT in obstetric emergencies are summarised in Figure 31.1.

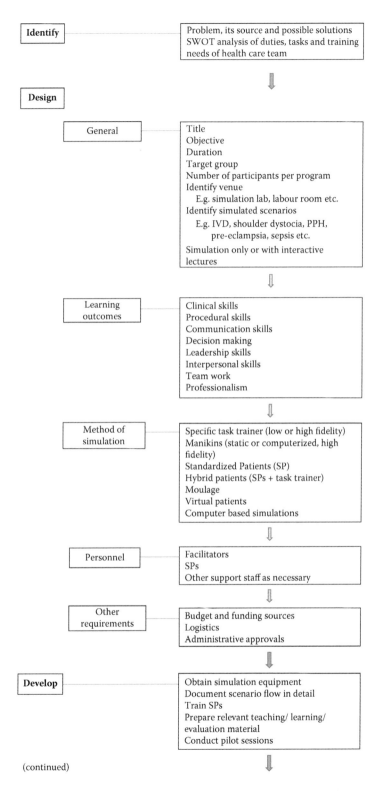

(continued)

FIGURE 31.1 Features of an SBT programme in obstetric emergencies (SWOT- strengths, weaknesses, opportunities and threats, IVD – instrumental vaginal delivery, PPH – postpartum haemorrhage).

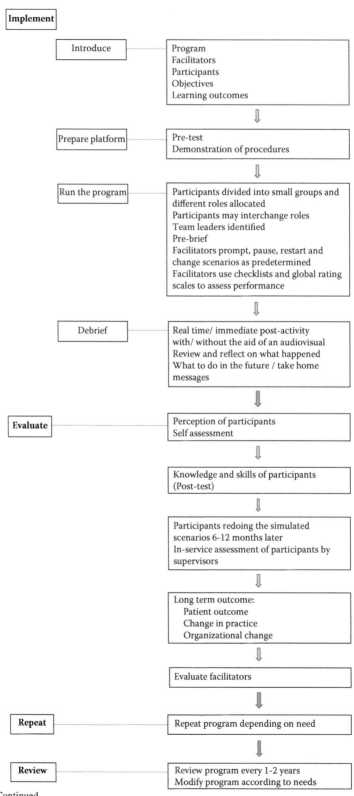

FIGURE 31.1 Continued.

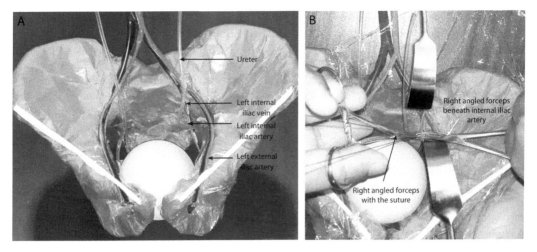

FIGURE 31.2 A Model Used to Practise Internal Iliac Artery Ligation; A – Model, B – Simulation of the Procedure.

Simulation-Based Training in Resource-Poor Settings

Financial restraints, lack of expertise and time and deficiencies in the infrastructure of a maternity unit make it difficult to provide simulation in resource-poor settings, where it may be even more essential than in well-resourced settings.

There are challenges faced in resource-poor settings that are usually not encountered in well-resourced settings.

- Non-availability of massive transfusion blood products, uterotonic agents or balloon tamponade of uterus
- Lack of essential medication such as rapidly acting intravenous antihypertensives and magnesium sulphate
- Lack of facilities for electronic fetal monitoring
- Non-availability of anaesthesia for assisted vaginal breech delivery and management of shoulder dystocia or umbilical cord prolapse
- Non-availability of additional skilled personnel for maternal or neonatal resuscitation

Therefore, simulation in these settings should be custom-made to the specific problems faced by both healthcare providers and patients. In addition, it is important to design and conduct SBT using local resources within a cost-effective model. A low-cost model devised by the first author in order to practise internal iliac artery ligation is shown in Figure 31.2.

The Future

One drawback of most of the simulators available in the market today is that there is more room for manoeuvres than in actual patients. There is a need to devise simulators that closely mimic the anatomy of the pelvis of real patients. As the use of ultrasound in the management of abnormal labour is a new entity, its incorporation into SBT needs to be assessed. Simulation has to be directed against conditions that could possibly pose challenges in the future with increasing maternal age, such as obesity and medical conditions. The experience gained through cardiorespiratory arrest simulation provides a platform to launch simulation in the field of critical care obstetrics. Wireless features that provide real-time feedback, as well as multiplex communication between the operator and learner, are emerging in the world of simulation. Questions on the cost, minimum standards, type of manikins, human resources and the frequency of drills required to achieve learning objectives remain unanswered and may possibly differ among various units.

Randomised controlled trials on the management of obstetric emergencies are not feasible due to impracticability and ethical restraints. Therefore, simulation may shed light on what may be the most suitable approach for the management of obstetric emergencies, and more research would be feasible in the future. What is happening in simulation at the present time may represent only the tip of the iceberg, and there is a lot more that we can adopt into simulation in obstetric emergencies. Maternity units and faculties all over the world, which still rely on traditional teaching and evaluation methods, should incorporate SBT into their curricula. It is likely that simulation in obstetrics, a major part of which is emergencies, will be increasingly incorporated into assessments, examinations and credentialing programmes in the future. However, it should be noted that negative learning or a false sense of confidence is also possible after SBT. Although SBT may play a pivotal role in training healthcare personnel in managing obstetric emergencies in the future, it should be complementary to rather than a substitute for a proper apprenticeship and clinical experience.

Key Points

- Simulation is the ideal tool used to train individuals as well as teams of healthcare personnel involved in maternity care in accomplishing specific tasks as well as managing emergencies that occur infrequently, without causing discomfort to or endangering patients.
- Simulation can be categorised into low, medium and high fidelity, depending on the degree to which it resembles reality and includes SPs, manikins and interactive computer-based delivery systems.
- A well-designed curriculum, competent and dedicated facilitators and homegrown, low-cost manikins can generate an excellent SBT programme.
- Comprehensive debriefing at the end of the simulation is the key to the learning process.
- Simulation in obstetric emergencies, potentially an indispensable educational tool, is likely to be increasingly integrated into curricula of various faculties, as well as licensing, certification and credentialing programmes in the future. However, SBT should be complementary to and not a substitute for a proper apprenticeship and clinical experience.

BIBLIOGRAPHY

1. Bullough AS, Boland T, Waters TP, Adams W. Obstetric team simulation program challenges. *J Clin Anes* 2016;35:564–70.
2. Cornette JM, Erkamp JS. Internal podalic version and breech extraction: enhancing realistic sensations in a simulation model. *Obstet Gynecol* 2018;131(2):360–3.
3. Deering S, Auguste TC, Goffman D, eds. Comprehensive Healthcare Simulation: Obstetrics and Gynecology. Switzerland: Springer, 2019.
4. Draycott TJ, Crofts JF, Ash JP, Wilson LV, Yard E, Sibanda T, Whitelaw A. Improving neonatal outcome through practical shoulder dystocia training. *Obstet Gynecol* 2008;112(1):14–20.
5. Merien AER, van de Ven J, Mol BW, Houterman S, Oei SG. Multidisciplinary team training in a simulation setting for acute obstetric emergencies: a systematic review. *Obstet Gynecol* 2010;115(5):1021–31.
6. Merriel A, Ficquet J, Barnard K, Kunutsor SK, Soar J, Lenguerrand E, Caldwell DM, Burden C, Winter C, Draycott T, Siassakos D. The effects of interactive training of healthcare providers on the management of life-threatening emergencies in hospital. *Cochrane Database Syst Rev* 2019;9:CD 012177.
7. Paige JB, Morin KH. Simulation Fidelity and cueing: a systematic review of the literature. *Clin Simul Nurs* 2013;9(11):e481–9.
8. Satin AJ. Simulation in obstetrics. *Obstet Gynecol* 2018;132(1):199–209.
9. Smith A, Siassakos D, Crofts J, Draycott T. Simulation: improving patient outcomes. *Semin Perinatol* 2013;37(3):151–6.

Index

For Product Safety Concerns and Information please contact
our EU representative GPSR@taylorandfrancis.com Taylor & Francis
Verlag GmbH, Kaufingerstraße 24, 80331 München, Germany

T - #0268 - 160425 - C0 - 254/178/16 - PB - 9780367543648 - Gloss Lamination